Law and Nursing

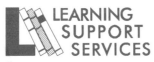

Commissioning editor: Mary Seager
Desk editor: Deena Burgess
Production controller: Chris Jarvis
Development editor: Caroline Savage
Cover designer: Helen Brockway

Law and Nursing

Second edition

Jean McHale LLB, MPhil
Professor of Law, Faculty of Law, University of Leicester, UK

John Tingle BA, Cert Ed, MEd
Barrister; Reader in Health Law; Director of the Centre for Health Law,
Nottingham Law School, The Nottingham Trent University, UK; Visiting
Professor of Law, Loyola University, Chicago, USA

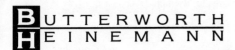

BUTTERWORTH
HEINEMANN

OXFORD AUCKLAND BOSTON JOHANNESBURG MELBOURNE NEW DELHI

Butterworth-Heinemann
Linacre House, Jordan Hill, Oxford OX2 8DP
225 Wildwood Avenue, Woburn, MA 01801-2041
A division of Reed Educational and Professional Publishing Ltd

A member of the Reed Elsevier plc group

First published 1998
Second edition 2001

British Library Cataloguing in Publication Data
McHale, Jean V. (Jean Vanessa), 1965–
 Law and nursing. – 2nd ed.
 1. Nursing – Law and legislation – England
 2. Nursing – Law and legislation – Wales
 I. Title   II. Tingle, John, 1954–
 344.4′2′0414

ISBN 0 7506 4806 6

Typeset by Avocet Typeset, Brill, Aylesbury, Bucks
Printed and bound in Great Britain by Biddles Ltd. *www.biddles.co.uk*

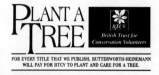

Contents

Preface

The law, and its relationship with nursing practice, has increased in scope and complexity in recent years, at a time when the role of the nurse has been evolving and the subject of many changes. From both within and without the profession nurses have been encouraged to expand their role and also to develop as specialists in clinical practice. Such developments are set to continue with the implementation of the Government's new 'NHS Plan'. However, such an expanded role brings with it enhanced accountability, with the risk of consequent litigation should something go wrong. At the same time nurses are also being encouraged to act as advocates for their patients, to safeguard standards of care and to speak out where those standards may be at risk. Many nurses have expressed concern regarding the scope of their legal obligations at a time when the structure of health care provision and their own role within it is subject to such shifting dynamics.

This book explores the legal regulation of nursing practice today and sets it in the context of recent developments, from the impact of the Human Rights Act 1998 to the development of clinical guidelines and protocols and the growth of nurse prescribing. The volume is not intended to be a substitute for specialist legal advice on specific problems that may arise in individual cases. Furthermore it should be noted that, as this field is so vast, it is the case that in some areas the account provided must be seen in context as a 'taster' for further more extensive reading of specialist legal sources.

As with our first edition, our very special thanks go to the editorial team at Butterworth-Heinemann and in particular to Mary Seager, Carrie Savage and Deena Burgess for their great help during the book's development and production. Thanks also to Marie Fox for reading drafts at an earlier stage. John Peysner was involved in the first edition of this text and his inspiration and insight into civil litigation issues provided an invaluable basis for our treatment of these issues in this book. All comments expressed and any errors that remain are, of course, the responsibility of the authors.

The law is as stated on 1 August 2000, though we have attempted to incorporate certain developments subsequent to this date.

Case list

Numbers in **bold** are page numbers in this book

Cases

AC	Law Reports, Appeal Cases
All ER	All England Law Reports
BMLR	Butterworths Medico-Legal Reports
CA	Court of Appeal
Ch D	Chancery Division Law Reports
CMLR	Common Market Law Reports
CR App R	Criminal Appeal Reports
Crim LR	Criminal Law Review
DLR	Dominion Law Reports
ECJ	European Court of Justice
ECR	European Court Reports
EHRR	European Human Rights Reports
ELR	Education Law Reports
Fam Law	Family Division Law Reports
FCR	Family Court Reports
FLR	Family Law Reports
KB	Law Reports, Kings Bench
Lloyd's Rep Med	Lloyd's Medical Law Reports
Med LR	Medical Law Reports
NLJR	New Law Journal Reports
PIQR	Personal Injuries and Quantum Reports
QB	Law Reports, Queen's Bench Division
RTR	Road Traffic Reports
SJ	Solicitors Journal
WLR	Weekly Law Reports

Australian cases:

Canadian cases:

European cases:

USA cases:

Health Service Commissioner decisions:

Practice Notes:

Statutes and statutory instruments

SI Statutory Instrument

Acts of Parliament:

Miscellaneous:

Chapter 1

Introduction: the nurse and the legal environment

Jean McHale

The role of the nurse is the subject of constant evolution. Today, nurses perform tasks that would in the past have been undertaken by doctors, an initiative encouraged by the government (DOH, 2000a). Many nurses are developing their practice to become clinical nurse specialists. At the same time the nurse – doctor dynamic has been changing, and there are new models of collaboration and of co-operation (Davies, 2000; Salvage and Smith, 2000). As has been noted by the Department of Health in the new NHS plan (DOH, 2000a, para 9.2):

> Throughout the NHS the old hierarchical ways of working are giving way to more flexible team working between different clinical professionals. Midwives, for example, are leading more responsive childbirth services in many parts of the country. In many accident and emergency departments nurses are treating patients with minor injuries and ailments, freeing up doctors' time and so delivering shorter waits for treatment. In some community clinics teams made up of occupational therapists, district nurse, physiotherapists and social care staff working flexibly together across traditional boundaries have halved the length of stay for orthopaedic patients and enabled more frail people to stay at home.

At the same time nurses are also being encouraged to act as advocates for their patients, to safeguard standards of care and to speak out where those standards may be at risk. Such an expanded role is accompanied by enhanced responsibilities, and some considerable debate and indeed controversy (see Chapter 4). In recent years, legal issues in relation to the nurse's role have never been far from the headlines – for example: 'Nurse performs operation'; 'Nurse blows the whistle on poor standards of care'; 'Nurses to prescribe drugs'. Many nurses have expressed concern regarding their legal obligations at a time when the structure of health care provision and their own role within it is subject to such shifting dynamics.

The legal environment affects nurses in many ways, from the law of negligence concerning breaches of the legal duty of care to patients and others, to the nursing professions' governing body, the United Kingdom Central Council for Nursing, Midwifery and Health Visiting (UKCC), which is established under statute (Nurses, Midwives and Health Visitors Act 1997). In recent years the courts have been faced with many issues relating to health care practice, such as the decision to withdraw treatment from patients in a persistent vegetative state, consent to treatment, negligence actions brought when patients have suffered harm during operations, and prosecutions where mercy killings have taken place. The structure of health care provision has been affected by legislation, notably the Health Act 1999, and the pace of change of law in this area has been rapid. Recent developments considered in this book include the reforms regarding the conduct of clinical malpractice litigation introduced as a consequence of Lord Woolf's report on civil justice (Woolf, 1996), the development of clinical governance, the proposals concerning nurse prescribing and the Human Rights Act 1998. There has been an increase in the number of negligence actions brought against health care practitioners. The scope of liability in negligence is considered below. Accompanying this has been the development of risk management practices aimed at reducing the prospect of litigation.

This book attempts to provide nurses with an account of their legal obligations, whether studying law as part of diploma or degree courses, or as busy practitioners seeking clarification of their legal position. This is a book on nursing law, written by lawyers for nurses. Although many ethical issues do arise in relation to the health care law matters in this book, the ethical debate is not addressed specifically; for that the reader is referred to the many health care ethics texts available (e.g. Tingle and Cribb, 2001). While it illustrates some of the legal dilemmas that arise, this book should not be seen as a substitute for the need to obtain specialist legal advice if particular problems occur.

This introductory chapter considers the framework of law and regulation within which the nurse practices. First, the structure of the English legal system and the nature of law, legal proceedings and court system are considered, then the structure of the NHS, and finally the role of nurses in relation to their professional body. The professional obligations of nurses have been affected by the publication of a number of guidance documents on the scope of the nurses' professional practice. This guidance is considered in detail in this book and reproduced in the appendices.

Law and the legal system

Types of law

The legal system is divided into two main branches: criminal and civil law. Criminal law is a system for the state punishment of offences. In a criminal law case, the action is usually brought by the Crown against the defendant. An individual may bring a private prosecution, but in practice these are very rare. A criminal law case is referred to as Regina versus Smith, which means the Crown against Smith or, as it is usually written, *R* v. *Smith*.

Civil law is the term given to an action brought by a person (the claimant or, before 26 April 1999, the plaintiff) who has suffered some harm or loss, against another person or organization (the defendant). A civil law case is normally referred to as *Bloggs* v. *Smith*. The types of civil law action with which the nurse is most likely to be concerned are claims for breach of contract and actions in 'tort'. A tort is a civil wrong. Examples of torts include undertaking surgery without obtaining any form of consent from the patient (a battery), and failing to monitor oxygen levels during an operation with the patient consequentially suffering brain damage (negligence). Other civil law actions include the action for breach of confidence, in which the patient claims that there has been unauthorized disclosure of confidential information entrusted to another in confidence. In civil law actions the claimant seeks a remedy, usually in the form of financial compensation (damages). In addition, the claimant may claim an 'injunction' to stop a particular type of conduct (an injunction being an order stopping the party performing the unjustified act). A contract is a legally enforceable promise, enforceable because both parties have given something of value. Examples include contracts of employment and contracts for sale of goods.

Public law

In some situations a person may want to challenge a decision of a government body, health authority or other public body. The person may claim that the body went beyond powers given to it by statute, or that it has wrongly exercised a discretion granted under statute. Claims against public bodies in such situations should usually be brought through a special procedure known as 'judicial review'. Judicial review is not an appeal; the court cannot substitute its own view as to how the public authority should have behaved. Instead, the court determines whether the public body has acted legally.

A number of special remedies are available against public authorities through judicial review. An action can be brought seeking a 'declaration' from the court – asking the court to declare the law on a specific point. So, for example, in *Gillick* v. *West Norfolk and Wisbech AHA* ([1986] 1 AC 112), Mrs Victoria Gillick went to court to ask for a declaration as to whether guidance given to health authorities that doctors could give contraceptive advice and treatment to girls under 16 years of age without parental consent was lawful. There are a number of what are known as 'prerogative writs'. One prerogative writ is the order of 'certiorari', which is obtained to quash an improper decision. The court may issue an order of 'mandamus' to require a public body to undertake its statutory duties. Perhaps the most well-known prerogative writ is that of 'habeas corpus' in relation to criminal proceedings, which is the requirement that the defendant be released from custody and the 'body' delivered to the applicant.

The nurse in the courtroom

When are nurses likely to appear in court? They may be a party to an action – for example, a nurse may be a claimant in a civil claim bringing an action for damages against his or her employer on the grounds of the employer's negligence. In a claim brought by a patient, the nurse may be called to give evidence; this may be regarding what the nurse saw happen to a patient who is claiming that he or she was given negligent treatment. In addition, the nurse may be called to give expert evidence, for example in a negligence action, as to the standard of practice that would be expected of a responsible nursing professional in that situation (see below).

Types of court

Criminal courts

The magistrates' court is a local court. Magistrates try minor criminal offences, and in addition they hear evidence in relation to more serious criminal offences before committing these cases for trial at the Crown Court. In the Crown Court cases are heard by a judge, usually sitting with a jury of 12 lay persons selected at random from people drawn from the electoral register in the local community.

Civil courts

The court in which a civil law case is heard usually depends upon the amount of damages claimed, which relates to the degree of harm caused and to the complexity of the case (see below). Use of juries in civil cases is very rare today; the most notable exception is that of libel cases. The whole civil justice system was subject to radical reform in 1999 following the report of Lord Woolf.

Court structure – the upper courts

High Court

There are three divisions of the High Court; the Chancery and Family Divisions hear exclusively civil law matters, and the Queen's Bench Division hears criminal law and public law matters. Each division is headed by a senior judge: in the case of the Chancery Division, the Vice-Chancellor; in the case of the Family Division, the President; and for the Queen's Bench Division, the Lord Chief Justice. These judges also sit in the Court of Appeal. The High Court may hear cases taken on appeal from the lower courts. Alternatively, cases may be heard for the first time in the High Courts. As noted above, such cases include serious negligence cases.

Court of Appeal

Above the High Court is the Court of Appeal. This is composed of senior judges known as Lord Justices of Appeal. It hears appeals in both civil and criminal cases. The civil division is headed by the Master of the Rolls, and the criminal division by the Lord Chief Justice.

House of Lords

The highest court within the United Kingdom is the House of Lords. It is composed of senior judges known as Law Lords. The Lord Chancellor presides over the House of Lords; this is a political appointment and the incumbent is also a member of the Cabinet. This court bears the same name as the second chamber of Parliament, the House of Lords. Peers who have a right to sit in the House of Lords do not have the right to sit as judges in the court, but the Law Lords may participate in parliamentary debates.

Civil procedure and the Woolf reforms

The legal system has long been criticized for its antiquated procedure, delays and use of complex language. In 1996 Lord Woolf was given the task of looking at the operation of the civil procedure rules, and this led to a much more wide-ranging enquiry into the operation of the civil justice system itself.

Lord Woolf recommended that the civil justice system should:

- be just in results delivered
- be fair in the way in which litigants are treated
- offer appropriate procedures at reasonable cost
- deal with cases at reasonable speed
- be understandable to those who need it
- be responsive to the needs of those who use it
- provide as much certainty as the particular case allows
- be effective/adequately resourced/organized.

The government accepted the majority of Lord Woolf's recommenda-tions, and these were implemented, with the bulk of the reforms becom-ing operational on 26 April 1999.

A new body, the Civil Justice Council, was created, with the task of keeping civil justice under review. Its chair is Lord Woolf, and the Vice-Chair is Sir Richard Scott. It considers how to make the civil justice system more accessible, fair and efficient. It advises the Lord Chancellor and the judiciary on the development of the civil justice system, and refers proposals for changes in the civil justice system to the Lord Chancellor and the Civil Procedure Rules Committee. It also makes pro-posals for research. New civil procedure rules were brought into opera-tion alongside Practice Directions, forms and protocols (Civil Procedure Act 1997), such as the Pre-action Protocol for the Resolution of Clinical Disputes. As a result of the reforms, the use of legal language has been considerably amended – for example, the word 'plaintiff' has now been replaced by the term 'claimant'.

Parties are encouraged to resolve their differences through the use of alternative dispute resolution mechanisms. There is a new power to stay (or halt) proceedings pending the parties being referred to alternative dispute resolution (Civil Procedure Rules, rule 1.4(2)(e)), and this has the aim of removing many issues from the scope of the courtroom and encouraging parties to resolve their differences. How effective this process actually is remains to be seen, particularly in view of the fact that lawyers have traditionally been somewhat sceptical regarding the use of alternative dispute resolution mechanisms. There are also issues such as whether at the point that parties approach lawyers to pursue litigation they are simply too polarized, such that alternative dispute resolution cannot really operate effectively. Nonetheless, evidence of use of mediation in pilot schemes in two NHS regions (Anglia and Oxford, and Northern and Yorkshire) has been encouraging, although the number of cases referred to the scheme was limited. It provided more flexible remedies – expla-nations, apologies, and the assurance that systems would be changed (DOH, 2000b).

The aim of the hearing is that matters are dealt with 'justly'. This includes in rule 1(1)(2) of the Civil Procedure Rules:

Dealing with a case justly includes, so far as is practicable:

a.   Ensuring that the parties are on an equal footing
b.   Saving expense
c.   Dealing with the case in ways which are proportionate
     – to the amount of money involved
     – to the importance of the case
     – to the complexity of the issues; and
     – to the financial position of each party
d.   Ensuring that it is dealt with expeditiously and fairly; and

e.   Allotting to it an appropriate share of the Court's resources while taking into account the need to allot resources to other cases.

The division of civil litigation

Civil proceedings today fall into three broad categories. The first is the 'small claims track'. There is a limit of £5000 on such cases, and of £1000 in personal injury cases. These cases are allocated to what were known as the 'small claims' courts. This referred to the procedure used in county courts for claims of low value. Cases regarded as suitable for such hearings include consumer disputes, accident claims, disputes regarding the ownership of goods, and most landlord and tenant disputes (other than those for possession). Secondly, there is what is known as the 'fast track', where there is a limit of £15 000 on cases. Such cases will usually be heard in the county court. Here claims will be subject to a fixed timetable, judicial monitoring, and only limited use of oral evidence. Failure to comply with case management directions will be the subject of sanctions. Cases involving claims of larger value (over £15 000) and of greater complexity are dealt with under the 'multi-track'. Here there is greater flexibility given to the court in the way in which a case will be managed appropriate to the particular needs of that case. A major feature of the reforms is the role of the procedural judge in 'managing' the case – guiding the proceedings through the court (CPR rule 14). There is now tight use of timetables and control of costs, and failure to comply with the rules/protocols may result in the parties being subject to sanctions – for example, the defence may be struck out or this may have an impact upon the costs to be awarded.

Medical negligence litigation and Woolf: specific issues

In Chapter 15 of his report, Lord Woolf directed considerable attention to medical negligence litigation. The report identified a number of problems in such litigation: there was disproportion between the costs awarded and the damages given; in many instances there were unacceptable delays in resolving cases; and the success rate was lower in medical negligence actions than in other personal injury cases. The report also commented that that there was a perceived lack of trust and openness between health care professionals and patients, and doctors/hospitals were traditionally unwilling to admit negligence.

Lord Woolf believed that patients had a number of aims. They wanted impartial information and advice, including independent medical assessment. They also wanted fair compensation for losses suffered, the dispute to be resolved quickly by fair and independent adjudication, and (sometimes) a day in court. Health care professionals also wanted speedy resolution and discreet (private) adjudication. They wanted an expert of their own or their solicitors' choice, and an economical system that did not encourage trusts to settle disputes over their heads regardless of liability. Lord Woolf considered the possibility of a new non-pecuniary remedy from the courts – a formal statement from the hospital explaining the incident of alleged negligence. The need for more open communication between the parties was emphasized in the report.

The Woolf Report and the subsequent civil justice reforms suggest that professionals and patients should adopt a constructive approach to complaints and claims. Guidance is now provided to the parties in the conduct of such cases through the operation of pre-action protocols. The aim of the protocols is to maintain or restore the patient–health care provider relationship, and to resolve as many disputes as possible without litigation. Sufficient information should be disclosed by the parties to enable each of them to understand the other's viewpoint. While the guidance in the protocols does not make specific reference to adverse outcomes, reporting provides that health care providers should have procedures in place for this. The role of clinical risk management is acknowledged in the pre-action protocols, but is left as a matter for specific health authorities. It is suggested that clinical risk management systems should be established, and also that health care providers should ensure that key staff are trained in an appropriate manner with some knowledge of health care law and complaints procedures. Information regarding adverse incidents and complaints should be used in a positive manner. Patients should be advised regarding an adverse outcome, and should on request be given information on what actually happened and information on other steps that could be taken.

Role of expert evidence

One of the major generators of costs in civil litigation that Woolf identified was the use of expert evidence (see Chapter 13 of the Woolf Report, and also Chapter 15 para 63 onwards). The Woolf reforms aim to reduce the use of expert evidence to where necessary, and today calling experts requires the permission of the court. There is great emphasis placed upon the use of written evidence. Where experts are to be called, then experts from the opposing sides will be encouraged to meet prior to the trial to identify the pertinent issues where consensus may be achieved and those issues where there is disagreement between the parties. In some areas there is provision for the use of a single expert, although in practice it appears to be the case that use of the single expert is unlikely in the majority of clinical negligence cases. This is because of the operation of the *Bolam* principle, and the fact that the test for negligence is that of the responsible body of professional practice, which necessitates the calling of evidence regarding the professional practice concerning that particular issue (see Chapter 2). Nonetheless, the Woolf Report does identify various areas in clinical negligence actions where the use of a single expert may indeed be appropriate – for example:

- The assessment of quantum of damages such as future care costs
- Regarding those medical issues which are uncontroversial, such as the precise nature of a tumour
- In relation to such matters as condition and prognosis in straightforward claims
- On matters of liability in claims under £10 000.

It will be interesting to see how restrained parties become through judicial intervention in reducing the number of experts called before the courts.

Specialist courts/tribunals

In addition to the two main categories of courts outlined above (civil and criminal), there are also a number of specialist courts dealing with issues such as family law or, in the case of coroners' courts, examinations into unexplained deaths. Hundreds of different bodies known as tribunals hear matters ranging from unfair dismissal claims in the context of employment tribunals to immigration appeals. A tribunal chairperson is normally legally qualified. In employment tribunals, for example, the chairperson usually sits to decide the case along with two other persons; one is drawn from the employer's organization and the other from a trade union organization. Tribunals are less formal than the courts, with more flexible procedures in relation to calling witnesses and hearing evidence. There is also no automatic right to legal representation or to legal aid.

Sources of law

There are a number of sources of law – first, Acts of Parliament (also known as statutes); second, case law (derived from cases decided in the courts of law). In addition, English law is in some situations governed by laws laid down in Europe through our participation in the European Union (see p. 11). A number of rules considered below govern how we assess which source of law contains the appropriate legal ruling in a situation.

Statutes

English law is to be found in Acts of Parliament. There are many Acts of Parliament relevant to nursing practice, such as the Human Fertilization and Embryology Act 1990 regulating infertility treatment, or the Abortion Act 1967. In addition, the nurse is affected by those statutes that apply more generally to the population as a whole, such as the Health and Safety at Work Act 1974. Statutes are being continually passed to govern new problems as they arise. A new statute may repeal an earlier statute, or it may amend it either in whole or in part. Statutes may also codify a particular area of law that was previously to be found in a large number of cases, or consolidate both earlier statute law and later case law in one statute.

To become an Act of Parliament, legislation must receive the approval of both Houses of Parliament (Lords and Commons) and it must also receive Royal Assent. A statute is presented to the House of Commons as a Bill. These take two forms. The first category involves Bills sponsored by the government, which almost certainly will result in legislation if the government has a majority. MPs are generally constrained to vote along party political lines. In addition, government-sponsored legislation is allocated a greater amount of parliamentary time. Alternatively, there may be Bills on which the government allows its supporters a free vote so that they can make their decision on a point of conscience. An example is the Abortion Act 1967. The second main category is Private Members' Bills. These, as the name suggests, are Bills introduced into Parliament that do not have the sponsorship of the government. These Bills will usually only become law if they have government support.

A statute may provide an outline of the legal position but then leave provisions to be defined by later secondary legislation known as 'statutory instruments'. This enables the legislation to have a more rapid passage through Parliament. For example, the Human Organ Transplants Act 1989 set down a regime for undertaking transplants from living organ donors, but the detailed procedure for undertaking those transplants was laid down in subsequent statutory instruments.

Government departments, such as the Department of Health, issue circulars. While such documents do not have the force of law, they may provide guidance as to what conduct constitutes accepted practice.

Statutory interpretation

A statute may state general legal obligations, but where disputes later arise, the statute will require interpretation. A court will examine the statute to see how it applies in a particular situation. A word or phrase within the statute may be ambiguous and require construction by the court. There are a number of rules of statutory interpretation that the court may apply. The court may look at the words of the statute and apply them literally, but it is more likely that the court will construe a word or phrase in the light of the 'purpose' of the statute (Bailey and Gunn, 1996).

Common law

In some situations there is no legislation governing a particular area, or if there is room for interpretation of the statute then it may be necessary to look elsewhere for guidance as to what is the current law. The relevant law may be found in common law, the term given to describe law that has arisen from previous decisions of the courts on that issue.

Precedent

Some cases are more important than others. Case law operates through a system of precedent. A later court may be obliged to follow the decision of an earlier court. The decisions of the highest court of the land, the House of Lords, are binding on all lower courts. Decisions of the Court of Appeal are also very important, and generally bind lower courts. Where a case arises involving a very important point of law, it may be referred up to the House of Lords in order to obtain a definitive ruling as to the legal position in this area. For example, the famous case of *Gillick* v. *West Norfolk and Wisbech AHA*, which concerned the legality of providing children under 16 years of age with contraceptive advice and treatment without parental consent, was heard in the High Court, the Court of Appeal and then in the House of Lords ([1985] 2 All ER 545).

The decisions of some lower courts do not act as binding precedents, for example, decisions at magistrates' court level. As far as tribunals are concerned, in theory each case is decided on its own facts. But tribunal decisions are frequently reported and as a consequence general principles have become established.

Interpreting cases

While there may not be a previous case with precisely the same facts, this does not mean that there are no previous cases that can be followed. Lawyers, when trying to discover the current law from previously decided cases, are primarily concerned not with the facts of a particular case, but with the point of law that was decided in that case – the ratio decendendi. They then use that point of law in order to argue by analogy to the particular case before them. In a particular case a judge may make a suggestion as to his or her view of the law, a statement which is not directly related to the decision in that case. That statement, known as the obiter dictum, does not bind lower courts. However, an obiter statement may be referred to in a later case as providing a helpful judicial view on the point of law in question.

European law

In 1973 the United Kingdom signed the Treaty of Rome and entered the European Economic Community (EEC). Since then, UK law has been increasingly affected by European law. In 1993 the Treaty of European Union was passed, which created a new body – the European Union. This is composed of the states of the European Community, but is broader in scope than the EEC.

The European Communities Act 1972 provides that rights created by or arising out of the Community Treaties shall have effect in UK law (s2(1) European Communities Act 1972). There is no general competence to regulate health matters as such across the European Union, but there is provision for certain specific regulation (Hervey, 1998). For example, Article 129 EC, which was introduced by the Treaty on European Union, provides that 'the Community shall contribute towards a high level of human health protection by encouraging co-operation between Member States and, if necessary lending support to their action'. A number of particular health matters are included, such as major health scourges and research into the cause and transmission of those diseases. Also included is the provision of information and education relating to health. In addition, UK citizens are affected by European secondary legislation; this is made up of regulations, directives and decisions. Regulations are binding and are directly applicable in English law, which means that the English courts are required to apply such regulations in English cases. Directives are also binding, but generally each state is left to determine the manner in which they apply. However, directives do apply to state authorities without further incorporation, and this includes NHS bodies (*Marshall* v. *Southampton and SW Hampshire AHA* [1986] ECR 723). There are many directives that have had a considerable impact upon nursing practice, such as the Control of Substances Hazardous to Health regulations (1988) and the mutual recognition of nursing qualifications (Directives 77/452/EEC and 77/453/EEC OJ 1977 L 176).

The European Court of Justice sits in Luxembourg. If in an English case point of law arises and a UK statute appears to be in conflict with European law, European law is supreme (*Van Gend en Loos* v. *Netherlands Belastingens-administratie* [1963] CMLR 105 ECJ). If there is uncertainty as to the extent to which, for example, a European directive applies in English law, then a reference can be made to the European Court of Justice under a procedure known as Article 177, asking for their opinion on this case. Decisions made by the European Court of Justice may be directly binding on English courts, and at the very least English courts will take notice of them (s2(1) European Communities Act 1972). Provisions of EU law have been used in litigation concerning access to health care services – for example, free movement principles under Article 59 EC have been successfully argued in relation to abortion services by EU citizens (*Grogan* [1991] ECR 4685), and regarding access to infertility services by Diane Blood, who sought to travel to Belgium in order that she could be artificially inseminated by her deceased husband's sperm (*R* v. *Human Fertilisation and Embryology Authority ex parte Blood* [1997] 2 All ER 687) (see further discussion in Chapter 9).

European Convention on Human Rights

We are also party to the European Convention on Human Rights (ECHR). This is totally separate to our membership of the European Union. The European Convention on Human Rights came into force on 3 September 1953, and individual citizens of the UK have had a right to petition under the Convention since 1966. The Convention contains a list of what are regarded as fundamental human rights. If a person believes that one of his or her fundamental rights has been violated and the claim is not upheld in the English courts, he or she can seek to bring the case before the European Commission of Human Rights in Strasbourg. Actions have been brought, for example, challenging a woman's decision to have an abortion (*Paton* v. *UK* [1980] 3 EHRR 408). Where a claim is upheld before the European Court of Human Rights, the English courts have in the past not been bound to follow it, nor has Parliament been bound to change the law on that matter. However, the role of human rights is likely to change radically following the enactment of the Human Rights Act 1998, which came into force in October 2000.

Human Rights Act 1998
The Human Rights Act 1998 is the first comprehensive bill of rights to be enacted in this country, and incorporates rights contained in the European Convention of Human Rights into English law. As noted above, individuals could bring claims direct to the European Court of Human Rights in Strasbourg, but this was a protracted process. Bringing such a claim could take several years and ultimately, while the English government might decide to act upon the findings of the Court, this was not invariably the case. The Human Rights Act 1998 therefore enacts a radical change. From October 2000, where an English court is determining a matter 'in connection with' a right under the Convention then it must, as far as is applicable, take account of Strasbourg case law (section 2). All primary and secondary legislation must be construed consistently with the 1998 Act. Where legislation is inconsistent, the court may disapply subordinate legislation. This applies as long as the legislation does not debar this. What the court cannot do is strike down primary legislation – in effect, act as a 'Supreme Court' in that situation. The word of Parliament as expressed through statute ultimately prevails. Certain courts, such as the House of Lords, High Court and County Court, have the power to make what is called a 'declaration of incompatibility' (section 4). As a consequence of such a declaration of incompatibility a government minister may make a 'remedial order' in relation to a particular piece of legislation, and this may also lead to remedial action in a particular case, although this is not automatic. There is a new right of action provided against a public body acting in a public capacity, such as an NHS body, which acts in a manner that is incompatible with a right under the ECHR (ss6(1), 7(1) Human Rights Act 1998).

Access to justice

One of the main restrictions upon use of the court process is the cost involved in bringing a case. For many years there was a system of state-funded legal advice, assistance and representation known as legal aid ((s1) Legal Aid Act 1988). Generally, applicants seeking legal aid were subject to a means test of their income and disposable capital to determine their eligibility. There was considerable criticism of the scheme, and it was argued that the threshold for disposable income and capital above which there was no entitlement to free legal aid was very low. In a situation in which a person's income and disposable capital were higher than the levels of eligibility, then he or she could be required to make contributions in accordance with income levels. The threshold set for those eligible to receive legal aid gradually decreased. Many cases were funded by legal expense insurance – for example, individuals involved in road accident cases and trade union members have access to legal support.

The operation of the funding system was altered by the Access to Justice Act 1999 (and see Modernising Justice, 1998). This establishes a new Legal Services Commission, which is a non-departmental public body that has the task of creating and developing the Community Legal Service and the new Criminal Defence Service (ss1 – 3). There are regional legal services committees, which work to ensure that needs for legal services and regional priorities are correctly identified. The previous civil and family legal aid budget is replaced by a Community Legal Services Fund. The changes in funding in legal services were partly driven by concerns that unmeritorious claims were being funded, that the previous system had been too heavily biased towards court-based solutions, and that lawyers, because they were paid according to the amount of work undertaken, had no incentive to undertake cases expeditiously.

The Fund is obliged to obtain the best value for money, and will contract for legal services with solicitors' firms. This is an extension of the scheme of legal aid franchising, under which firms who wanted to obtain legal aid work had to satisfy various quality control thresholds before obtaining a legal aid franchise, which gave them the ability to obtain more work. There is to be a 'quality mark', and applications for this can be received not only from solicitors' firms but also from other advice agencies, etc. The government has also encouraged the development of 'Community Legal Service Partnerships' between bodies such as local authorities, charities and advice providers. The aim is to widen access to legal advice.

Persons making applications to the Fund must satisfy the Funding Code (ss8 and 9), which replaces the civil merits test. The Code is more restrictive than the previous system. Applicants for funding from the scheme will be subject to a 'funding assessment', and relevant factors include whether there is another way of resolving the dispute or if there are alternative sources of funding for litigation, and also whether a reasonable person would be prepared to spend his or her own funds to pursue the litigation. The majority of personal injury claims will now be funded through what is known as a 'conditional fee' system rather than through state aid.

Conditional fees

'Conditional fees' for civil law cases were introduced by the Courts and Legal Services Act 1990 (s58 Courts and Legal Services Act 1990). These allow lawyers to take on cases without the client incurring any cost for representation, but the lawyer can recover a higher fee offset against the damages awarded in a successful action. This is different to the scheme of 'contingency fee' common in the USA, where a lawyer takes on a client's case without requiring any initial financial contribution to the legal fees, but if the client's case succeeds, then the lawyer can recover an agreed percentage of the damages. The scope of conditional fees was extended in 1998 to apply to a range of civil proceedings, but not in relation to family proceedings. Following the 1999 reforms the conditional fee has an enhanced importance, because state-funded legal assistance will not be available to those persons who are bringing personal injury actions (although clinical negligence actions are excluded from this restriction). The conditional fee system has been amended so that successful litigants can recover success fees and insurance fees from their opponents (Access to Justice Act 1999). Such a funding scheme may widen access to litigation and provide enhanced financial incentives for lawyers to undertake litigation; however, the danger for litigants is that those cases where there is considerable uncertainty may never be pursued because lawyers do not want to take the risk. This is one reason why clinical negligence actions still receive state-funded assistance.

Criminal Defence Service

In criminal cases there is not a set budget for funding litigation, and the crucial issue is the merits of the case. There is a new 'Criminal Defence Service', which has the aim of ensuring that persons 'have access to such advice, assistance and representation as the interests of justice require'. As with civil procedure, if solicitors wish to provide this service they must 'contract' to do so with the new Legal Services Commission. There will also be lawyers who will be directly employed by the Commission to undertake representation in criminal cases. One of the criticisms of this scheme is that it will result in a reduction in the availability of legal services, because far fewer law firms will be offering this type of representation.

Settlements

While a dispute may lead to parties seeking legal advice and beginning legal proceedings, this does not mean that a case will ultimately go to court. The majority of cases are settled before proceedings in court have begun. Indeed, the threat of legal proceedings may operate as a negotiating tool, encouraging parties to settle their differences.

The structure of the National Health Service

Most health care in England is provided the NHS, although nurses may of course work outside the NHS — for example, in nursing homes and residential care homes. In this section, the structure of health care provision within the NHS is examined. The Secretary of State for Health is accountable to Parliament for the operation of the health service, and controls NHS expenditure through the use of cash limits. Day-to-day management of the Health Service is undertaken by the NHS Executive (NHSE), which is largely based in Leeds.

The structure of the NHS has been altered by the Health Authorities Act 1995. Prior to 1 April 1996, below the NHSE in England were regional health authorities (RHAs). After that date RHAs were abolished, with their statutory functions being transferred to eight 'regional outposts' of the NHSE (Health Authorities Act 1995). These bodies are responsible for overseeing the efficient operation of the NHS.

Prior to 1 April 1996, below regional level, health care was regulated through district health authorities (DHAs) and family health service authorities (FHSAs). The Health Authorities Act 1995 introduced amendments to this structure and, as of 1 April 1996, DHAs and FHSAs were merged to form new unitary health authorities. This is part of a movement towards a greater focus on primary health care provision. General practitioners are under an obligation to provide care to those patients who are on their list. In addition, they are required to provide care to other persons seeking treatment where treatment is 'immediately required' (Terms and Conditions of Service, paragraph 4(1)b).

In 1990, the National Health Service and Community Care Act created an 'internal market' in health care. Health care provision was to be purchased from 'providers'. Purchasers were to be DHAs and general practice fundholders (GPFH), and providers were to include the new National Health Service trusts (NHSTs) and also private hospitals. Parties within this internal market in health care entered into contracts, and the contracts between NHS purchasers and private sector providers took a conventional legal form and were enforceable in the courts in the usual way. This meant little change from the position prior to 1990, as for many years DHAs had been buying some services from independent hospitals; however, after 1990, dealings between bodies within the NHS itself were to be operated via contracts. Contracts were placed between NHS bodies that had no direct management relationship, covering arrangements such as those between a GPFH and a hospital and an NHST. The Act called these 'NHS contracts'. Confusingly, despite their name, these contracts were not enforceable in the courts, and instead a special procedure was established to which these disputes could be referred (s4(3)). The Labour government was opposed to the internal market, which has now been replaced. While contracts are still at present operational within the NHS, the emphasis today is on partnership and co-operation. Primary Care Groups are being formed, which are larger groups of primary care purchasers, to commission services. The Health Act 1999 provides for the development of new bodies known as 'primary care trusts', which will eventually take over the commissioning of services – initially of health and later, it is envisaged, also of social care. Fund-holding practices have been abolished (s1 Health Act 1999).

Clinical governance

Emphasis is being placed upon the need to maintain standards in health care. An early example of such emphasis on standards was the Patient's Charter. While this document is essentially a list of guidelines, and breach of Patient Charter requirements are not directly enforceable in the courts, the movement towards stating acceptable standards of health care has continued in recent years. In the White Paper 'The New NHS', the concept of clinical governance was discussed. This was further explored in the consultation paper on quality, issued by the Department of Health in 1998 (DOH, 1998), which defined 'clinical governance' as being 'a framework through which NHS organizations are accountable for continuously improving the quality of their services and safeguarding high standards of care by creating an environment in which excellence in clinical care will flourish'. The Health Act 1999 made provision for the NHS trusts and primary care groups to be placed under a new statutory duty of quality in section 18. Clinical governance will be promoted through the operation of the Commission for Health Improvement and the National Institute for Clinical Excellence.

The Commission for Health Improvement

The Commission for Health Improvement was established under section 19 of the Health Act 1999. It is headed by Dame Deidre Hine, a former Chief Executive for Wales. The Commission is composed of 13 members, and there are eight lay members. It is concerned with the implementation of clinical governance, National Service Frameworks and the guidelines issued by the National Institute of Clinical Excellence. The aim of National Service frameworks is to ensure clear national service standards to facilitate quality and consistency in care and treatment provisions. The Commission also has the role of assisting the NHS in the identification of serious or persistent clinical problems, and will have responsibility for the oversight and assistance of external NHS incident inquiries. They are also producing benchmarks for good practice. In their role in relation to clinical governance they have the task of visiting each NHS trust, primary care trust and health authority every 4 years.

National Institute for Clinical Excellence

Another new body, the National Institute for Clinical Excellence (NICE), has also been established. This is a special health authority, and provides guidance as to 'best practice' to patients, health professionals and the public. Such guidance covers the clinical management of specific conditions, and also individual health technologies such as medicines, diagnostic devices and procedures. NICE is involved in the development of clinical audits with the aim of enabling health professionals to monitor their practice, and will be involved in assessing how a particular technology has been used nationally through the merger of clinical audit findings. NICE's important role in the development of clinical guidelines is discussed further in Chapter 4. Nurses need to be aware of the role and operation of such organizations, and of the increasing emphasis on both clinical accountability and quality in health care practice.

Challenges to failure to provide health services

The Secretary of State for Health has various statutory duties. Section 1 of the National Health Service Act 1977 states:

> It is the Secretary of State's duty to continue the promotion in England and Wales of a comprehensive health service designed to ensure improvement:
>
> (a) in the physical and mental health of the people of those countries and
> (b) in the prevention, diagnosis and treatment of illness and for that purpose to provide or secure effective provision of services in accordance with the Act.

Section 3 of that Act states:

> It is the Secretary of State's duty to provide throughout England and Wales to such extent as he considers necessary to meet all reasonable requirements – (a) hospital accommodation ... (c) medical, dental, nursing and ambulance services ... (f) such other services as are required for the diagnosis and treatment of illness.

Can the Secretary of State be held liable if services are not provided? In a number of cases persons have challenged a failure to provide health care services in the courts. For example, patients in Birmingham challenged the Health Authority's refusal to provide a unit for orthopaedic services (*R* v. *Secretary of State for Social Service ex parte Hincks* (1980) (1979) 123 Sol J 436). The application failed. In the Court of Appeal, Lord Denning, agreeing with the judge at first instance, stated that the Secretary of State's duty needed to be read in the light of the financial resources available. Subsequently, in two cases, both concerning surgery required on an infant, the courts again rejected the claim that in refusing to provide these facilities the Secretary of State had acted in breach of duty.

In the second case, Stephen Brown L.J. stated that:

> This is a hearing before a court. This is not the forum in which a court can properly express opinions upon the way in which national resources are allocated or distributed. [There] may be very good reasons why the resources in this case do not allow all the beds in the hospital to be used at this particular time. We have no evidence of that and indeed ... it is not for this court or for any other court to substitute its own judgment for the judgment of those who are responsible for the allocation of resources.

It might have been thought that the advent of the NHS internal market would have led to more parties 'chancing their arm' and challenging resource allocation decisions. However, litigants have not been flocking to the courts.

The question of allocation of resources arose in the context of a well-publicized case involving a young child. B, a 10-year-old child, suffered from leukaemia. Treatment was undertaken involving chemotherapy and a bone marrow transplant, which was initially successful; however, the cancer recurred. Cambridgeshire Health Authority refused to authorize a further course of treatment. Doctors stated that a third course of chemotherapy and a further transplant would not be in the child's best interests, and that overall the success rate of the procedure was 1 – 4 per cent. The child's father sought to challenge the decision to refuse treatment. The case was heard first in the High Court and then on appeal in the Court of Appeal (*R* v. *Cambridge District Health Authority ex parte B* [1995] 2 All ER 129). Both hearings took place on the same afternoon.

At first instance in the High Court, Laws J. said that, in determining whether to give treatment, the Health Authority must act reasonably. This meant that, in making the decision, the Health Authority should have regard to all relevant considerations. In this case he said the Health Authority had not taken into consideration the views of B's family. He was also of the view that in a situation where, as here, a patient was at risk of death, the Health Authority had to explain why it had decided not to fund the treatment.

However, his judgment was overturned in the Court of Appeal. Sir Thomas Bingham, the Master of the Rolls, held that, while the Finance Director of the Health Authority had not spoken directly to the family, he had noted the interests of the family. In addition, difficult issues concerning resource allocation had to be weighed in the balance. He stated that:

> Difficult and agonising judgments had to be made as to how a limited budget could best be allocated for the maximum advantage of the maximum number of patients. That was not a judgment for the court.

Sir Thomas Bingham held that the Authority had weighed up the various factors in reaching the decision and had not acted unreasonably. Relevant factors were that the treatment was untested and that it could almost be regarded as being experimental in its nature. There was only around a 1 – 4 per cent success rate. In addition, the court noted the fact that there were potentially dehabilitating side effects. The court held that in these circumstances the decision of the Health Authority was not unreasonable.

However, subsequently the courts have indicated greater willingness to scrutinize decisions concerning the allocation of resources. In *R* v. *North Derbyshire Health Authority, ex parte Fisher* [1997] 8 Med LR 327, a High Court judge held that North Derbyshire Health Authority had acted unlawfully in that a patient with multiple sclerosis had been denied treatment with an expensive new drug, Beta inferon. The Authority adopted a policy to the effect that the drug would not be made available outside a clinical trial, even though they were informed of the fact that clinical trials of this drug had been the subject of indefinite postponement. Dyson J. held that the Health Authority had imposed what amounted to a blanket ban on the drug, although there was NHS guidance in existence regarding its use. He said that:

> A blanket ban is the very antithesis of national policy, whose aim is to target the drug at patients who could most benefit from the treatment.

In *R* v. *North West Lancashire HA ex parte A, D and G* ([2000] 1 W.L.R. 977), Lancashire Health Authority's refusal to fund gender reassignment surgery for transsexuals was challenged successfully. The Authority had a policy which stated that they would not fund such treatment unless there was overriding clinical need or other exceptional circumstances. The Court of Appeal held that while the Authority was entitled to establish a policy, the operation of the policy by the Council was closer to a blanket application of a policy rather than the legitimate recognition of a policy subject to individual exceptions.

The issue of guidelines in relation to the prescribing of Viagra by general practitioners was challenged successfully in *R* v. *Secretary of State for Health ex parte Pfizer Ltd* ([1999] *Lloyds Rep Med* 289). Here the Secretary of State issued a Health Service circular with the aim of limiting the prescription of Viagra by general practitioners. The NHS terms of service for general practitioners had provided that:

> … a doctor shall order any drugs or appliances which are needed for the treatment of any patient to whom he is providing treatment under these terms of service by issuing to that patient a prescription form.

The action for judicial review succeeded. It was held that the doctor was entitled to give such treatment as was considered necessary and appropriate.

On what basis should such matters be left to the courts? The approach taken by Laws J. in the Child B case has considerable relevance for those who are arguing for health rights and exploring this in the context of litigation deriving from the Human Rights Act 1998. It is undeniable that resources are, and indeed always will be, limited. In an analogous area, the provision of care under the Chronically Sick and Disabled Persons Act 1970 (section 2), the House of Lords confirmed that when assessing needs under the Act this could not be divorced from the costs involved in the supply of those needs (*R* v. *Gloucester CC ex parte Barry* [1997] AC 584). Thus while the Human Rights Act 1998 provides the prospect for further challenges regarding resource allocation decisions, with claims likely to be centred upon rights such as the right to life, when it comes to actually intervening with clinical decision-making processes the extent of judicial involvement in practice may still be limited. The procedure for judicial review is precisely that – review and not appeal. The court cannot substitute its judgment for that of the body which has made the initial decision. Moreover, even if courts were prepared to intervene, it is arguable that they do not provide an appropriate forum for such scrutiny. The whole question of rationing in health care needs to be addressed at national level rather than on a case-by-case basis as matters are referred to the courts. We may profit from consideration of the model adopted in Oregon, USA, where rationing has been put on a statutory footing (Newdick, 1995). Here, public consultation was undertaken before a list of treatment priorities was enacted in statute. The role of the National Institute for Clinical Excellence in the public prioritization of health care resources is thus likely to prove of some considerable importance here in the future.

Professional accountability

The United Kingdom Central Council for Nursing, Midwifery and Health Visiting

The work of nurses in this country is overseen by their professional governing body, the UKCC, which is established by the Nurses, Midwives and Health Visitors Act 1997. The UKCC is composed of a council containing a maximum of 60 members (s1 Nurses, Midwives and Health Visitors Act 1997). Two-thirds are registered nurses, midwives or health visitors elected from their professional peers, and one-third are appointed by government ministers after consultation with bodies including professional organizations and consumer groups. They are health professionals or persons with experience in other fields, such as education, which are believed by the Secretary of State to be appropriate.

The professional register

The UKCC keeps a register of nurses, midwives and health visitors (s7 Nurses, Midwives and Health Visitors Act 1997). There are 15 subcategories to the register, e.g. children's nurses and mental illness. It establishes rules regarding entry, removal and reinstatement from the register. Qualifications obtained in other European Community countries are recognized, and the UKCC also recognizes other qualifications. Nurses may be entered on the register if they have an appropriate professional qualification and are of good character. The UKCC is also concerned with nurse training, both at entry into the profession and post-qualification (s2, 1997 Act). The UKCC provides guidance as to what are acceptable standards of professional conduct through its Code of Conduct and other statements such as its *Guidelines for Professional Practice* (UKCC, 1996a). As will be seen later, nurses may face a difficult dilemma if their obligations under the professional ethical code and under the contract of employment are at variance.

Misconduct

If a nurse is found to have behaved in a manner which constitutes 'misconduct', then he or she is liable to disciplinary action (s10 Nurses, Midwives and Health Visitors Act 1997). The Rules define misconduct as being (UKCC, 1998) 'conduct unworthy of a nurse, midwife or health visitor (Rule 1(2))'. Examples of misconduct are the physical and sexual abuse of patients, stealing from patients, failing to care for patients properly, failure to keep proper records, failing to administer records safely, deliberately concealing unsafe practices, and committing serious criminal offences.

Initial allegations are screened by an officer of the UKCC. There may be a short investigation by a solicitor to establish whether there is a case to answer, and the matter may then be referred to the Preliminary Proceedings Committee, which 'screens complaints'(UKCC, 1998).

The Preliminary Proceedings Committee

The Preliminary Proceedings Committee examines allegations made against practitioners. If it finds that these are trivial, it may 'decline to proceed'. If, however, it takes the view that the allegations concern a matter that is probably misconduct, then this can be referred for a formal public hearing. Alternatively, the Committee may direct the Registrar to issue a formal caution (s11 Nurses, Midwives and Health Visitors Act 1997, and rule 4 SI 1993) if the charges are admitted. Cautions are given in a situation in which misconduct has been proven and admitted, but where there are strong mitigating circumstances such that in this particular situation removal from the register is not appropriate in a particular case (UKCC, 1998). A caution will remain on the register for up to 5 years, and is something that would be disclosed automatically in a situation in which, for example, an employer or member of the public contacted the UKCC in relation to registration matters. The Committee may also convene a hearing as a matter of urgency and order that a practitioner be suspended prior to a formal hearing before the Professional Conduct Committee (rule 3 of Professional Conduct Rules (SI 1993 No. 893)).

Professional Conduct Committee

Serious matters are referred to the Professional Conduct Committee. This Committee considers cases and makes findings on the basis that professional misconduct has been proven beyond all reasonable doubt. Hearings are held in public, save where by hearing the issue in private the patient's anonymity is safeguarded, or the case regards medical information of a confidential nature (UKCC, 1998). The practitioner may choose to be represented by a lawyer/trade union officer, etc. (Rule 13(5)). Where allegations are not admitted, a hearing with cross-examination of witnesses is undertaken. The Committee has a number of powers. A case may be held to be 'not proven' or that, while the facts are proven, this does not constitute professional misconduct in a particular case.

Sanctions

Where the case is found proven, a name can be removed from the register, the practitioner may be issued with a caution (rules 9 and 18), the Committee may postpone judgment for a fixed period (rule 18), or a decision may be made to take no action. It should be noted that, after a finding of misconduct has been made but before sanction is determined, the committee should hear evidence as to the nurse's general record and the nurse may cross-examine witnesses and challenge any new allegations (Rule 18(3)). Grounds for removal include abuse of patients, breach of confidentiality and 'reckless and wilfully unskilled practice' (UKCC, 1990); also failure to provide training to a nurse who requested it, and breach of other managerial responsibilities. If evidence of ill health has emerged, this may be referred to the Health Committee of the UKCC (UKCC, 1998).

The nurse has the right to appeal from either of these committees to the High Court (s12 Nurses, Midwives and Health Visitors Act 1997). However, in practice the court is unlikely to overturn the decision, as they are more prepared to accept the judgment of the professional body (*Slater v. UKCC*, unreported 18 May 1988 (QBD)). In addition, the conduct of proceedings of the committee may be subject to judicial review. The committees are under a duty to act fairly, and must give nurses an opportunity to present their case and to answer the charges made against them. If they fail to do so, this may lead to a challenge that the conduct of the hearing was contrary to the rules of natural justice (*Hefferen v. The Committee of the UKCC* (1988); *The Independent,* 11 March).

Illness

If a Committee examining a claim of professional misconduct believes that the matter raised concerns a question of ill health, then it may be referred to a separate panel, the Health Committee (Rule 29). Initially, such a claim is considered by a panel of screeners who are UKCC council members (Rule 9(3) and UKCC, 1998). They may refer the claim to the Health Committee, or decide that it concerns matters outside the remit of that Committee and that it should be referred back to the Professional Conduct Committee. The nature of the hearing before the Health Committee usually means that such a hearing will be held in private (UKCC, 1998). The Health Committee examines whether the nurse's ability to practise has been seriously impaired by a physical or mental condition, and whether he or she is a danger to the public. They may close the case, refer it back to the PPC or PCC, or remove/suspend registration.

Restoration to the register

A nurse who has been removed from the register may later apply to be restored (Rule 22). A hearing is held at which the nurse is entitled to be present. The nurse must nominate two persons to act as referees, and these must be persons with knowledge of the facts and who have known the nurse since he or she was removed from the register. In 1996 the UKCC indicated that it was tightening up the grounds on which individuals may be restored to the register; this followed controversy over the restoration of two persons who had originally been removed when they had been convicted for rape. Applications to restore to the register will be heard every 4 months by a panel of four, usually chaired by the president of the UKCC and generally with two panel members drawn from a consumer organization (UKCC, 1998). Individuals are required to show that they understand/accept the reason for their removal from the register, that appropriate steps have been taken to address the problems leading to their removal (for example by counselling), that they have been working in a field which is related for a significant period of time, and that they have demonstrated 'exemplary standards of conduct during that period'. Finally, their application must be supported by impeccable references from their current employer and, if appropriate, by a medical practitioner (UKCC, 1998). The UKCC has stated that (UKCC, 1996b):

> ... for certain offences such as murder, rape, child abuse and serious physical assault, the applicant will not be restored to the register if this is likely to undermine public confidence in the professions regulated by the UKCC.

Midwives

Midwives are also subject to further regulation through local supervisors, who are appointed by the local supervising authority (s15 Nurses, Midwives and Health Visitors Act 1997). Midwives are required to inform supervisors of where they intend to practise. Supervisors can investigate or suspend midwives if they present a risk to public health because they could spread illness or because of misconduct (Rule 38).

The National Boards

In addition to the UKCC, bodies known as National Boards appointed by the Secretary of State have a role in regulating nursing. There are three Boards, one each for England, Wales and Scotland. The Boards comprise a chief executive and six appointed members, including one representative from each of the professions (s5, 1997 Act). In the past they were involved in regulating misconduct, but today their role is more limited. They have the task of approving institutions that provide training courses for nurses, midwives and health visitors (s6, 1997 Act).

The nature of nurse training is currently under evolution under the government's 'Making a Difference' strategy. There is a movement towards joint training across the professions in issues such as communication skills and NHS principles and organization (DOH, 2000a, para 9.18). It will be interesting to see if this facilitates the breaking down of boundaries between the professions.

Reforming nursing regulation

The operation of the UKCC has been the subject of some considerable criticism. A firm of consultants, JM Consulting, was commissioned to examine the nature of nursing regulation in the form of the Nurses, Midwives and Health Visitors Act. It proposed that a new Nursing and Midwifery Council should be established, and that this should be composed of between 24 and 27 members. There should be a majority of professional members, and a minimum of one-third of the committee should be lay members. The government is now consulting on their proposals for a new Council to replace the UKCC and the four national Boards in their document *Modernising Regulation the New Nursing and Midwifery Council* (DOH, 2000a). The Council will be required to:

- Treat the health and welfare of patients as paramount
- Collaborate and consult with key stakeholders
- Be open and pro-active in accounting to the public and the professions for its work.

The new body will have wider powers than the existing bodies to deal with practitioners who pose a risk to patients. It will be a smaller body, consisting of some directly elected practitioners and also lay practitioners. The professional register is to be streamlined, and registration is to be linked to evidence that there is continuing professional development of the practitioner. It is envisaged that these reforms are to take place by Order under the Health Act 1999, section 69.

Conclusions

This chapter has set out the framework of legal regulation within which nurses undertake their practice. In subsequent chapters the operation of the law is considered in a number of areas that are particularly pertinent to nursing practice.

References

Bailey, S. H. and Gunn, M. J. (1996). *Smith and Bailey on the English Legal System*. Sweet and Maxwell, Chapter 6.

Davies, C. (2000). Getting health care professionals to work together. *Br. Med. J.*, **320**, 1021–2.

Department of Health (1998). *A First Class Service – Quality in the New NHS*. DOH.

Department of Health (2000a). *Modernising Regulation: The New Nursing and Midwifery Council*. DOH.

Department of Health (2000b). *Mediating Medical Negligence Claims: An Option for the Future?* DOH.

Modernising Justice (1998). HMSO.

Hervey, T. (1998). *European Social Law and Policy*, Chapter 7. Longmans.

Newdick, C. (1995). *Who Should We Treat?* Oxford University Press, pp. 30–36.

Salvage, J. and Smith, R. (2000). Doctors and nurses; doing it differently. *Br. Med. J.*, **320**, 1019–1020.

Tingle, J. and Cribb, A. (eds) (2001). *Nursing Law and Ethics*, 2nd edn. Blackwell Scientific Publications.

UKCC (1990). *With a View to Removal from the Register*. UKCC.

UKCC (1996a). *Guidelines for Professional Practice*. UKCC.

UKCC (1996b). UKCC tightens its rules on restorations to the register. *Register*, **17**, 3.

UKCC (1998). *Complaints Against Professional Misconduct*. UKCC.

Woolf, Lord (1996). *Access to Justice*. HMSO.

Chapter 2

Nursing negligence: general issues

John Tingle

Introduction

Nurses are not only professionally accountable to patients through the United Kingdom Central Council for Nursing, Midwifery and Health Visiting (UKCC) Code of Professional Conduct, but like all other professionals they are also accountable in law, and malpractice may lead to a civil action or a criminal prosecution. A nurse is under a legal duty to act carefully towards the patient. If a nurse fails to exercise sufficient care and by so doing causes injury or harm to the patient, he or she will be held liable in the tort of negligence.

The next section considers liability in tort for negligent conduct; later sections consider liability in criminal law, where actions are gravely negligent, and some issues regarding reform of the law of negligence. The present chapter focuses upon general principles of liability. Various related negligence issues are examined in later chapters, including liability under certain statutes for negligence. Questions of liability in relation to childbirth and conception are considered in Chapter 9.

Liability in tort for negligent conduct

Accidents sometimes happen

A nurse is not negligent if he or she acts in accordance with a practice accepted as proper by a responsible body of nursing opinion. The nurse is not expected to take precautions against unforeseeable risks, and even if risks are foreseeable they may still be justified in the particular circumstances of the case.

Accidents, untoward incidents or adverse treatment outcomes may occur without any findings of fault being made against the nurse. For example:

1. A competent nurse, following the correct procedure for venipuncture, may still cause the patient to develop a haematoma or bleed after the removal of the needle if the patient is on anti-coagulant therapy. This may happen occasionally even though the nurse has ascertained that the patient is taking anticoagulants, and has applied pressure to the site of venipuncture personally. Bruising can be reduced if pressure is applied by the nurse or phlebotomist, but can still occur in the older patient along with, occasionally, slight pain and discomfort.
2. Ribs have been known to fracture when a patient receives external cardiac massage when the nurse has carried out the procedure correctly.

Elements of the tort of negligence

Generally speaking, the claimant (the person bringing the court action) must prove negligence against the nurse or the nurse's employers. The claimant will normally have to prove his or her case on the 'balance of probabilities' (Foster, 2001). The elements of the tort of negligence must be established.

The basic elements are:

- Duty
- Breach
- Damage
- Remoteness.

Duty

The claimant must first establish that the defendant (nurse, health authority or trust) owed him or her a legal duty of care. In the health care context this is usually not a problem, as Jones (1992) commented when defining the tort:

In cases of medical negligence the existence of a duty owed to the patient is usually regarded as axiomatic, and attention normally focuses on whether there has been a breach of duty or whether the breach caused damage.

However, the issue of duty could be problematic where a nurse acts as a 'Good Samaritan' and causes further injury by negligently administering first aid to the accident victim. The duty issue in relation to accident victims was raised in the Court of Appeal in *Kent* v. *Griffiths and Others* ([2000] 2All ER 474). It was held that, in appropriate circumstances, an ambulance service could owe a duty of care to a member of the public on whose behalf a 999 call was made if, due to carelessness, it failed to arrive within a reasonable time. The acceptance of the call by the ambulance service established the duty of care, and the ambulance in this case was delayed through no good reason, taking 40 minutes to arrive. The claimant, an asthmatic, suffered an asthma attack and eventually went into respiratory arrest. Had the ambulance arrived in a reasonable time there was a high probability that the arrest would have been averted. The delay caused the claimant further injuries. The defendant's appeal was dismissed.

The courts are unlikely to find an express legal duty to rescue a stranger; the nurse could walk past a victim with legal impunity (Tingle, 1991). However, if the nurse stops and acts then a legal duty of care will flow from his or her actions. The nurse could now be sued if he or she practises first aid negligently and causes further injury. In contrast, it appears that in some instances the UKCC would expect the nurse to act as a Good Samaritan and assist if this could easily be done. Examples 2 and 3 given by the UKCC in their advisory document (UKCC, 1996) provide useful illustrations of the UKCC approach to the nurse as a Good Samaritan. In Example 3 (see Appendix 1, section 14), a distinction is made between legal and professional duties. A nurse would be expected to make some response in the emergency situation postulated, at the very least comforting and supporting the injured patient. There is a risk, however, that if the nurse does act and makes a mistake, then legal consequences may follow. However, it should be remembered that the likelihood of a Good Samaritan being sued is fairly remote, and that the public interest is better served by doing and encouraging Good Samaritan acts.

Duty questions

The first issue is whether a person has in fact become a patient of a health care professional or a hospital. This question is discussed in sections 11–14 of UKCC (1996), and some useful illustrations are given. Considering the situation described below may also help to explain the issue.

> An injured, confused man wanders into a hospital after a road traffic accident and is unable to locate the accident and emergency department. He requires urgent medical treatment. A hospital security guard passes him in a corridor in the hospital and does not challenge or question him. A nurse hurrying home after finishing her shift also passes him without stopping. Should the guard and the nurse have stopped and questioned him?

Can the guard and the nurse be said to have owed a duty of care to the accident victim, which would have required such action? Furthermore, what about the position of the hospital? Were there any organizational failures, such as failure to erect a signpost properly or to man a reception desk, that would make the hospital directly liable for any negligence?

Much depends on the circumstances of the case and on answers to factual questions such as: how ill did the victim look? what was the time of the incident? etc. It will be seen that Example 2 of section 14, UKCC (1996), is similar in facts to the problem discussed. The UKCC states that in its example the nurse would be expected to take some action, comforting and supporting the patient and calling for expert help.

Breach

The second step is for the claimant to prove that the nurse was negligent in breach of a legal duty of care. The nurse's conduct would be viewed from the perspective of what 'the ordinary skilled nurse in her speciality would have done in the circumstances of the case'. The nurse would also have been expected to take precautions against reasonably known risks only.

Legal standard of nursing competence

In determining the legal standard of care if litigation was being brought, lawyers would have to take advice from other nurses in the same speciality. If the case went to trial, the judge would hear expert evidence and would draw conclusions from this as to the standard of professional practice. The legal principles stated come from the well-known *Bolam* case (*Bolam* v. *Friern Hospital Management Committee* [1957] 1 WLR 582). In this case, the Judge, Mr Justice McNair, stated what has become known as the *Bolam* test:

> The test is the standard of the ordinary skilled man exercising and professing to have that special skill. A man need not possess the highest expert skill; it is well established law that it is sufficient if he exercises the ordinary skill of an ordinary competent man exercising that particular art ...

The judge went on to say that a professional would not be liable in negligence:

> ... if he has acted in accordance with a practice accepted as proper by a responsible body of medical men skilled in that particular art. ... Putting it the other way round, a man is not negligent if he is acting in accordance with such a practice, merely because there is a body of opinion who would take a contrary view.

Sections 15 and 16 of UKCC (1996) provide a discussion of the concept of reasonableness with reference to the *Bolam* principle. If a nurse is a trainee, he or she is still expected to accord with the standard of a qualified practitioner (*Nettleship* v. *Weston* [1971] 2 QB 691). Nurses who are unsure of what to do should get advice from a more experienced practitioner. By doing so, not only are they acting in accordance with good practice, but this is also likely to absolve them of liability in negligence (*Wilsher* v. *Essex AHA* [1986] 3 All ER 801).

Reasonable differences of opinion

There may be legitimate differences as to what constitutes a body of responsible professional practice. Take, for instance, the issue of nurses using cot-sides. One nurse may decide to use cot-sides while another nurse may refuse to have them on the ward because it is known that patients can roll over the sides and fall from a higher level. Another nurse may decide not to take any of these courses of action and choose to nurse the patient on a mattress on the floor. Nursing experts advising lawyers and the court would say that, generally speaking, all the above nursing actions are reasonable, and that there are competent bodies of nursing opinion which would support such practices. Applying the *Bolam* test, the courts would usually accept the nursing experts' views and would not choose between competing views and practices. A small number of medical practitioners could constitute a responsible body of medical opinion (*De Freitas* v. *O'Brien and Another* [1993] 4 Med LR 281).

The courts have not totally handed over the task of determining the standard of care to the nursing and medical professions. While expert evidence as to nursing or medical practice will usually be accepted, the courts could still overrule a body of professional practice. Nevertheless, the courts would not easily condemn accepted nursing or medical practice as negligent (Jones, 1996). The question of what happens when professional opinion differs was considered by the House of Lords in a case involving a nurse plaintiff (*Maynard* v. *West Midlands Regional Health Authority* [1984] 1 WLR 634). Staff Nurse Maynard consulted a physician and a surgeon experienced in the treatment of chest diseases. Tuberculosis was considered to be the most likely diagnosis, but there were symptoms that also suggested Hodgkin's disease, carcinoma and sarcoidosis. Unless there was early treatment of Hodgkin's disease it would prove fatal (as treatment was understood in 1970), so the doctors decided upon a mediastinoscopy, which would provide them with a biopsy that they could have examined immediately. The operation involved a risk of damage to the left laryngeal nerve, even if carried out correctly, and unfortunately this occurred. The biopsy proved negative and it was later confirmed that the plaintiff was suffering from tuberculosis and not Hodgkin's disease. She sued in negligence, alleging, amongst other things, that it was a negligent decision to carry out the mediastinoscopy rather than await the results of the sputum test. Her action failed. Lord Scarman stated:

> A case which is based on an allegation that a fully considered decision of two consultants in the field of their special skill was negligent

clearly presents certain difficulties of proof. It is not enough to show that there is a body of competent professional opinion which considers that theirs was a wrong decision, if there also exists a body of professional opinion, equally competent, which supports the decision as reasonable in the circumstances. It is not enough to show that subsequent events show that the operation need never have been performed, if at the time the decision to operate was taken it was reasonable in the sense that a responsible body of medical opinion would have accepted it as proper. ... Differences of opinion and practice exist, and will always exist, in the medical as in other professions. There is seldom any one answer exclusive of all others to problems of professional judgment.

These legal principles can be applied to another controversial nursing issue; the Edinburgh University solution of lime (Eusol) wound care dressing debate (Tingle, 1990). Many nurses are reluctant to use Eusol, with some arguing that they have a professional duty not to do so because they believe it is ineffective as a promoter of wound healing. Some consultants like to use Eusol and ask nurses to use it. There have been a number of publicized disputes as nurses face a conflict between the consultant's request and their own professional view on Eusol. Applying the principles set out in *Bolam* and *Maynard*, it can be seen that, generally speaking, it is not negligent to use Eusol because there is a competent body of medical opinion which would support its use (Burton, 1993).

Developments in health care practice generally may influence the manner in which the *Bolam* test may operate, and assist in defining what amounts to a responsible body of professional practice. It is interesting to speculate the extent to which concepts such as evidenced-based medicine/nursing and clinical guidelines and protocols will push the standard of care, from reasonable practice in the *Bolam* sense, to best practice. Evidence-based medicine is practice based on a clear body of research and agreed principles.

The Bolitho case

In the case of *Bolitho* v. *City and Hackney Health Authority* (1997) [1998] Lloyd's Rep Med 26, a 2-year-old boy was being treated for breathing difficulties in hospital. He suffered two episodes of acute shortness of breath on one day, and a doctor was summoned urgently by the ward sister. The doctor failed to attend or to arrange for another doctor to attend. Later that day, the boy suffered a respiratory and cardiac arrest. He was resuscitated and was found to have brain damage, and the Health Authority was sued for negligence. It was alleged that the plaintiff's brain damage was caused by the negligent failure of medical staff to attend. Negligence was admitted by the defendant as medical staff should have attended when summoned, but that was not the end of the matter. Intubation of an infant is not an easy or completely safe procedure. The doctor who had been summoned and failed to attend said that she would not have intubated him even if she had attended. Expert opinion was divided on the necessity of intubation. This case was referred to the House of Lords, and the issues of breach of duty and causation were key issues of discussion. The *Bolam* case was discussed, and Lord Browne-Wilkinson's speech contains the contemporary view on how *Bolam* is to be applied. To an extent, we can see a movement away from reasonable to best or evidenced-based practice as the legal benchmark for the standard of care to be sought:

> The use of these adjectives responsible, reasonable and respectable all show that the court has to be satisfied that the exponents of the body of opinion relied upon can demonstrate that such opinion has a logical basis. In particular in cases involving, as they so often do, the weighing of risks against benefits, the judge before accepting a body of opinion as being responsible, reasonable or respectable, will need to be satisfied that, in forming their views, the experts have directed their minds to the question of comparative risks and benefits and have reached a defensible conclusion on the matter.

Expert reports in cases must be evidence-based. In Chapter 4 (*Penney and Others* v. *East Kent Health Authority* (*The Times*, 25 November, 1999 (C.A.)), we will see how the courts can approach national clinical guidelines and the *Bolitho* and *Bolam* cases. It is also unclear whether nurses will be subject to the same degree of scrutiny as doctors, or indeed whether the courts would be willing to undertake a more rigorous review than is the case as regards medical decision making. (Kennedy and Grubb, 1993).

Departing from accepted practice

A nurse would not necessarily be viewed as being negligent if he or she departed from accepted nursing practice in a particular situation. For example, a wound care specialist might decide, on the basis of a recent research study, to mix two types of topical wound care solutions together and apply them to a patient's wound, arguing that recent research has shown that when the solutions are mixed together they became more effective. This is not, however, the conventional way to apply the solutions. If problems do occur and the patient then takes legal action, the nurse would have to justify the departure from conventional practice. There is a clear danger in accepting claims made by one research paper only. There is a need for confirmation and exploration of the implications of changing practice, and there must be critical appraisal of new research.

If a nurse is given instructions by a doctor but is of the view that these are wrong, what should he or she do? It is suggested that it would be good practice to raise the concerns with the doctor. However, if the doctor disagrees and the nurse goes along with the doctor's instructions, then if harm results the nurse may be held not to be negligent because the action taken was on the doctor's orders (*Gold* v. *Essex County Council* [1942] 2

All ER 237; Montgomery, 1995 and Montgomery, 1997), although this may be an approach that the courts are less willing to take as the nurse's role in clinical practice increases still further.

Assessing risk

The nurse in the above example might have felt that there were no real significant adverse risks to the patient in the proposed course of action, the benefits outweighing any treatment risks. Whether the nurse was correct in this assessment would be an important issue for the experts to determine in their reports to the lawyers.

Taking precautions against foreseeable risks

The defendant's conduct in a negligence case is viewed from the date the incident occurred, and not from the time of the court hearing. The defendant would be expected only to guard against events that could reasonably be foreseen at the time of the alleged negligence. *Roe v. Ministry of Health and Others, Woolley v. Same* ([1954] 2 All ER 131) illustrates this point. Two patients underwent an operation, and prior to the operation a spinal anaesthetic consisting of Nupercaine was administered to them by lumbar puncture. The plaintiffs developed spastic paraplegia after the operation and were paralysed from the waist down. Their injuries were caused by the injection of contaminated Nupercaine. The Nupercaine was in glass ampoules which, prior to administration, were immersed in a phenol solution. Unknown to the anaesthetist, the phenol had percolated into the glass ampoules by means of invisible cracks or molecular flaws in the glass. At the time of the incident, the risk of percolation in the manner that occurred was not generally appreciated by competent anaesthetists. It was an unforeseeable occurrence, and the defendants were not legally expected to anticipate the danger. Denning L.J. expressed the following sentiment in the case, which can equally be said to be applicable to all health care professionals today:

> Every surgical operation is attended by risks. We cannot take the benefits without taking the risks. Every advance in technique is also attended by risks. Doctors, like the rest of us, have to learn by experience; and experience often teaches in a hard way. Something goes wrong and shows up a weakness, and then it is put right. That is just what happened here ... we must not look at the 1947 accident with 1954 spectacles.

Legal duty to keep up to date

A nurse could breach his or her legal duty of care by not keeping up to date with major developments in his or her speciality. Consider the following example:

A new wound care dressing has been created which is very effective and is becoming widely used. A district nurse is unaware of the new dressing because she feels she has no time to read the professional journals or to attend study days, which are put on by her employer at regular intervals. One of her patients has a wound that will not heal. Another district nurse attends the patient and uses the new dressing, and the wound heals very quickly. The patient asks why the new dressing was not used before by the regular district nurse.

This issue is addressed by the UKCC in the Code of Professional Conduct (1992):

As a registered nurse, midwife or health visitor, you are personally accountable for your practice and, in the exercise of your professional accountability, must ... maintain and improve your professional knowledge and competence.

The nurse in the wound care example, as well as possibly being in breach of her duty of care to her patient, could also be viewed as being in breach of clause 3 of the Code of Professional Conduct (UKCC, 1992): blind indifference to her professional duty of personal updating and development. She should try to keep reasonably up to date.

Within the nursing profession, the UKCC Post-Registration Education and Practice Project (PREP) provides an important professional impetus for personal updating. To help their organizations support the clinical governance initiative, nurses should practise reflectively (UKCC, 2000).

The issue of professional updating has been considered by the Court of Appeal in *Crawford* v. *Board of Governors of Charing Cross Hospital* (1953) (*The Times*, 8 December, 1953). The plaintiff Mr Robert Joseph Crawford was admitted to Charing Cross Hospital for an operation for the removal of his bladder. The plaintiff's left arm was extended at an angle from his body so that a blood transfusion could be given. After the operation the plaintiff complained of paralysis in his left arm; brachial palsy had developed. He sued alleging negligence. The main issue was whether the anaesthetist was negligent in missing an article that had appeared in *The Lancet* in January 1950; the operation was performed in July 1950. The article warned about the risk of brachial palsy when the arm was kept in an extended position. The plaintiff did not succeed as no negligence was found. Denning L.J. states that all reasonable care was taken by the hospital and that it would amount to imposing too high a burden on the doctor to require that he read all articles in the medical press.

The judgment on the facts makes sense; nobody can read all the professional articles that appear in the numerous journals. Nonetheless, while ignorance of one warning in the professional press may be acceptable, missing a number of warnings could well lead to a finding of negligence. Mason and McCall Smith (1999), referring to the *Crawford* case, feel that a less charitable view would be taken if the same facts occurred today:

> The practice of medicine has, however, become increasingly based on principles of scientific elucidation and report, and the pressure on doctors to keep abreast of current developments is now considerable. It is no longer possible for a doctor to coast along on the basis of long experience; such an attitude has been discredited not only in medicine but in many professions and callings.

The courts have recently affirmed health care professionals' obligation to keep themselves up to date by familiarity with mainstream literature (*Gascoine* v. *Ian Shendan and Co and Lathan* [1994] 5 Med LR 437).

The nurse must thus remember the professional and legal duty to keep up to date with developments in nursing practice.

Damage

The plaintiff must prove that the defendant's breach of duty caused or materially contributed to his or her damage. A direct link has to be made between the two elements of breach and damage. The plaintiff must be 'able to prove that the negligence has made a difference, that it has adversely affected the condition in some way'. A first step is to prove factual causation: the cause in fact of the plaintiff's condition.

Causation in fact

Lawyers use a test known as the 'but for test'. Jones (1996) summarizes this test as follows:

> If harm to the plaintiff would not have occurred 'but for' the defendant's negligence, then the negligence is a cause of the harm. It is not necessarily the cause, however, because there may well be other events which are causally relevant. Putting this another way, if the loss would have been incurred in any event, the defendant's conduct is not a cause.

The application of this principle can be illustrated by the case of *Barnett* v. *Chelsea and Kensington Hospital Management Committee* ([1968] 1 All ER 1068). The plaintiff, William Barnett, was a nightwatchman at a college hall of residence. He was drinking some tea with two other nightwatchmen. Soon afterwards they all started vomiting and went to the defendant's casualty department. They were seen by a nurse, who telephoned the casualty officer, Dr Banerjee, who unfortunately was not feeling well himself. He did not see the men, saying that they should go home and see their own doctors. Mr Whittall, one of the men, was asked by Dr Banerjee to stay for an X-ray. He had seen Dr Banerjee on another matter sometime before. All the men went away and, some hours later, the plaintiff died. It was discovered later that the cause of death was arsenical poisoning. His widow claimed that the hospital had been negligent in not treating her husband. The casualty officer was found by the court to be in breach of his legal duty of care in not examining and treating Mr Barnett, but the legal action failed. Element 3, Causation in Fact, had not been proved; death had been inevitable for Mr Barnett. Had he been seen and admitted to hospital he would have died before the antidote could have been given, and the defendant's breach of duty had, therefore, not caused his death; they could not have done anything to save him in time.

The plaintiff has the burden of proving that the defendant's actions or omissions have caused or materially contributed to the damage suffered. This can be a difficult task in medical and nursing negligence cases where there can often be a number of biological causes, natural causes of a plaintiff's condition. The burden of proof is on the plaintiff to establish that the breach of duty was a material contribution to the damage caused (*Wilsher* v. *Essex Area Health Authority* [1986] 3 All ER 801). A nurse who is expert in the relevant speciality would be called to give evidence. A number of reported cases involve allegations of both medical and nursing negligence, and in such circumstances both types of experts will be used.

Clinical negligence: general issues

The case of *Kay* v. *Ayrshire and Arran Health Board* ([1987] 2 All ER 417) illustrates key causation principles. Andrew Stuart Kay was aged 2 years and 5 months when he was admitted to the Seafield Children's Hospital, Ayr. His GP admitted him because she thought he may have been suffering from meningitis, and this diagnosis was later confirmed by the hospital. The consultant paediatrician in charge of the case instructed that 10 000 units of penicillin be administered intrathecally. By mistake, a senior house officer injected 300 000 units of penicillin instead of the required 10 000 units. Andrew went into convulsions and later developed a degree of paralysis on one side of his body. Immediate action was taken to remedy this negligent mistake, and Andrew recovered and appeared to suffer no immediate ill effects of the overdose. He made a rapid recovery from meningitis. However, some time after his discharge from hospital his parents noticed that he appeared to be suffering from deafness; this was later confirmed. An action for negligence was commenced, alleging that the overdose of penicillin had caused his deafness. The action failed because factual causation was not established; it could not be proven that the overdose caused or materially contributed to Andrew's deafness. The weight of evidence in the case pointed to the deafness being caused by the meningitis.

As well as being instructive on the issue of experts and evidence-based health care, *Bolitho* is also a leading authority on causation. The facts of *Bolitho* were stated earlier. A key issue in the litigation was the possible relationship of the *Bolam* principle to causation; Lord Browne-Wilkinson in the case said that there were two questions for the judge at first instance to decide on causation:

(1) What would Dr Horn have done, or authorized to be done, if she had attended Patrick? and (2) If she would not have intubated, would that have been negligent? The Bolam test has no relevance to the first of those questions but is central to the second.

Bolam therefore does seem to have some relationship to causation.
Jones (1998) argues:

In reality Bolitho is about whether the failure to intubate, for whatever reason (non-attendance or conscious professional judgment), was negligent. The defendant's evidence that she would not have intubated simply moved the focus of the argument about negligence, i.e breach of duty, from the non-attendance to the non-intubation.

Remoteness

Having established what factually caused the plaintiff's damage, there may still be a need to consider the cause for attributing legal responsibility, often termed remoteness, causation in law or proximate cause. A defendant generally cannot be held liable for everything that happens to a plaintiff; the damage may be too remote, outside the bounds of what can be legally recovered. Instances would be where the damage would be much more extensive, or of a different type, or occur in a different way, to that normally expected.

Consider the following example:

A district nurse makes regular visits to an elderly patient to change dressings. The elderly patient lives alone and looks forward to the nurse's regular visits. The nurse gives her company and spends some of her time talking generally to the patient. Due to promotion the nurse needs to move districts, with another nurse taking over her visits. The patient appears to take this news well, but the next day is found dead with a suicide note. The patient, unable to face the change in nursing routine, has committed suicide. The patient's relatives blame the nurse, saying that she should have anticipated the patient's reaction and taken preventative steps.

A key issue would be the foreseeability of the patient's action. Was there any existing evidence of psychiatric illness, and was this passed on to the nurse? If there was no such evidence, then it could be argued that the patient's actions would not have been reasonably foreseen by the nurse.

She would not have been expected to act to prevent the suicide; the event would have been legally too remote.

In some situations there is more than one cause of harm that a patient suffers. Consider a patient who has been negligently knocked off his motorbike by a motorist. He is seriously injured, with damage to the spine. The doctor in casualty causes further injury and paralysis through negligent medical treatment. In ascertaining legal liability, the court would have to consider evidence as to what caused the ultimate injury. It may be the case that both the motorist and doctor could be negligent and liable to some extent.

Where there are two or more defendants liable for the same damage to the plaintiff, the Civil Liability (Contribution) Act 1978 allows them to claim contributions from each other for any damages awarded.

Damages for loss of chance

What if there is a delay in providing treatment and the patient later seeks to bring an action, claiming that it was this delay that resulted in an incomplete recovery? In effect, the claim is that the negligence led to the 'loss of a chance' of recovery in that situation. This issue arose in the case of *Hotson* v. *East Berkshire Area Health Authority* ([1987] 2 All ER 909). The plaintiff was 13 years of age when he injured his hip in a fall. He had sustained an acute traumatic fracture of the left femoral epiphysis, but this condition was not diagnosed at the hospital when he attended and he was sent home. He was in severe pain for 5 days. He returned to the hospital and his condition was correctly diagnosed. He suffered avascular necrosis of the epiphysis, and at the age of 20 years he had a major permanent disability.

The plaintiff claimed damages for negligence against the Health Authority, which admitted a breach of duty but denied that the resulting delay had adversely affected the plaintiff's long-term condition. When the action was tried, the trial judge found that even if the hospital medical staff had correctly diagnosed and treated the plaintiff on his first visit to the hospital there was still a 75 per cent risk of the disability developing. The medical staff's breach of duty had turned that risk into an inevitability. The plaintiff was in effect denied a 25 per cent chance of a good recovery. Damages were awarded, which included an amount that represented 25 per cent of the full value of the damages awardable for the disability. The Court of Appeal affirmed the judge's decision. The Health Authority successfully appealed to the House of Lords and the Court of Appeal's decision was reversed. The appeal was allowed on the narrow ground that the plaintiff failed to establish a cause of action in respect of the avascular necrosis and its consequences. The trial judge's finding of fact was that on the balance of probabilities the injury caused by the plaintiff's fall left insufficient blood vessels intact to keep the epiphysis alive. The fall was the sole cause of the avascular necrosis.

This case again graphically illustrates the practical difficulties in establishing causation. The broad issue raised by the case of the possibility of claiming for loss of chance in tort was left open by the House of Lords, and it remains to be seen whether such an action may succeed in the future.

Res ipsa loquitur

There are circumstances when the courts are prepared to infer from the facts that a defendant was negligent. Under this evidential rule the burden of proof is not formally reversed and the inference of negligence can be rebutted. Generally speaking, the principle will apply where it is obvious that there has been negligence – for example, where the doctor has amputated the wrong leg or a swab or forceps has been left in a patient, etc. An extreme example of *res ipsa loquitur* was noted in the *Yorkshire Evening Post*, 14 October, 1982:

> An enquiry has begun at a hospital in Vienna into how a man, suffering from a broken leg, was mistakenly given a heart pacemaker (Dixon, 1984).

Further examples of situations in which *res ipsa loquitur* may be pleaded are to be found in the following cases cited by Action for Victims of Medical Accidents (AVMA, 1984–1985):

> Foreign bodies were as varied as ever – ranging from swabs (14), insoluble sutures (5), clips (4), metal thread/wool (3), packs (3), bits of catheter apparatus (3), needles (2), clamps (2), gauze (2), scissors (1), forceps (1), and even part of a glass test tube. Most of these arose from abdominal surgery – 13 from gastroenterology cases.

The Medical Defence Union (MDU, 1993) noted a case where a patient received approximately £27 000 in compensation for an overlooked swab. This, in common with the other examples of the situation in which *res ipsa loquitur* might be used, can be seen to be of particular relevance to theatre nursing.

A number of conditions must be satisfied before the *res ipsa loquitur* principle can apply. The event, when it occurred, must have been under the control, supervision or management of the defendant, and the event would not normally have happened unless there was negligence. The whole circumstances of the case would be considered. The lawyers and the judge would consider, as a matter of common sense and common experience, whether such events could have occurred without negligence. The defendant must have offered no reasonable explanation of what has happened.

The principle has worked in a number of health care cases. *Cassidy* v. *Ministry of Health* ([1951] 1 All ER 574) and *Bull* v. *Devon Area Health Authority* ([1989] [1993] 4 Med LR 117, 22 BMLR, 79) are just two cases where the principle has been used. In *Cassidy*, the plaintiff was operated on for Dupuytren's contracture. He was suffering from a contraction of the third and fourth fingers of the left hand. After the operation, a nurse bandaged the plaintiff's hand and arm to a splint. The bandage was tested by a doctor to see if it was too tight, and circulation was judged to be satisfactory. The patient subsequently complained of exceptional pain, and was seen on occasions by medical staff. The splint and bandage were left intact and morphia was administered. The plaintiff continued to complain about excessive pain until the removal of the splint, when he discovered that he had lost the use of all four fingers. He sued for negligence in regard to the post-operational treatment he received. Even though he could not identify who in particular was negligent, the principle of *res ipsa loquitur* was applied. The evidence showed a *prima facie* case of negligence, and this evidence was not rebutted by the defendants, who were responsible for the medical and nursing staff.

Bull v. *Devon Area Health Authority* ([1989] [1993] 4 Med LR 117) demonstrates a controversial application of the principle; not all the judges in the case agreed to it being used. The case concerned the negligent organization of maternity services. Mrs Bull was in premature labour, carrying uniovular twins. The twins were sharing the same placenta. The first twin, later named Darryl, was spontaneously delivered at 7.27 pm; he was born healthy. The second twin, later named Stuart, was born 68 minutes later with severe brain damage; he suffers from cerebral palsy and is a quadriplegic spastic. Experts at the trial agreed that he should have been born as soon as reasonably practical after his brother, and in any event within 20 minutes. Stuart did receive £750 000 compensation (Miles, 1990). The delay in securing the attendance of senior medical staff capable of dealing with the emergency situation was too long, and therefore there was a breach of duty. The call system had broken down.

Lord Justice Slade agreed with the submission made by counsel for the appellants and the judge at first instance: that the Health Authority had to justify the delays if it could under the *res ipsa loquitur* principle. He said:

> In my judgment, however, all the most likely explanations for this failure point strongly either (i) to inefficiency in the system for summoning the assistance of the registrar or consultant ... or (ii) to negligence by some individual or individuals in the working of that system. This is, in my judgment, accordingly a case where the res ipsa loquitur principle had to be applied. ... (4 Med LR 132).

Dillon L.J. did not expressly deal with the desirability of using the principle. Mustill L.J. did not see the case as warranting the application of the principle.

On the issue of *res ipsa loquitur*, the case is notable for a number of reasons. The fact that the judges in the case were not united in their view over the application of the principle illustrates the degree of uncertainty that can surround it. Furthermore, the principle was being used in a novel situation: in the organization of health care services. In practice, *res ipsa loquitur* is thus only likely to be applicable in exceptional situations – for example, in *Glass* v. *Cambridgeshire AHA* ([1995] 6 Med LR 91), where the plaintiff suffered brain damage consequent upon a heart attack under general anaesthetic. It was held that this was not something that would normally be expected to occur in all the circumstances. As a consequence of this, the burden moved to the defendant to explain that this was consistent with an absence of negligence. More recently the Court of Appeal subjected the maxim *res ipsa loquitur* to a very detailed examination in *Ratcliffe* v. *Plymouth and Torbay HA and Devon and Exeter HA* ([1998] Lloyds Rep Med 102).

Who pays the compensation?

The law of tort can be seen as the legal mechanism for the recovery of compensation by the patient. The issue of who is actually responsible for the payment of the compensation is important for nurses. Many worry that if they are negligent they may be personally liable to pay the patient compensation, and others worry that if their employers pay the compensation to the injured patient their employers may seek to recover the money from them personally. In the NHS, damages are paid by the employer of the negligent nurse. A number of schemes and organizations help trusts and health authorities deal with clinical negligence damages claims. These are the Clinical Negligence Scheme for Trusts (CNST), the Existing Liabilities Scheme (ELS) and the National Health Service Litigation Authority (NHSLA). The ELS provides financial assistance where claims exceed £10 000 (including costs), and applies to matters that arose prior to 1 April 1995. The CNST is a voluntary scheme. NHS bodies can pool the costs of claims which will be honoured by the CNST will then satisfy claims. This is subject to an excess. The aim of the scheme is to ensure that one particular trust is not crippled by a single negligence action. The NHSLA co-ordinates these schemes, and it also looks at proposals to settle cases and has an advisory role in cases in which the claim is of a high value or will have policy implications across other NHS bodies. The NHSLA also determines standards of risk management for CNST members (and NHS bodies generally).

Vicarious liability

Employers are liable, along with their employees, for non-authorized acts performed in the course of their employment. This principle is known as 'vicarious liability', and it makes the employer jointly and severally liable even when not at fault; it is a form of strict liability. It is a necessary condition that the employees were acting in the course of their employment when they committed the tort, and that the action complained of was one that the employee was authorized to undertake. The injured patient can sue the nurse, the hospital and the nurse, or just the hospital.

Whatever course is taken, the nurse who committed the negligent act always remains personally responsible and accountable for his or her negligence, and it is possible that the employer could seek to recover from the nurse the compensation which has been paid out. However, recent NHS guidance states that attempts should not be made to recover costs from employees in this manner (NHS Executive, 1996). The nurse has broken an implied term in the contract of employment that he or she will exercise reasonable care and skill. There is also a statutory provision that would allow the employer to recover any compensation paid out on the negligent nurse's behalf (Civil Liability (Contribution) Act 1978).

Generally speaking, lawyers proceed against the employer and not the employee. If, however, the employer can establish that the nurse was not acting in the course of employment when the negligence occurred, then the lawyers acting for the injured patient could bring an action against the nurse directly. However, in practice such an action is unlikely to go ahead, because it is questionable whether the individual nurse would have the financial resources to pay the compensation. It is not an easy legal task to determine what constitutes action taken in the course of employment. There are many cases on this point, and some are quite difficult to reconcile; there is no definitive test.

Direct liability

If a patient was injured, not by the acts or omissions of a nurse, but because of a defect in machinery or because the system of care in the hospital failed, then the hospital could be held directly liable to the injured patient (*Cassidy* v. *Minister of Health* [1951] 1 All ER 574). This is because of what is termed a 'non-delegable duty'. The issue of a health authority or trust's direct liability for medical or nursing negligence is a controversial one, but one that has been affirmed by the court in recent years in *M* v. *Calderdale and Kirklees HA* ((1998) Lloyds Rep Med 157) and see *Robertson* v. *Nottingham Health Authority* [1997] 8 Med LR 1. Here the plaintiff underwent an abortion performed by a private clinic, which was acting under contract to the defendant Health Authority. It was held that the Health Authority had a non-delegable duty in this situation for the actions of the private clinic. The Health Authority had not taken steps such as ensuring that there was indemnity insurance, ensuring the competence of the staff of the clinic etc. This was a decision of Judge Garner, at the first instance at Huddersfield County Court. Nonetheless, the concept of direct liability may yet have a greater effect as more services are contracted out to the private sector. Where negligence is alleged, the injured patient could proceed against the NHS body, claiming that it was directly liable for the injury caused.

Product liability

If a nurse is injured when a piece of equipment she is using fractures or a patient claims that he or she has been harmed through the administration of a defective drug, he or she may bring an action claiming damages for the harm suffered under the Consumer Protection Act 1987. This statute allows an action to be brought against producers and suppliers of defective products where the defect in the product led to damage. The legislation was introduced following a European Directive on Products liability. Guidance issued within the NHS as to the operation of the legislation states that a health authority may be liable under the 1987 Act in a number of situations (HN(88)3, HN(FP)(88)5). First, they may be liable as a producer of medicines, appliances or pharmaceutical products. Second, they may be liable unless the producer or supplier can be identified. Finally, they may be liable as a 'keeper' if the supplier or producer shows that the product has not been used according to instructions, or has not been sufficiently maintained.

The important difference between the 1987 Act and a negligence action at common law (as outlined above) is that fault does not have to be shown; it is sufficient to establish that the defect caused the damage. In considering what amounts to a defect, section 3(2) outlines a number of factors to be taken into account:

> ... the manner in which, and the purposes for which, the product has been marketed, its get-up, the use of any mark in relation to the product and any instructions for, or warnings with respect to, doing or refraining from doing anything with or in relation to the product.

If the injured nurse had, for example, not followed the instructions, then she could not bring an action under the statute.

An action may only be brought against a producer of the product within 10 years of the product having been supplied. There is a defence to actions under the legislation if, at the time the product was produced, scientific and technical knowledge was not such that (s4(1)):

> ... a producer of products of the same description as the product in question might have been expected to have discovered the defect.

While use of this statute remains theoretically possible, establishing liability may be practically difficult. The fact that the product is defective needs to be shown, which can be as difficult as establishing negligence in a standard common law claim (see Jones, 2000).

Criminal liability and negligent conduct

While in most situations grave carelessness by the nurse will lead to civil proceedings, in some instances a criminal prosecution may result. If a nurse's actions are gravely careless and if death ultimately results, then the nurse may be prosecuted for manslaughter. While there have been no notable prosecutions of nurses for gross negligence or manslaughter, there have been criminal prosecutions of doctors. In *R* v. *Adomako* ([1994] 3 All ER 79), a patient died after an anaesthetist, during an eye operation, failed to notice that the endotracheal tube assisting the patient's breathing had become disconnected. Evidence at the hearing was to the effect that the conduct of the plaintiff was 'abysmal', with 'gross dereliction of duty'. He was found guilty of manslaughter. Lord MacKay set out in his judgment the basic test for manslaughter in criminal law:

> ... the principles of the law of negligence apply to ascertain whether or not the defendant has been in breach of a duty of care towards the victim who has died. If such a breach of duty has been established the next question is whether that breach of duty caused the death of the victim. If so, the jury must go on to consider whether that breach of duty should be characterized as gross negligence and therefore as a crime. This will depend on the seriousness of the breach of duty committed by the defendant in all the circumstances in which the defendant was placed when it occurred. The jury will have to consider whether the extent to which the defendant's conduct departed from the proper standard of care incumbent upon him, involving as it must have done a risk of death to the patient, was such that it could be judged criminal.

Application of this test is unlikely to be easy; in effect, assessment of what amounts to culpability has been left in the hands of the jury. It is not clear whether the same principles apply to situations in which the defendant has failed to act as those that apply when the defendant has acted. There is a further issue where a nurse makes a mistake and a death of a patient results, but the nurse claims that the negligence results from working in a situation in which there are severe financial constraints and underfunding. Where does liability lie? One possibility is that the trust could be held to be liable on the basis of what is known as 'corporate manslaughter'. This means that the managers are held responsible for the actions of the organization (see *R* v. *P&O European Ferries (Dover) Ltd* [1991] 93 Cr App R 72).

Reform

Concern over the increase in litigation involving health care professionals has led to discussions of alternatives. One approach adopted in Sweden and New Zealand is to enable individuals to claim compensation through a no-fault scheme (Brazier, 1993; McLean, 1993). Under such a scheme they would not have to establish fault by a health professional; merely that the actions of the health professional caused the harm suffered. It appears unlikely that such a scheme would be adopted in this country, at least in the near future. Many are concerned as to the costs of such a compensation scheme, both in its initial establishment and subsequent operation, pointing to the experience of New Zealand, which prompted various limitations to be imposed on the scheme (Oliphant, 1996).

However, there is increasing emphasis upon settling matters without recourse to litigation in this country (see Chapter 1). The reforms introduced consequent upon the Woolf Report (1996) into civil procedure have had a considerable impact upon the conduct of clinical medical negligence litigation. As described in Chapter 1, cases will be tightly managed by the judge, and parties will be encouraged to settle their differences prior to trial and make use of alternative dispute resolution mechanisms. There will be more restrictive use of expert evidence, and experts will be encouraged to narrow down their differences prior to trial through the use of pre-trial meetings.

Conclusions

Nurses do not have to practise to an impeccable standard; only as ordinary skilled nurses would have acted in the circumstances of the case. The legal accountability of the nurse is set by the *Bolam* test. In following chapters, specific questions of liability in relation to negligence are considered.

References

AVMA (1984–1985). *Action for Victims of Medical Accidents. Annual Report*. AVMA, p. 7.
Brazier, M. (1993). The case for a no-fault compensation scheme. In: *Compensation for Damage: An International Perspective* (S. McClean, ed.). Aldershot, Dartmouth.
Burton, J. (1993). Skin complaint. *Nursing Times*, **89(7)**, 76.
Dixon, E. (1984). *The Theatre Nurse and the Law*. Croom Helm.
Foster, C. (2001). Negligence. In: *Nursing Law and Ethics*, 2nd edn (J. H. Tingle and A. Cribb, eds). Blackwell Science.
Jones, M. A. (1992). Medical negligence. In: *Doctors, Patients and the Law* (C. Dyer, ed.). Blackwell Scientific Publications.
Jones, M. A. (1996). *Medical Negligence*, 2nd edn. Sweet and Maxwell.
Jones, M. A. (1998). *Textbook on Torts*, 6th edn. Blackstone Press.
Jones, M. A. (2000). *Textbook on Torts*, 7th edn. Blackstone Press.
Kennedy, I. and Grubb, A. (1993). Commentary, *Bolitho* v. *City and Hackney Health Authority. Med. L. Rev.*, **1**, 241.
Mason, J. K. and McCall Smith, R. A. (1999). *Law and Medical Ethics*, 5th edn. Butterworths, p. 227.
McLean, S. (ed.) (1993). Can no-fault analysis ease the problem of medical injury litigation? In: *Compensation for Damage: An International Perspective*. Aldershot, Dartmouth.
MDU (1993). Case histories: delay in diagnosis of retained surgical swab. *J. Med. Defence Union*, **9**, 6.
Miles, K. (1990). Health authority liable for negligent organisation of maternity services – *Bull* v. *Devon Health Authority. AVMA Med. L. J.*, **1**, 11.
Montgomery, J. (1995). Negligence. In *Nursing Law and Ethics* (J. H. Tingle and A. Cribb, eds). Blackwell Science.

Montgomery, J. (1997). *Health Law*. Oxford University Press.

NHS Executive (1996). *NHS Indemnity Arrangements for Clinical Negligence Claims in the NHS.* 96 HR 0024, DOH.

Oliphant, K. (1996). Defining medical misadventure; lessons from New Zealand. *Med. Law Rev.*, **3**, 1–31.

Tingle, J. H. (1990). Eusol and the law. *Nursing Times*, **86**, 70.

Tingle, J. H. (1991). First aid law. *Nursing Times*, **87**, 48.

UKCC (1992). *Code of Professional Conduct.* UKCC, (i) clause 3.

UKCC (1996). *Guidelines for Professional Practice.* UKCC.

UKCC (2000). *The Contribution of Professional Self Regulation and Clinical Governance.* Clinical Governance Pack. UKCC.

Woolf, Lord (1996). *Access to Justice. Final Report to the Lord Chancellor on the Civil Justice System in England and Wales.* HMSO.

Chapter 3

Patient complaints

John Tingle

More people than ever before are complaining about the care they receive in the NHS. In many instances when something goes wrong patients are likely to want to know what went wrong and why it went wrong, rather than necessarily being concerned about obtaining some degree of financial compensation for what has taken place. An effective complaints system has come to be regarded as an essential part of good health care management. This chapter attempts to explain the complaints procedures in the NHS. It should be noted that the complaint system is separate from the health care professional disciplinary system. (For discussion of the United Kingdom Central Council for Nursing, Midwifery and Health Visiting (UKCC) disciplinary procedures, see Chapter 1). The patient may not be the only person who seeks to complain. Health professionals may want to voice their concerns as to the standard of care being provided to patients. Staff complaints are treated separately from patient complaints, and this issue is returned to in Chapter 7, where the question of whistleblowing is considered.

Complaints are an inevitable aspect of professional life. Despite the very best intentions and efforts of nursing staff, something will at some time or other go wrong, and some patients will always complain. Patients are now much more aware of how to complain, and to whom, and of the fact that in appropriate circumstances they can sue. There is evidence of an increase in the number of complaints made about treatment in the NHS. The DOH (1998) published the first detailed information on monitoring of NHS complaints since the implementation of the new system of NHS complaints procedures in April 1996.There were 92 974 written complaints received about hospital and community health services in 1996–1997, a fall from 1994–1995. Recent figures released by the DOH (DOH, 2000a) show a continuing decrease in the number of written complaints received about hospital and community health services. Complaints decreased by 3 per cent to 86 013 between 1997–1998 and 1998–1999, an overall decrease of some 8 per cent since the implementation of the complaints procedure in April 1996. However, the number of written complaints received about general medical and dental services and Family Health services administration increased by 2 per cent to 38 857, an overall increase of 5 per cent since the implementation of the complaints procedure. The Health Service Commissioner, William Buckley, stated in evidence to the House of Commons Select Committee on Health (House of Commons, 1999a) that complaints to his office have been going up very quickly for the last 10 years. His Annual Report for 1998–1999 notes an 8 per cent increase in complaints during the year (HSC, 1999a). According to the source consulted, complaints can be seen to be rising in some sectors and falling in others.

A rise in complaints may not necessarily be directly attributable to a general deterioration in the quality of the Health Service, but rather to a much more informed, consumer-orientated and less deferential public, which maintains high expectations of the Health Service. A more vocal public is increasingly holding all types of professionals to account. Initiatives such as *The Patient's Charter* (DOH, 1995a) and the government's health quality reforms (Command Paper 3807, 1997; DOH, 2000b), which are intended to forge a quality-driven NHS, have raised patient expectations and helped draw attention to the patients' right to complain. The Shipman (Beecham, 2000) and the Wisheart Bristol Heart Surgery scandals (Dyer, 1999), widely reported by the media, have also kept medical and nursing matters well in the public eye and have inevitably driven up care expectations. Berrington and Barnwell (1995) discussed the Central Statistical Office publication *Social Trends* (Volume 25), and noted:

> Britons have become healthier, sometimes wealthier and more likely to own their own homes; higher expectations mean we are also increasingly dissatisfied.

Health complaints can be seen in a much broader and more generalized context; we live now in a much more complaining and litigation-conscious society. Health professionals may in some respects be at a disadvantage in that complaints made against them are more likely to attract media attention because of the 'human interest' factor. Finally, where a complaint is made in the context of health care it is not simply a matter of ensuring that a fault is remedied. There is an important issue of public accountability in the context of the NHS (Simanowitz, 1985).

Health care provision is a matter of public funding and of public concern. There is an expectation that health care providers should be accountable. Nurses need to be aware of the complaints process and the fact that they may be the subject of complaints made, whether at informal or formal level. It is also important that the nurse is aware of what rights patients have in this area regarding her or his role as patient advocate.

Complaints and patient confusion

Frequently a patient's complaint may arise from confusion, anxiety and frustration at not receiving a satisfactory explanation of why something has gone wrong – frustration that may result in anger and trigger off a complaint (Medical Defence Union, 1993). Litigation or a formal complaint might never have taken place had the patient been given an understandable explanation of what had gone wrong and the steps being taken to remedy matters. Vincent *et al.* (1994) surveyed 227 patients and relatives who were taking legal action through five firms of plaintiff solicitors. They found that the decision to take legal action was determined not only by the original injury, but also by insensitive handling and poor communication after the original incident.

> Vincent *et al.* (1994) identified the following four main factors in the analysis of reasons for litigation:
>
> • Accountability
> • Explanation
> • Standards of care
> • Compensation and admission of negligence.

Patients and relatives wished to see staff disciplined and called to account. They wanted an explanation, and felt ignored or neglected after the incident. They also wanted to make sure that the same problem did not happen to anybody else.

Complaints can arise from what may seem to the health carer to be trivial matters. The diabetic clinic may have been very busy and short staffed at a particular time, and as a result a patient may have had a long wait for treatment. An overworked nurse may have been a little abrupt when the patient asked how much longer he was going to have to wait, and the patient then took offence at what he saw as a personal insult and complained. However, some matters are more complex and may raise issues of such gravity that monetary compensation is required as well as an explanation.

Complaints may or may not have a reasonable basis. Truelove (1985) states:

> Some people complain only reluctantly and as a last resort, when prompted by a deep emotion. Some complain reasonably on reasonable grounds. Some complain 'unreasonably' on reasonable grounds. Some complain 'reasonably' on unreasonable grounds. A few (usually with a history of psychological disturbance) complain unreasonably on unreasonable grounds. A few seem to be 'born complainants' who relish a battle and will complain on any grounds whatsoever.

Nevertheless, while some complaints may be unjustifiable it is important that an effective complaints procedure is established and in operation. The importance of complaints systems is emphasized in Department of Health clinical governance, controls assurance and clinical risk management documentation. The NHS Litigation Authority, which manages the CNST (NHSLA, 2000), has Risk Management Standard No. 4 requiring that an 'agreed system of managing complaints is in place', and with a number of areas of assessment. The NHS Executive (1999a), in *Guidelines for Implementing Controls Assurance in the NHS: Guidance for Directors*, lists in the core standards the requirements for risk management (see below).

NHS Executive (1999a) core standard requirements for risk management include the following:
Criterion 8
There is a designated complaints manager who is readily accessible to the public, and well-publicized arrangements are in place for making a complaint.
Criterion 9
Front line staff are empowered to deal with complaints on the spot.
Criterion 11
There is a designated claims/litigation manager who is knowledgeable about health care law, civil litigation practices and procedures, and the organisation's complaints procedure.

The importance of having an effective complaints system can be seen to be firmly emphasized and recognized by the DOH.

Complaint processes in the NHS have changed gradually over the last 10 years, and will continue to change in the light of experience. The most significant reform, however, took place on 1 April 1996. New, unified complaints procedures for dealing with complaints about hospitals, community health services and family health services came into effect. The previous procedures were regarded by many as unsatisfactory. As Simanowitz (1995) commented:

If someone of negative intent had sat down to create a system for patients to complain about health care they would have been unlikely to have come up with anything as unhelpful as the present system, if that is what it can be called.

Different complaints procedures were to be followed depending on where the treatment took place. Each set of procedures had different rules. Fundamentally, there was no common ethos. Not surprisingly, many patients were confused by the complaints procedures. The government established a committee to examine the issue. The Wilson Committee

Report (1994) carefully considered the existing procedures, and recommended major reform. The government response to Wilson, *Acting on Complaints* (DOH, 1995b), was positive, and the Wilson Committee recommendation for a two-stage complaints procedure within the NHS, overseen by the HSC (Ombudsman), was accepted. A new simplified procedure, which recognized the NHS patient as a consumer and embodied the principles recommended by the Wilson Committee, came into effect in April 1996. Complaints about hospitals, community health services and family health services are now dealt with in similar fashion at two clear levels, with the HSC sitting at the apex of the complaints system.

Handling complaints

Whatever the complaint, it must be correctly handled. Hospitals should have established standards and protocols on complaint handling. All staff should be aware of these, and they should reflect a number of basic principles. The NHS Training Division (1995), in the *Local Resolution Training Resources Pack for the NHS Complaints Procedure*, states that the foundation principles of complaints procedures are those found in the Wilson Committee Report (1994), set up by the DOH to review complaints procedures (see below).

The foundation principles of complaints procedures (Wilson Committee Report, 1994) are:

- Responsiveness
- Quality enhancement
- Cost effectiveness
- Accessibility
- Impartiality
- Simplicity
- Speed
- Confidentiality
- Accountability

Complaints and a culture of communication

The new complaints procedures were designed to produce a system and culture that helped develop the communication processes between staff and patients, to enable staff to:

- Elicit comments in relation to service provision
- Listen to and understand the complaint
- Find out what the complainant wants
- Eliminate adversarial situations

- Acknowledge complainants' feelings
- Be seen to act on matters raised.

These principles will result in improvement in the communication process between patients and health carers, which should, in time, help to avoid formal complaints and litigation.

The UKCC (1996), in sections 22 and 23 of their *Guidelines for Professional Practice*, discuss the issue of patient and client communication and recognize that communication is an essential part of good professional practice. A useful communication strategy is outlined, which includes an emphasis on the importance of listening. Hill (1991) of the Medical Defence Union (MDU) also offers some useful guidance on complaint handling:

> When dealing with patient's complaints remember the four S's; complaints should be handled SPEEDILY, with SYMPATHY, to the patient's SATISFACTION, and (if indicated) with an expression of SORROW. Conciliation, not confrontation, should be the goal.

It is important to remember that a complaint could result in litigation.

Complaints should also be analysed for trends. The success of risk management, quality assurance, controls assurance and clinical governance strategies is dependent on complaints and claims analysis.

A patient may wish to complain and asks a nurse about appropriate channels. To function effectively as a patient advocate, the nurse must have a reasonable working knowledge and understanding of the complaints system and protocols (Tingle, 1990), in particular those of his or her own local hospital. Minor complaints can often be handled by the nurse as they arise, and this is encouraged by DOH guidance. More significant complaints should be referred promptly to a line manager.

Guidance issued by the NHS Executive (1996a) places great emphasis on resolving complaints as quickly as possible and informally through front-line staff, called 'local resolution'. The guidance is not designed to be all-embracing. Individual complaint models can be developed, but they must take account of the legal framework, directions and regulations that have been issued.

Local resolution

The trust/health authority must establish a clear local resolution process. According to DOH guidance, the process should be open, fair, flexible and conciliatory. Its primary purpose should be to give a comprehensive response that satisfies the complainant.

Time limit

There is a time limit on initiating complaints. Normally, a complaint should be made within 6 months from the incident that caused the problem, or within 6 months of the date of discovering the problem, provided that this is within 12 months of the incident. There is discretion to extend this time limit. The complaint can be made orally or in writing, by an existing or former patient or by somebody acting on the patient's behalf.

Complaints manager

Trusts and health authorities must have a designated complaints manager who oversees the complaints procedure. The manager will receive the complaints from patients and should be readily identifiable to staff and public. If a complaint is not resolved at this informal stage, then the complainant can make a request to a convener for an independent review.

Independent review

Trusts and health authorities must appoint at least one person, who may not be one of its own employees, to act in the role of convener. At least one of the persons appointed must be a non-executive of the trust or health authority. There is no automatic right to an independent review of a complaint. A complainant can request an independent review to the convener, either orally or in writing, within 28 calendar days from the completion of the local resolution process. The convener has the discretion to consider requests made outside the time period.

Action by the convener

The convener must obtain a signed written statement from the complainant setting out the complaint and why the complainant is dissatisfied with the investigation of the initial complaint. In deciding whether to convene a panel, the convener considers a number of factors in consultation with an independent lay chairman from the regional list. Where the complaint concerns a matter of clinical judgment, then clinical advice must be obtained.

Issues examined include whether further action can be taken by the trust or authority towards satisfying the complainant without appointing a panel to investigate the complaint. Alternatively, the trust or health authority may have taken all the action that is practical towards satisfying the complainant, and no further benefit would be achieved by appointing a panel. Although advice must be sought, the decision as whether or not to set up a panel is ultimately one for the convener to make.

Where an independent review has been refused, the complainant and any person complained against should be advised of this decision in writing, with reasons, and of whether or not the convener believes there is further action the trust or health authority can take. The complainant must also be advised of his or her right to complain to the HSC. If a panel is to be set up, the terms of reference should be stated. If a complainant is dissatisfied following reference back to the trust or health authority, he or she may ask the convener to reconsider whether an independent review panel should be set up. The NHS Executive (1999b) has published a good practice guide for conveners (HSC 1999/193).

The panel

The panel consists of three members, one of which, the chairman, is nominated by the Secretary of State. The trust or health authority should also appoint a member to act as convener, and there should be a member representative from the purchaser. The panel has discretion over the nature of the procedures adopted for dealing with the complaint. If there is disagreement as to these procedures, then the chairman of the panel has the power to make the ultimate decision. A legally qualified person may accompany a participant and speak to the panel or assessors with the chairman's consent; however, this person must not speak as an advocate for the participant.

Assessors

If the complaint concerns or partly concerns the exercise of clinical judgment, then at least two assessors must be appointed. Their role is to advise and make a written report to the panel regarding matters related to clinical judgment. The assessors are nominated by the Secretary of State from an approved list.

Report of the panel

There are certain matters that must be included in the panel's report (see below).

> The report of the panel must include the following matters:
> 1. Findings of fact relevant to the complaint
> 2. The opinion of the panel on the complaint having regard to the findings of fact
> 3. The reasons for the panel's opinion
> 4. The assessors' report
> 5. Where the panel disagrees with any matter included in the report of the assessors, the reason for its disagreement.

The report may also include suggestions that would improve trust or health authority services and the steps that might be taken to satisfy the complainant. It cannot, however, suggest that disciplinary proceedings be taken against any person. The final report will have a restricted circulation, and among those who will receive a copy are the complainant, any person named in the complaint, clinical assessors, chairman, chief executives, etc.

End of proceedings

When chief executives receive the reports, they must write to the complainants informing them of any action that is going to be taken or the reasons for taking no action. A complainant's right to apply to the HSC must also be stated.

Practice-based complaints procedures

All family health service practitioners (persons undertaking to provide general medical services, general dental services, general ophthalmic services or pharmaceutical services under the National Health Service Act 1977) were required to establish their own practice-based procedures for dealing with patient complaints by 1 April 1996 (NHS Executive, 1996b). The aim of the new system is to try where possible to resolve most complaints at practice level – local resolution. If the complainant does not wish to complain directly to the practice, matters can go to Family Health Services Conciliation. Independent review procedures can be requested where matters remain unresolved.

The complaints procedure is not concerned with practitioner discipline; there is a completely separate and distinct procedure for these matters. The terms of service of GPs and other family health service practitioners have been amended to include the setting up of practice-based complaint systems and the requirement to co-operate with health authority procedures. GPs have discretion in the nature and operation of their practice-based complaints system; however, their system must reflect the national criteria.

National criteria

The national criteria for a practice-based complaints system include the following:

- Practice-based procedures should be practice owned and managed
- One person should be nominated to administer the procedure, although how this is done is for the practice to decide
- Practices must give the procedure publicity and make written information available to anyone who asks for it
- Complaints should normally be acknowledged within 2 working days
- An explanation should normally be provided within 10 working days.

Guidance is given on a model procedure, which includes information on initial contact, the interview, leaflet, acknowledgement, etc. An in-house complaints procedure should be:

- Simple and responsive
- Accessible and well-publicized
- Confidential
- Understood by all practice staff so that they can advise patients on how to use it
- Speedy yet thorough.

A complainant may be unhappy with the outcome of the local practice-based procedure, and may request an independent review. Independent review procedures, as discussed above, are applicable to complaints made against GPs. The convener again has responsibility for looking at the complaint in consultation with an independent lay chairperson and deciding whether to agree to a request for independent review. The old formal service committees, as they were known, have gone. It will be recalled that the convener has a number of available options open, which include referring the complaint back to the practice for further consideration (if it appears that the practice-based procedure has not been fully exhausted), or arranging conciliation if it appears that that course would be helpful.

Family health services conciliation

A complainant may not, for some reason, wish to have his or her complaint dealt with by the GP practice complaints procedure. The complainant may not feel it is sufficiently independent, or may be experiencing difficulties getting the complaint dealt with. In these circumstances the health authority can act as an 'honest broker' and try to resolve the complaint through lay conciliators at local resolution. If the complainant remains dissatisfied, then he or she can request an independent review. If a complainant remains dissatisfied after the independent review, or has been denied an independent review, he or she will be able to ask the HSC or Ombudsman to consider investigating the complaint.

Health Service Commissioner (Ombudsman)

The Health Service Commissioner (HSC) is an official who is independent of the NHS and government. He is accountable to Parliament for his work, which is overseen by the Select Committee on the Parliamentary Commissioner for Administration. The HSC presents an annual report to both Houses of Parliament, and periodically produces volumes of selected investigation reports. The HSC can also issue reports on particular cases or issues. A special report was made on investigation of complaint handling by Salford Royal Hospitals NHS Trust (HSC, 1996a), and reports on

Investigations of Complaints about Clinical Failings (HSC, 1999a) and *Investigation of Complaint about Treatment by Deputising Doctors* (HSC, 1999b) (all these publications are available from The Stationery Office). The HSC now sits at the apex of the complaints system, and can investigate complaints about the NHS. The Health Service Commissioner's (Amendment) Act 1996 extended considerably the HSC powers of investigation, which now include the power to investigate matters involving the clinical judgment of health care professionals and to investigate complaints about the family health services provided by GPs, dentists, pharmacists and opticians. Section 43 of the Health Act 1999 has amended the power of the HSC to release information, and the HSC can now share information with regulatory bodies like the UKCC even when he or she has not investigated the complaint – for example, information could be passed to the UKCC regarding a discernible pattern of complaints in relation to a particular nurse. It would then be up to the UKCC to decide whether to take action or not.

Matters the HSC cannot investigate

The HSC is unable to investigate a number of matters, including:

- Personnel issues such as staff appointments, discipline or pay
- Complaints about local disciplinary arrangements for family health service providers
- Commercial or contractual matters, unless they relate to services for patients provided under an NHS contract
- Situations where the complainant could take legal proceedings. An example would be a clinical negligence claim or a right of appeal reference or review before a tribunal. The HSC can still investigate these matters if satisfied that in the particular circumstances it is not reasonable to expect the complainant to follow this course.

Maladministration

The HSC investigates matters where there has been maladministration or a failure of service. The HSC and staff subscribe to the following statement of purpose (HSC, 1995):

> To investigate impartially and expeditiously complaints about maladministration or failure in service leading to injustice or hardship, and about refusal of access to official information by NHS authorities; to obtain appropriate redress for the complainant; and to promote fairness, integrity and practical improvements in public administration and the quality of service provided to users of the National Health Service.

What is maladministration?

The term maladministration is a key concept to the understanding of the work and jurisdiction of the HSC. Before a discretionary decision of a trust, health authority or other body or person can be challenged, there must be evidence of maladministration. The term acts as a trigger for the involvement of the HSC. The term is not defined in a statute, but is discussed by the HSC (1996b).

The term maladministration includes:

- Bias
- Neglect
- Inattention
- Delay
- Incompetence
- Ineptitude
- Perversity
- Turpitude
- Arbitrariness
- Rudeness (though that is a matter of degree)
- Unwillingness to treat the complainant as a person with rights
- Refusal to answer reasonable questions
- Neglecting to inform a complainant on request of his or her rights or entitlements
- Knowingly giving advice that is misleading or inadequate
- Ignoring valid advice or overruling considerations that would produce an uncomfortable result for the overruler
- Offering no redress or manifestly disproportionate redress
- Showing bias, whether because of colour, sex, or any other grounds
- Omitting to notify those who thereby lose a right of appeal
- Refusal to inform the complainant adequately of the right of appeal
- Faulty procedures
- Failure by management to monitor compliance with adequate procedures
- Cavalier disregard of the guidance which is intended to be followed in the interests of equitable treatment of those who use a service
- Partiality
- Failure to mitigate the effects of rigid adherence to the letter where that produces manifestly inequitable treatment.

The list given is illustrative and not exhaustive. This HSC focus on mal-administration does not apply when a complaint relates to a decision taken in the exercise of clinical judgment (HSC, 1996b):

... the Ombudsman may uphold the complaint without having regard to considerations of maladministration because the test of maladminis-tration is not apt for clinical decisions.

The HSC has assessors who are able to advise whether the actions com-plained of were based on a reasonable and responsible exercise of clinical judgment of a standard that the patient could be reasonably entitled to expect in the circumstances.

Access procedures

Generally speaking, complaints must be made to the HSC by the person directly concerned within 1 year of the matter coming to the person's notice. It is possible that another person or organization could complain on the patient's behalf. The complaint can even be made after the death of the complainant by the next of kin or by some other person or organiza-tion.

The HSC has indicated that complaints brought by hospital staff on the patient's behalf will be received. The HSC will not normally consider a complaint until the local review stages have been completed. The HSC has provided a special complaint form, which is available on the Internet at: http://www.health.ombudsman.org.uk/form/healthfm.htm (Office of HSC, 1996). Staff employed by NHS bodies, independent providers, family health services practitioners and those working for them can com-plain to the HSC if they consider that they have suffered hardship or injus-tice through the complaints procedure operated by trusts or health author-ities. Established local grievance procedures must be completed before approaching the HSC.

Investigation

The HSC has assistants, including investigating and screening officers. The HSC also has specialist health care professional advisers for com-plaints on clinical judgment. The investigation is conducted in private, and the procedure is informal. Comments are sought from hospital staff on the complaint. The HSC has the same powers as a High Court judge to obtain information and documents, and if staff do not want to co-operate they can be compelled to testify. The production of documents and reports can also be formally ordered. Relations between the HSC and health authority staff are normally good, and these formal measures would only be used as a last resort.

Report

When the investigation is complete, the HSC sends a report to the complainant, the relevant NHS authority and to any individual who has had allegations made about him or her in the complaint. The report states whether the complaint or any part of it has been upheld, and recommends a remedy. This may take the form of an apology from the health authority and the other parties involved. The HSC report cannot be enforced in a court of law, and HSC investigations and findings are separate and quite distinct from court proceedings.

HSC investigations and findings of maladministration have also led the HSC to make detailed recommendations, which have included:

- Changes in procedures
- The creation of training programmes
- Improvements in record keeping, etc.

The HSC cannot award compensation, but does sometimes recommend that an *ex gratia* payment be made to cover a complainant's expenditure or financial loss. An example can be seen in case W.525/91–92 (HSC, 1992a). Damage was caused to the complainant's property by a mentally ill patient jumping naked from a hospital window into the complainant's house. The complainant was dissatisfied with the health authority and hospital's response to the incident. The HSC recommended that the district health authority, as an act of grace, make an *ex gratia* payment without admission of liability to cover the complainant's uninsured loss. The district health authority promised to make a payment to cover half of the complainant's loss.

Errors and failures

HSC reports reveal a wide catalogue of errors and failures which, generally speaking, could have been easily avoided. A large number involve communication failures; the HSC (1992b) commented:

> ... some topics – such as record keeping, complaints handling and observation of patients – feature regularly in ... annual reports.

Seven years on, the same problems still persist (HSC, 1999c):

> Communication difficulties lay at the heart of a significant number of complaints about clinical care. Sometimes the problem was poor communication between professionals, and sometimes between professionals and patients (or their relatives). In other cases, while I was satisfied that reasonable clinical care had been given, an opportunity to resolve the complainant's concerns had been missed because of poor communication and complaint handling.

Nurses do feature in a number of complaints to the HSC. For example (HSC, 1999c):

The service area with the largest number of complaints about clinical care (26) was, not unexpectedly, hospital inpatients: about 35 per cent were upheld. About 13 per cent of clinical grievances investigated primarily involved nurses and 19 per cent hospital doctors.

The following case investigation report (W.232/90–91) provides a good illustration of the problems that the HSC investigates, in a nursing context (HSC, 1992c). A woman was terminally ill with cancer and was also suffering from claustrophobia. She was nursed during the week in a surgical ward and, for hospital financial reasons, was moved at the weekend to other wards and sometimes a small side room. A decision was eventually made to transfer her to a hospice, where she died 3 days after the transfer. Her husband complained that the weekend ward transfers caused his wife unacceptable distress and that nursing staff in these wards were unaware that his wife suffered from claustrophobia. He said that there had been inadequate nursing care in one ward. He claimed that his wife had not been given help with washing, that pressure sores had been allowed to develop, and that her urostomy and ileostomy bags had not been changed regularly. He complained of insensitivity on the part of a ward sister, whom he stated had asked his wife to cut up an incontinence roll when supplies had run out. The roll was inadequate for his wife's needs, and he had to buy another one. The sister, he claimed, had also been unwilling to arrange for an ambulance to take his wife to the hospice. Some of the husband's complaints were upheld. The HSC found 'a deplorable lack of regard by management for patient's welfare'. The health authority apologized.

The investigation reports of the HSC provide a useful perspective from which to view the professional accountability of the nurse. The HSC (1995) Annual Report contains the following case (S.104/93–94, Tayside HB):

> A woman developed a pressure sore while in hospital and I considered that there had been an avoidable delay in taking preventative measures. I also criticized the poor standard of record keeping. I found that nursing staff had not communicated satisfactorily with the patient's daughter. Board to check that monitoring of pressure area care standards was operating effectively.

The HSC (1998) reported the following in Case No. E.189/97–98, which involved failures in medical and nursing care, delay in transfer to an intensive care unit (ICU) at another hospital, and unsatisfactory complaint handling. Findings include the following:

> The evidence indicates that Mr B's drip was out for about two hours. My assessors have said that that would not have had an adverse effect on his condition. I accept that. However, it is not satisfactory that Mr B was left with bloodstained pyjamas and bedding until the family asked for them to be changed.

Complaints to the HSC can cover a range of matters involving GPs, doctors, nurses, dentists and so on. The HSC investigates a wide range of matters, and a recent trend is that more clinically complex matters are being dealt with (HSC, 1999c). The HSC role is capable of further development and improvement. The Association of Community Health Councils for England and Wales (ACHCEW, 1999) has made a number of recommendations to reform the office of HSC, which include the following:

- The Ombudsman should name primary care groups and primary care trusts that have been the subject of his investigations
- Stronger mechanisms are required to ensure that the Ombudsman's recommendations are complied with
- The ability of a complainant to take a complaint to the Ombudsman's office should not be constrained by a time limit.

The reports and investigations of the HSC show that this office is providing a very valuable and important function. The HSC reports are always clear, thorough and incisive. The value of the HSC lies in independence from the NHS; the HSC reports to Parliament. The role of HSC does need to keep pace with the changes in the NHS, and should not be seen as static. Experience of the HSC shows that the role will change to meet new demands. The extension of the HSC's jurisdiction to cover clinical judgement is one example of how the role can develop positively.

Complaint handling: reform

Criticisms of the NHS complaints system have come from a number of influential quarters. The Association of Community Health Councils for England and Wales (ACHCEW, 1996) argues that local resolution of complaints requires a revolution in attitudes among NHS staff, and that the arrangements for training to bring this about are woefully inadequate. Some other misgivings have been expressed. Harris and Simanowitz (1996) argue that the newly overhauled NHS complaints system lacks true independence from the NHS, and places unnecessary restrictions on complainants. They express concerns as to the impartiality of the system where a complainant requests an independent review. Requests are screened by a member of the health authority or trust involved. They fear that the HSC, now placed at the apex of the system, will be overloaded with appeals from dissatisfied complainants who have been refused an independent review. They also argue that the 6-month time limit for bringing complaints under the new system is too restrictive. More recently, in evidence to the House of Commons Select Committee on Health (House of Commons, 1999b), the NHS complaints system was critically discussed by a number of witnesses and failings identified. The Health Committee summarized the criticisms in paragraphs 72–75 of its Sixth

Report (House of Commons, 1999c), and referred to patients' complaints of inconsistencies across the country regarding the way in which similar matters were dealt with. *Health Which?* (2000) published a survey that revealed high levels of dissatisfaction among patients complaining about the NHS. *Health Which?* investigators contacted 38 community health councils (CHCs), who forwarded their questionnaire to more than 2000 patients who had approached them between September 1998 and September 1999 with a view to making a complaint to the NHS. The report was based on the experiences of 712 people across the UK. The survey found that resolution of complaints at local level was deeply flawed, with most complainants preferring not to approach the staff who their complaint concerned, and few complainants getting the outcomes they had hoped for – 69 per cent had wanted action to prevent the problem happening again, but only 37 per cent said they had got this. Many complainants were not happy with the fairness of the process, and complaint time limits were not being met. Another report in this chapter also reveals patient dissatisfaction with the complaints system.

The Public Law Project (Wallace and Mulcahy, 1999), in their report on the NHS complaints system, also identified a number of failings in the handling of complaints and in the procedure itself. The authors argue that:

> Major changes need to be made to the complaints procedure in order to restore public confidence in its independence and effectiveness. Reform is needed to:
>
> - Ensure complaints are handled impartially and swiftly at local resolution
> - Enhance the independence and powers of the independent review process
> - Introduce tighter mechanisms for ensuring that lessons are learned from complaints to improve standards of care across the NHS.

The Health Committee (House of Commons, 1999c) made a number of recommendations, which included the abolition of the role of the convener as presently organized, and that IRPs (independent review panels) should consist of a majority of lay members and should not be connected with the trust or health authority that is the subject of the complaint. Furthermore, it recommended that IRPs should be funded by and accountable to the regional offices of the NHS Executive. A number of other important recommendations were made. The government has commissioned a 2-year evaluation of the complaints procedure (NHS Executive, 1999c), and an interim evaluation will be published in 2000. The NHS National Plan (DOH, 2000b) contains a number of far-reaching proposals dealing with patient satisfaction and complaints. The plan calls for patient advocates and advisers in every hospital, and it works from a notable patient-centred premise:

10.1 Patients are the most important people in the health service. It doesn't always appear that way. Too many patients feel talked at, rather than listened to. This has to change. NHS care has to be shaped around the convenience and concerns of patients.

There does seem to be a ground swell of opinion developing, which is saying that all is not right with the NHS complaints system. When the complaints system was introduced in 1996 the accompanying DOH documentation looked very promising, with clear advice on strategies to avoid and handle complaints being given. Experience with the system over time has revealed difficulties that do need to be resolved, and reform does now seem to be inevitable.

The question is, how far will reform extend? Will the system be scrapped and a new one introduced, or will certain 'rough edges' be trimmed? The final decision rests with the DOH and the government, who have enough expert literature to make informed and evidence-based determinations. Such determinations are going to have to take account of other initiatives in the NHS, such as controls assurance and clinical governance, and organizations such as CHI and NICE. A complaints system cannot exist in splendid isolation from these dynamic and focused health quality improvement initiatives. The links will have to be carefully thought through to avoid overlaps and inconsistencies.

References

ACHCEW (1996). *CHC Newsletter*, **Issue 1**, June.
ACHCEW (1999). *Health Perspectives: The Health Service Ombudsman: The Public's Perspective*. ACHCEW.
Beecham, L. (2000). Milburn sets up inquiry into Shipman case. *Br. Med. J.*, **320**, 401, http://www.bmj.com/cgi/content/full/320/7232/401/a.
Berrington, L. and Barnwell, R. (1995). Britain's moaning minnies who know their rights. *The Times*, 26 January.
Command Paper 3807 (1997). *The New NHS, Modern, Dependable*. The Stationery Office.
Department of Health (1995a). *The Patient's Charter*. DOH.
Department of Health (1995b). *Acting on Complaints: The Government Proposals in Response to 'Being Heard', the Report of a Review Committee on NHS Complaints Procedures*. DOH.
Department of Health (1998). *Handling Complaints: Monitoring the NHS Complaints Procedure, England, Financial Year 1996–97*. DOH.
Department of Health (2000a). *Publication of Handling Complaints: Monitoring the NHS Complaints Procedures, England, 1998–99*. Statistical Press Notice, 2000/0169, 23 March. DOH. Internet version of the report at http://www.doh.gov.uk/nhscomplaints.
Department of Health (2000b). *The NHS Plan*. Command Paper 4818-1. The Stationery Office.
Dyer, C. (1999). Bristol trust admits liability in baby heart surgery case. *Br. Med. J.*, **319**, 213. http://www.bmj.com/cgi/content/full/319/7204/213/a.
Harris, T. and Simanowitz, A. (1996). Letter. *The Times*, 13 April.
Health Service Commissioner (1992a). *Selected Investigations Completed, April–September 1992*. HMSO.
Health Service Commissioner (1992b). *Annual Report for 1991–92*. HMSO.

Health Service Commissioner (1992c). *Selected Investigations Completed October 1991–March 1992.* HMSO.

Health Service Commissioner (1995). *Annual Report for 1994–95.* HMSO.

Health Service Commissioner (1996a). *Investigation of Complaint Handling by Salford Royal Hospital NHS Trust.* Second Report for Session 1995–96. HMSO.

Health Service Commissioner (1996b). *A Guide to the Work of the Health Service Ombudsman.* Office of HSC.

Health Service Commissioner (1998). *Investigations Completed April–September 1998, First Report, Session 1998–99.* The Stationery Office.

Health Service Commissioner (1999a). *Investigations of Complaints about Clinical Failings, Fourth Report for Session 1998–99, HC 496.* The Stationery Office.

Health Service Commissioner (1999b). *Investigation of Complaint about Treatment by Deputising Doctors, Second Report for Session 1998–99, HC 341.* The Stationery Office.

Health Service Commissioner (1999c). *Annual Report for 1998–99.* The Stationery Office.

Health Which? (2000). NHS complaints. Consumers' Association.

Hill, G. (1991). *Complaints about Clinical Care: Correct Management.* Medical Defence Union.

House of Commons (1999a). HC 549-IV, Select Committee on Health, Minutes of Evidence for Thursday 8th July 1999, Question 548, *Procedures Related to Adverse Clinical Incidents and Outcomes Incidents and Outcomes in Medical Care.* The Stationery Office. http://www.publications.parliament.uk/pa/cm199899/cmselect/cmhealth/cmhealth.htm.

House of Commons (1999b). HC 549-II, Select Committee on Health, Sixth Report, 23 November, *Procedures Related to Adverse Clinical Incidents and Outcomes in Medical Care, Volume II – Evidence and Appendices.* The Stationery Office. http://www.publications.parliament.uk/pa/cm199899/cmselect/cmhealth/cmhealth.htm.

House of Commons (1999c). HC 549-I, Select Committee on Health, Sixth Report, 23 November, *Procedures Related to Adverse Clinical Incidents and Outcomes in Medical Care, Volume I – Report and Proceedings.* The Stationery Office. http://www.publications.parliament.uk/pa/cm199899/cmselect/cmhealth/cmhealth.htm.

Medical Defence Union (1993). *Talking to Patients.* MDU.

NHS Executive (1996a). *Complaints, Listening, Acting and Improving: Guidance on Implementation of the NHS Complaints Procedure.* All accompanying Executive Letter EL 96(19), Implementation of New Complaints Procedures: Final Guidance, 12 March. NHS Executive.

NHS Executive (1996b). *Practice-Based Complaints Procedures: Guidance for General Practices.* NHS Executive.

NHS Executive (1999a). *Guidelines for Implementing Controls Assurance in the NHS, Guidance for Directors.* NHS Executive. http://tap.ccta.gov.uk/doh/rm5.nsf/Publications?OpenView.

NHS Executive (1999b). *Good Practice Guide for Conveners,* HSC 1999/193. DOH. http://www.doh.gov.uk/coinh.htm.

NHS Executive (1999c). *Evaluation of NHS Complaints Procedure,* Circular, MISC (99)12. NHS Executive.

NHSLA (2000). *Clinical Negligence Scheme for Trusts (CNST): Risk Management Standards and Procedures, Manual of Guidance.* NHSLA.

NHS Training Division (1995). *Local Resolution Training Resources Pack.* NHS Executive.

Office of Health Service Commissioner (1996). *Do You Have a Complaint about the Service You have Received from the NHS?* Office of HSC.

Simanowitz, A. (1985). Standards, attitudes and accountability in the medical profession. *Lancet,* **2(8454)**, 546.

Simanowitz, A. (1995). Patients' complaints in health care provision. In: *Nursing Law and Ethics* (J. H. Tingle and A. Cribb, eds). Blackwell Science, pp. 59–76.

Tingle, J. H. (1990). Complaints and the law. *Nursing Standard*, **5(2)**, 44.

Truelove, A. (1985). On handling complaints. *Hosp. Health Serv. Rev.*, **(i)**, 229.

UKCC (1996). *Guidelines for Professional Practice*. UKCC.

Vincent, C., Young, M. and Phillips, A. (1994). Why do people sue doctors? A study of patients and relatives taking legal action. *Lancet*, **343**, 1609.

Wallace, H. and Mulcahy, L. (1999). The Public Law Project. *Cause for Complaint? An Evaluation of the Effectiveness of the NHS Complaints Procedure*. Birkbeck College, University of London.

Wilson Committee Report (1994). *Being Heard, The Report of a Review Committee on NHS Complaints Procedures*. DOH.

Chapter 4

Legal aspects of expanded role and clinical guidelines and protocols

John Tingle

This chapter focuses upon certain specific issues that have important ramifications regarding nursing accountability, such as expanded role, the operation of clinical care guidelines and protocols, and nurse prescribing.

Developments in nursing practice

Today, the number of tasks undertaken by nurses has increased. This is related to a number of factors, ranging from resource issues (such as the need to reduce junior doctors' hours) to the fact that nurses are being entrusted with wider responsibility as recognition of their role as independent practitioners. The government's published strategy for nursing, midwifery and health visiting, contained in *Making a Difference* (DOH, 1999a) is notable for its proactive stance on nurses taking on more advanced activities. The government would like nurses to extend their role and to make better use of their knowledge and skills. It also wants to make it easier for them to prescribe. Health Secretary Alan Milburn has laid down a 10-point challenge on nursing skills to be implemented throughout the NHS. This includes nurses being able to: order diagnostic investigations (e.g. pathology tests and X-rays); make and receive referrals direct to, for example, therapists or pain consultants; run their own clinics (e.g. ophthalmology or dermatology); and take a lead in the way local health services are organized and run (DOH, 2000a). The impetus for role expansion has been firmly set by the government; however, the momentum for role expansion has been growing steadily for a number of years, and now the government can be seen to be taking this forward. *The NHS Plan* (DOH, 2000b) further promotes the expanded role.

Nurses now undertake activities such as ECGs, defibrillation after a heart attack, verification of death (although not in cases of unexpected death), taking blood samples, and performing male catheterization (Eaton, 1993). There are nurse-led minor injury units (MIUs) where nurses carry out a variety of activities, including suturing, X-rays, plastering and referrals (Carlisle, 1995). There are also nurse endoscopists (Jowett *et al.*, 2000).

The growth of the nurse's work has been termed 'expanded role' by some commentators. In the past the term 'extended role' was used when discussing the issue of nurses carrying out activities traditionally carried out by doctors (Tingle, 1993). The position altered, however, in 1992 (DOH, 1992), following a report issued by the Standing Medical Advisory Committee and the Standing Nursing and Midwifery Advisory Committee (1989). The United Kingdom Central Council for Nursing, Midwifery and Health Visiting (UKCC) stated that the terms 'extended' or 'extending roles' are no longer favoured, as they '… limit, rather than extend the parameters of practice' (UKCC, 1992a).

The UKCC published a document in 1992 (UKCC, 1992a), *The Scope of Professional Practice*, which gives guidance to nurses regarding the expanded role.

The Scope of Professional Practice (UKCC, 1992a) states that:

The registered nurse, midwife or health visitor:
1. must be satisfied that each aspect of practice is directed to meeting the needs and serving the interests of the patient or client;
2. must endeavour always to achieve, maintain and develop knowledge, skill and competence to respond to those needs and interests;
3. must honestly acknowledge any limits of personal knowledge and skill and take steps to remedy any relevant deficits in order effectively and appropriately to meet the needs of patients and clients;
4. must ensure that any enlargement or adjustment of the scope of personal professional practice must be achieved without compromising or fragmenting existing aspects of professional practice or care and that requirements of the Council's Code of Professional Practice are satisfied through the whole area of practice;
5. must recognize and honour the direct or indirect personal accountability borne for all aspects of professional practice; and
6. must, in serving the interests of patients and clients and the wider interests of society, avoid inappropriate delegation to others which compromises those interests.

The UKCC have announced a review of this document, which will take place during 2000 (UKCC, 2000). Also being reviewed are the *Code of*

Professional Conduct (UKCC, 1992b) and *Guidelines for Professional Practice* (UKCC, 1996). Review is an essential process in fast-changing times; it is important that these documents are seen to be relevant and appropriate.

Many see role expansion as presenting an exciting opportunity to develop new specialisms. However, expanding the nursing role has been controversial, and there has been disagreement within the nursing profession as to what approach should be taken. There is no national standard or catalogue of expanded roles, and practices differ from region to region and even within hospitals (Standing Medical Advisory Committee and Standing Nursing and Midwifery Advisory Committee, 1989). The debate is still an intense one. Some nurses argue that nursing may as a result become too technical and less patient-centred (Giles, 1993; Shepherd, 1993; Healey, 1996). Eaton (1993) quotes Derek Dean (formerly Director of Policy and Research at the Royal College of Nursing (RCN)):

> The worry among nurses, many of whom welcome this additional responsibility, is that they are being asked to do extra work without anyone extra to take the load off them. A lot of members have expressed concern. They have said, 'We are being asked to do things and are rushed off our feet'.

Similarly, Waters (1996) quotes RCN community adviser Mark Jones, who presented at a conference a catalogue of cautionary tales illustrating the dangers of nurses overreaching themselves. The list included one case where a practice nurse with no formal midwifery training had taken over antenatal care and had missed a fetus dying *in utero*.

A report by Doyal *et al.* (1998) looked in detail at the development of four new nursing posts, where each post involved nurses taking over some part of the work previously done by junior doctors. This study explored the views of nurses themselves, and was quite revealing. While the study revealed excitement at the professional challenges they faced, it also indicated that practitioners received little support and there was considerable confusion surrounding their new roles. Some legal and accountability issues were also noted:

> ... there were many staff who admitted that they did not know about the arrangements for accountability. They included consultants, ward nurses and junior doctors who worked with the postholders. Certain factors seemed to contribute to the confusion about the understanding of the arrangements for the postholder's accountability. One of these was lack of clarity about the role. So for instance, at Site X, the doctors saw the postholder's role as a support worker for them and hence the postholders' accountability was described as being to the doctors. Senior nurses, however, interpreted the role as that of a nurse specialist with accountability identified within the nursing framework.

The authors make a number of recommendations for managers and postholders about the management of change, which include:

Areas of work should be identified which the postholder can take over completely with maximum autonomy and minimum dependency on junior doctors for completion of the work. Nurses and doctors should be equal partners in planning and managing such developments. The GMC, UKCC and NHS Executive need to clarify and harmonise relevant regulations concerning the scope and standards of new clinical roles, influence legal process and educate the public about changing professional roles.

This report provides a focused practical perspective on the many problems and benefits of extended role development. The authors of this report were also in a small working group, which looked in further detail at the accountability of changing nurses' roles. The analyses were published in the *British Medical Journal* (Dowling *et al.*, 1996). They noted that the resulting uncertainties about appropriate management for clinical roles evolving between the professions, coupled with a public increasingly going to court, put nurses and consultants at risk. These health care professionals faced the risk of complaints, litigation and possible disciplinary hearing. Recommendations to reduce risk included that doctors and nurses should be equal partners in planning the new roles, and that patients should be informed adequately of the postholder's role and relevant training. Guidance regarding such practices should also be drawn up by the professional organizations, the UKCC and the GMC, in conjunction with bodies such as the British Medical Association (BMA) and the Royal College of Nursing (RCN).

It would be helpful if all these organizations could reach an understanding on expanded role. The current advice, as will be shown, shows marked differences of approach The emphasis today is upon the nurses themselves making the decision as to whether to undertake an expanded role. If nurses believe that they have the necessary competence, then they may undertake a task themselves. The UKCC is opposed to the use of certificates of competence, which state that the nurse has undergone a training programme and thus may be competent to perform a particular task (UKCC, 1992a):

in order to bring into proper focus the professional responsibility and consequent accountability of individual practitioners, it is the Council's principles for practice rather than certificates for tasks which should form the basis for adjustments to the scope of practice.

It has been suggested that if nurses are given such certificates, this may give them a false sense of security and lead them to think that accountability for actions has shifted to their assessor. However, at the same time, before a nurse undertakes an expanded role appropriate training is advisable, and such knowledge needs to be sustained and updated. Nurses are under a duty to undertake a minimum of 5 days of study in each 3-year period to update their knowledge (an activity requirement). A key tool to ensure a safe environment of care may be through the use of guidelines for tasks that have been delegated by doctors to nurses, or where a new role has been developed. The issue of guideline development will be discussed later.

It is interesting to note that while the discourse in nursing practice is that of nurses themselves undertaking an expanded role, difficult issues remain as to the boundaries of practice and where ultimate responsibility lies. Nurses may take on an increased role because they are acting as independent practitioners. Alternatively, it may be because they have been delegated certain tasks to be performed by doctors. Guidance has been issued by the General Medical Council on the issue of delegation (GMC, 1998; see below).

Guidance on the issue of delegation (GMC, 1998):

Delegation and referral

39. Delegation involves asking a nurse, doctor, or medical student or other health care worker to provide treatment or care on your behalf. When you delegate care or treatment you must be sure that the person to whom you delegate is competent to carry out the procedure or provide the therapy involved. You must always pass on enough information about the patient and the treatment needed. You will still be responsible for the overall management of the patient.

40. Referral involves transferring some or all of the responsibility for the patient's care, usually temporarily and for a particular purpose, such as additional investigation, care or treatment, which falls outside your competence. Usually you will refer patients to another registered medical practitioner. If this is not the case, you must be satisfied that such health care workers are accountable to a statutory regulatory body, and that a registered medical practitioner, usually a general practitioner, retains overall responsibility for the management of the patient.

There is recognition that doctors can refer cases to nurses as opposed to delegating care; however, overall responsibility still usually lies with the GP.

Where tasks are delegated, then the doctor delegating the task should follow appropriate guidelines. Should the doctor fail to do so and harm results to the patient, the doctor may be held liable in negligence for the harm caused. It may also be the case that even where the delegation is properly undertaken, the doctor is held ultimately responsible in any event under what is known as the 'captain of the ship' approach (Montgomery, 1992). It is interesting to note that both the GMC and the BMA assume that where delegation takes place, the doctor retains ultimate accountability (BMA, 1996). It may, however, be questioned to what extent such an approach is appropriate as the role of the nurse develops and he or she is recognized as having greater personal autonomy, and indeed whether the courts would be more likely to hold that the nurse was solely liable where tasks have been legitimately delegated.

The boundaries between activities that are undertaken as part of expanded role and those that follow from delegation are unclear. Darley and Rumsey (1996) note that the use of language such as 'delegation' is indicative of hierarchy. They suggest that it would be better to talk in terms of 'shared care' or 'referral'; this would have the advantage of emphasizing the partnership and teamwork aspects. To avoid confusion, a co-ordinated approach on these matters is urgently needed from both the GMC and UKCC and from other bodies such as the BMA and RCN (see Dowling *et al.*, 1996).

In 1997, the UKCC commissioned independent research from Public Attitude Surveys Ltd, in conjunction with King's College, London, into the application and impact of its document, *The Scope of Professional Practice* (Jowett *et al.*, 2000). The report gives a real-time view of the *Scope* document in the context of professional practice, and will inform the UKCC review discussions. Almost one-third of respondents were not aware of the *Scope* document. However, among those who were, much interest was expressed and the key principles were seen to be widely endorsed:

> There were, however, concerns about what implementing *Scope* really means and such uncertainty may limit the extent to which staff are willing, or able, to innovate.

The report has implications for the UKCC, which include the need for them to improve awareness and understanding of the *Scope* document, and its marketing.

A key issue inherent with any code, protocol or guidance is the extent to which you can satisfactorily incorporate quite difficult concepts such as competence and accountability, without trivializing them or making them too simplistic. Codes can spell out the conventional wisdom of a group of people or an organization – for example, the UKCC – but the enforceability and absorption of that wisdom are more difficult questions. The *Scope* document seeks to change professional cultures, which is a hard thing to do, and therefore such change will be necessarily incremental and slow. Government initiatives such as the 10-point challenge on nursing skills and the NHS National Plan (DOH, 2000a) may, however, speed up the pace of change.

Clinical negligence and professional misconduct

Case study

A case involving a negligent practice nurse illustrates some of the difficulties regarding accountability (Parker and Wilson, 1992).

A 34-year-old man attended the doctor to have his right ear syringed. On examination, the GP suspected that he had an abscess and prescribed penicillin and asked him to return in 1 week to see the nurse and have his ear syringed then. When the patient returned his ear was syringed by a locum practice nurse, and the patient later admitted that during the procedure he had felt excruciating pain and dizziness. He returned to the surgery complaining of a sore ear, and the nurse referred him to the doctor. On examination he was found to have a perforated eardrum. He made a good recovery but sued alleging negligence, and the GP was found to have fallen below the acceptable standard of care in delegating the procedure to the nurse without first having established her competence. The nurse had not performed ear syringing for some 20 years. The Medical Defence Union (MDU) settled the claim.

The crucial issue for the employer, then, is to ensure that, first of all, the nurse is lawfully undertaking the task. The GP in the case above should have at least asked the nurse whether she had performed ear syringing before and, if so, how long ago. On the facts of the case, the GP could be viewed as wrongfully assigning the procedure to the practice nurse. This may mean that the GP was acting negligently. Can the present system deal with the nurse who feels that he or she will 'have a go' at an expanded role, taking a very liberal view of her or his own competence and experience? Last *et al.* (1992) raised the same point:

> How can chief nurses, directors of nursing services and nurse managers be sure that all practitioners are safe to enlarge the scope of their practice? How can managers allow those who are able to fly to do so, yet provide a safety net to those who could never fly, or even worse, those who think they can but cannot, from falling down?

Expanding the nurse's role and stress at work

Managers, doctors and nurses have to be trusted to operate the system satisfactorily and in a way that does not compromise patient safety. Overloading nurses may also have implications for the management should the nurses be unable to perform their role because they have developed some form of stress-related illness. Nurses who fall ill and claim that this was caused by unduly high stress levels in the workplace may bring legal proceedings claiming compensation for the harm suffered.

The fact that a contract of employment may stipulate stressful working conditions does not by itself mean that a nurse who suffers physical or psychological harm consequent upon that stress cannot bring a claim for damages. This was made clear by the case of *Johnstone* v. *Bloomsbury AHA* ([1991] 2 All ER 293). Here, a junior hospital doctor brought an action claiming that his employer had broken an implied duty to take reasonable care for his safety and had broken his contract of employment. He was required by his contract to work a basic week of 40 hours and to be available for up to 48 hours per week overtime. In the Court of Appeal, a majority of the judges held that he had an arguable case. Stuart Smith L.J. held that the Health Authority was under a duty to provide a safe system of work. While the obligation to work up to 88 hours per week was contained in a junior doctor's contract, this had to be set against an employer's duty to take reasonable care for the employee's safety.

One difficulty in bringing such actions is that of showing that stress-induced psychiatric injury is foreseeable. Much depends on the circumstances of the individual case. In some instances, employers can justifiably argue that they were not aware that their employee had been subject to excessive stress levels. However, where an employer is put on notice that an employee is susceptible to such a breakdown and then that employee returns to work and suffers a second nervous breakdown due to stressful working conditions, then an action consequent upon the second breakdown may meet with more success (*Walker* v. *Northumbria County Council* [1995] 1 All ER 737). A nurse would also have to establish that it was the stressful working conditions themselves that amounted to a material cause of a breakdown. This may itself be problematic; in many situations stress levels are influenced by factors external to the employment relationship itself, such as home and family life. It is also the case that the assessment of stress levels is a matter that would fall under the employee obligations under the Health and Safety at Work Act 1974 and the Management of Health and Safety at Work Regulations 1992.

Legal standard of care to be exercised by a nurse performing an expanded role

Where a nurse performs traditional nursing duties, the standard of practice required is that of the ordinary skilled nurse in his or her particular speciality in the circumstances of the case – the *Bolam* principle. But what is the standard of care the nurse must reach if performing an expanded role? Guidance can be taken from the case *Wilsher* v. *Essex Area Health Authority* ([1986] 3 All ER 801).

The Wilsher case

The plaintiff, Martin Wilsher, was an infant child born about 3 months early. He was very ill, and was placed in a special care baby unit where a junior and inexperienced doctor monitoring the oxygen in the plaintiff's bloodstream made a mistake and mistakenly inserted a catheter into a vein rather than an artery. The junior doctor asked a registrar to check what he had done, but the registrar failed to notice the mistake and, when replacing the catheter himself some hours later, made the same mistake himself. The catheter monitor failed to register correctly the amount of oxygen in the baby's bloodstream, and he was given excess oxygen. It was alleged that the excess oxygen in his bloodstream had caused an incurable condition of the retina, retrolental fibroplasia. Martin is now completely blind. A key issue discussed by the Court of Appeal was the standard of legal care to be exercised by the junior doctor in the case. Mustill L.J. stated (p. 813):

> In a case such as the present, the standard is not just that of the averagely competent and well-informed junior houseman (or whatever the position of the doctor) but of such a person who fills a post in a unit offering a highly specialized service.

Glidewell L.J. stated (p. 831):

> In my view, the law requires the trainee or learner to be judged by the same standard as his more experienced colleagues. If it did not, inexperience would frequently be urged as a defence to an action for professional negligence.

On the facts before the court, the junior doctor was not found negligent – he had done the reasonable thing and asked his superior. However, the registrar was found to be negligent. The case went on appeal to the House of Lords on the issue of causation, and was eventually set down for retrial. The case was settled for £116 724.40 (Kerry, 1991). (This case is quoted by the UKCC (1996) in Section 16 of their Guidelines, in Appendix 1.) The key point to be taken from the *Wilsher* case is that a nurse is liable to be judged by the professional standard of the post that he or she is performing at that time. This means that if the nurse is performing an expanded role, he or she is expected to operate at the level of skill and competence outlined in the expanded role. A further point is that, as Kloss (1988) argues:

> If a nurse undertakes a task for which she knows she has insufficient training, this in itself may constitute negligence, even if she is acting on the orders of a doctor. … If a nurse takes on the doctor's role she will be judged by the standard of the reasonable doctor.

There is much older legal authority (*Philips* v. *William Whitley Ltd* ([1938] 1 All ER 566) that could be used to argue against the *Wilsher* elevated legal standard of care proposition. It appears that the *Wilsher* approach is more likely to be followed. The case of *Djemal* v. *Bexley Health Authority* ([1995] 6 Med LR 269) supports the *Wilsher* approach.

The issue of the appropriate standard of legal care to be exercised by nurses performing medical tasks has been brought into sharp focus by a number of recent initiatives where new health care professional posts have been created that involve the performance of some medical activities – for example, transplant clinicians' assistants and cardiac surgeons' assistants. These posts can be occupied by nurses or other health care professionals. If a negligence case involving one of these staff occurred, the court would have difficulty in assessing the appropriate standard of care to be exercised by the professional because the posts are so new and there may be only one or two in existence. The court could look at the nature of the tasks performed and determine who normally performs those tasks. If doctors normally undertake them, then a medical standard of care and skill will be expected (Caine, 1993; Naish, 1995; Peysner, 1995). Dowling *et al.* (1996) highlights some useful criteria that a court considering an expanded role case might take into account in determining the standard of care. These include the nature of the task and the way the nurse 'holds himself or herself out' to patients. With regard to the second of these criteria, relevant factors would include dress, name badge, language, socialization, and the way the nurse is perceived by patients.

Conclusions

If a nurse undertakes a role previously undertaken by a medical practitioner, then his or her competence to perform that role is that of the level of the medical practitioner. The courts may be looking for the nurse to exercise and maintain medical knowledge, and if the nurse cannot demonstrate this he or she could be found negligent and in breach of the UKCC Professional Code of Conduct (UKCC, 1992b). Inexperience is not a defence to a nursing negligence action. It is very important that nursing staff closely adhere to the UKCC (1992a) *Scope of Professional Practice* principles, particularly principle 9:3, which relates to taking steps to remedy deficits in knowledge.

Advanced practice situations

Clinical guidelines, protocols and the law

The setting of guidelines or protocols is fast becoming an increasingly important aspect of nursing and health care as strategies to ensure quality and avoid risk take effect. The development of clinical guidelines is a government priority, and an important aspect of its commitment to enhance the quality of patient care, and this is identified in the NHS National Plan (DOH, 1999b, 2000b). A Special Health Authority, NICE (the National Institute for Clinical Excellence), has been set up to promote best health care practice. It was set up on the 1 April 1999 to provide the NHS, patients and the public with authoritative, robust and reliable guidance on current 'best practice'(NICE, 1999).

NICE is now a key player in clinical guideline creation in the NHS in England and Wales. It has established a Clinical Guidelines Secretariat, led by a Head of Guidelines and Audit. A Clinical Guidelines Committee consisting of experts drawn from the health professions, patient organizations, health economists and NHS management has also been created. The Secretariat will initially assess clinical guidelines. The Committee meets six times a year, and its role includes advising on commissioning briefs, signing off completed guidelines, advising on audit benchmarks and giving advice on the audit methodologies underpinning the guidelines. The Committee also considers appeals from interested parties against the advice contained within individual clinical guidelines on grounds of either failure of 'due process' or that the guidelines are perverse (NICE, 2000).

The establishment of NICE and its clinical guidelines focus have created a momentum for guideline development. Clinical guidelines can now clearly be seen to be operating at a national (macro) level and a local (micro) level.

At the macro level, NICE and other health care organizations, such as professional nursing and medical groups, universities' professional associations and the Royal Medical Colleges, create clinical guidelines. At the local micro level, wards and care teams in hospitals, primary care groups and trusts, GPs and individual care practitioners can also be seen to produce guidelines.

A nurse may be working with national and locally produced clinical guidelines. It is important to remember that clinical guidelines at the national and local level are advisory only; they should never be used automatically and without proper regard to the care of the patient.

NICE lists 10 key principles for NHS clinical guidelines (NICE, 2000):

- The objective of guidelines is to improve the quality of clinical care by making available to health professionals and patients well-founded advice on best practice
- Quality care is based on clinical effectiveness – the extent to which the health status of patients can be expected to be enhanced by clinical interventions
- Quality of care in the NHS necessarily includes giving due attention to the cost effectiveness of health care interventions
- NHS guidelines are relevant to the care provided by the NHS throughout the NHS in England and Wales
- NHS clinical guidelines are advisory

- NHS clinical guidelines are based on the best possible research evidence, expert opinion and professional consensus
- NHS clinical guidelines are developed using methods that command the respect of patients, the NHS and NHS stakeholders
- While guidelines are focused around the clinical care provided by clinicians, patients are to be treated as full and equal partners along with the relevant professional groups involved in a guideline development
- All those who might be affected by a clinical guideline deserve consideration within the guideline development (usually including clinicians, patients and their carers, service managers, the wider public, government and the health care industries)
- NHS clinical guidelines should be both ambitious and realistic in nature, they should set out the clinical care that might reasonably be expected throughout the NHS

These principles underpin NICE clinical guideline development and appraisal. It is logical also to suggest that they should underpin local clinical guideline development.

It is stated in the key principles that clinical guidelines are advisory. This is a common sense principle, and reflects the legal position of guidelines. Clinical guidelines do not suspend clinical autonomy; nurses remain reflective and autonomous practitioners and a patient's condition may clearly contraindicate the application of a clinical guideline. The patient's condition should always be assessed before applying a clinical guideline. However, if a clinical guideline is not followed, a proper reason should be advanced as an explanation. This principle will be explained further later in this chapter.

Clinical guidelines are care management tools that broadly set out the procedure to be followed by the nurse in an advanced practice situation – for example, the MIU or the Well Women clinic. A GP may develop, with the practice nurse, a guideline or a protocol for the giving of inoculations. The practice of setting guidelines or protocols raises important professional and legal issues, some of which have already been noted. It should be said at the outset, however, that the use of terminology by authors in the literature is not consistent or clear. As well as clinical guidelines or protocols, a variety of other terms, such as practice parameters, clinical pathways and algorithms, are used, often to describe the same tool.

Guidelines or protocols can be seen to be guidance statements based on sound practice. For ease of reference, the term 'clinical guidelines' will be used. Protocols are generally regarded as being more directive than guidelines. The law relating to guidelines applies equally to protocols.

The DOH (1996a) defines clinical guidelines as 'systematically developed statements, which assist the individual clinician and patient in making decisions about appropriate health care for specific conditions'. NICE have a similar definition (NICE, 1999, p. 15).

Legal issues

Fundamentally, the existence of clinical guidelines may impact upon the operation of the *Bolam* test (see Chapter 2). If a guideline is in existence and a nurse has failed to follow it, then this may be a factor that a court takes into consideration when discussing the legal duty of care and whether this has been breached. Nonetheless, the fact that a guideline exists does not mean that the court will accept the guideline. As noted in the previous chapter, the court may overrule the decision of a responsible body of professional practice.

Reasonable clinical guidelines

The *Bolam* principle will apply to the creation and use of clinical guidelines. The case of *Early* v. *Newham Health Authority* ([1994] 5 Med LR 214) illustrates the application of the case to clinical guidelines.

The plaintiff, aged 13 years, was having an appendectomy. The anaesthetist gave an intravenous injection of thiopentone (100 g phentonyl and 100 mg of suxamethonium). Unfortunately he was unable successfully to intubate the plaintiff. The effect of the thiopentone wore off before the effect of the short-term paralysing drug, suxamethonium, wore off, and the plaintiff came to in a state of panic and distress, as she was still partly paralysed by the drug. She alleged that the anaesthetist was negligent in failing to intubate her the first time and that the Health Authority's failed intubation guidelines were faulty. No negligence was found.

The judge considered the guidelines and found them reasonable. He was not satisfied that the guidelines were such that no reasonably competent authority would have adopted them. Before the hospital had adopted the guidelines they were put before the Division of Anaesthesia, and the consultants discussed them. They decided that this was the proper procedure to adopt and minutes of the discussion were kept. The key point was that the judge found that a responsible body of medical opinion in the *Bolam* sense would have adopted the failed intubation guidelines that were used. The standard of legal care was therefore satisfied in the case.

In order to satisfy the legal standard of care under *Bolam*, nurses, in drafting and using clinical guidelines, have to act as ordinary skilled nurses in their speciality would have acted. There must be a responsible body of opinion, albeit perhaps a minority opinion, which regards their practice as proper. The *Bolitho* case, *Bolitho* v. *City and Hackney Health Authority* ((1997) [1998] Lloyd's Rep Med 26), can be said to add a gloss to *Bolam* in that it is clear from the speech of Lord Browne-Wilkinson that this opinion should be evidence-based, it must have a logical basis, and a risk–benefit analysis should have been performed (p. 33).

Foster (1998) argues:

> Although *Bolitho* did not change the law, many people think it has, and so it is likely to alter in a few respects the way that litigation is conducted. Experts will have to appear not only respectable but also reasonable. The defendant will be judged not only by the cut of his expert's suit. Experts will have to be prepared to say not only that they do something a particular way, but why? Reports will have to be more carefully reasoned and referenced. … If the published evidence makes a wholly one-sided case against a particular medical practice, it will be difficult for any expert to say that its adoption by the defendant was reasonable, even though he or she is in august medical company in doing so.

Furthermore, the decision of the Court of Appeal in *Penney and Others* v. *East Kent Health Authority* (*The Times*, 25 November 1999; Tingle and Rodgers, 1999) is notable. This case hints at the possible future for clinical negligence, with more reliance on clinical guidelines than on the clinicians themselves. A judge may disagree with the experts and prefer other expert evidence (see Chapter 2).

Inappropriate use of clinical guidelines

Situations change, and a clinical guideline drafted some months previously may not now fit into the appropriate clinical care setting. Resource levels may have deteriorated, or there may have been staffing changes affecting the ward skill mix. The conventional wisdom on a ward may be that a particular clinical guideline is no longer appropriate. If there are reasonable concerns about the effectiveness and safety of a clinical guideline, then good practice dictates that it should be withdrawn and re-evaluated. It may be negligent not to do so, as health care professionals are required to keep up to date regarding the scope of their professional practice (see Chapter 2).

Not a substitute for professional judgment

When considering the NICE clinical guidelines programme it is worth emphasizing again that, when using clinical guidelines, nurses must always practice as reflective practitioners and responsibly exercise their clinical discretion. They must use their own professional judgment and skill, and assess the appropriateness of the clinical guidelines for the particular care situation. If they decide to deviate from a clinical guideline, then they should record on the notes their reasons for so doing. If unsure about the use of a clinical guideline, then advice should be sought from more experienced colleagues.

Clinical guidelines should be reviewed systematically

If a particular clinical guideline became an issue in a nursing negligence case, a key issue would be the review system in operation in the hospital or surgery. The court would want to be satisfied that a clinical guideline was being used appropriately and updated where necessary. Concepts of risk management clinical governance and quality assurance would also demand a systematic review system.

Clinical guidelines are legally discoverable

Clinical guidelines that were used in the care of a patient would be relevant documents for the purposes of a nursing negligence action. The clinical guideline would be subject to a fairly detailed examination in court. Having a clinical guideline based on reasonable criteria, good research and good practice would provide an indication that a reasonable and reflective care system was in operation. The key point would be to show that the clinical guideline was appropriate to the circumstances of the particular case and was followed by the staff involved. The fact that it was followed or not followed should always be recorded. A clinical guideline shows at the very least that there is a controlled environment of care.

Evidence-based clinical guidelines

The government pledge to improve the quality of health care in the NHS has seen a strong, centrally-led policy adherence to the concept of evidence-based care. This concept underpins the NICE work, and can be seen as an underlying judicial philosophy in cases such as *Bolitho*.

While this is controversial, it is certainly the case that if a particular approach was deemed to be appropriate after an evidence-based evaluation had taken place, then this may be held to be accepted professional practice. Again, however, that does not mean that there would be automatic judicial acceptance. A court examining a clinical guideline would be looking at the information underpinning the clinical guideline, the quality of research and clinical practice. This was done in the *Penney* case. Unrealistic clinical guidelines that tried to do too much, and those based on poor research, practice, etc. would be criticized by the NHS Executive (DOH, 1996a) and by NICE.

Conclusions

Clinical guidelines raise a number of important legal issues. They are being used in legal proceedings, and will be seen increasingly as an established quality improvement and clinical risk management tool in the health care environment. Clinical guidelines must be used reflectively; they are not substitutes for professional judgment. Effectively used, they have the potential to reduce the level of complaints and litigation in health care by improving communication processes and the quality of care.

Nurse prescribing

One way in which the role of the nurse appears set to develop in the future is in having a wider role in prescribing drugs and medical appliances (Jones, 1999). In 1986, the Cumberlege report stated that community nurses should have prescribing rights. This was followed by a Crown Report in 1989, which stated that health visitors and nurses should have the power to prescribe medication from a 'nurse's formulary' to benefit patients. Legislation was introduced in 1992 in the form of the Medicinal Products (Prescription by Nurses) Act of that year. By March 2001 some 23,000 district nurses and health visitors will be qualified to prescribe from the *Nurse Prescriber's Formulary*. Prescribing is different from the situation in which a nurse administers a drug under a protocol, as in this situation it is the doctor who has responsibility for the prescribing. Nurses must prescribe in accordance with the *Nurse Prescriber's Formulary*. Items included are dressings, appliances, paracetamol and carbaryl.

A Midwives Supply Order allows midwives to possess and use certain controlled drugs. Powers have also been given to enable occupational health nurses to administer prescription only drugs. This may be undertaken as long as they do so only in writing and under a doctor's supervision (Medicines (Products Other Than Veterinary Drugs) (Prescription Only) Order 1983 SI 1983 No. 1212 as amended; NHS Pharmaceutical Services (Amendment) Regulations SI 1996 No. 698 r8).

Nurses have also been administering medication in accordance with protocols produced by doctors, who themselves would actually prescribe the drug. Controversy arose in 1996 over this practice. Advice was given by union lawyers to the effect that this was illegal (Naish and Garbett, 1996); in contrast, the MDU stated that nurses could administer such medication as long as they were working to a protocol. This, it is argued, is in accordance with section 58(2)(b) of the Medicines Act 1968, which provides that:

No person shall administer (otherwise than to himself) any such medicinal product unless he is an appropriate practitioner or a person acting in accordance with the directions of an appropriate practitioner.

The appropriate practitioner would be the doctor in this instance. The arguments advanced by the MDU are in accordance with the guidance issued by the UKCC to the effect that:

Nurses can administer medicines according to the directions of a doctor and a detailed protocol would satisfy this requirement.

However, nurses cannot supply medicines for the patient to take away unless there is a signed prescription.

Nonetheless, there is one question mark regarding the status of administration under protocol (Mayor, 1997). It appears that the direction under the statute applies to a specified individual, and it has been argued that this would not cover administration to groups of patients. The whole issue of nurse prescribing was the subject of a review by the Department of Health, chaired by Dr June Crown (DOH, 1996b, 1998, 1999). Its purpose was to:

> ... develop a consistent framework to determine in what circumstances health professionals could undertake new roles with regard to the prescribing, administration or supply of medicines in the course of clinical practice; and to consider possible implications for legislation, and for professional training and standards.

The Review produced two reports. The first examined the supply and administration of medicines under protocol, and the second the wider prescribing issues. On the legal issues regarding administration under protocol, Crown commented that:

> Advice to the Department of Health is that group protocols may not meet the requirements in sections 55(1)(b) and 58(2)(b) Medicines Act 1968 for the supply and administration of medicines 'in accordance with the directions of a doctor' and that in order to meet the requirements of current legislation, protocols should leave the minimum of discretion to the health profession involved. Protocols which specify the patient by name (patient specific protocols) are more likely to be within the law than those which apply to groups of patients.

It recommended that the use of protocols should continue, but that this should be subject to certain guidelines. The content should deal with the clinical condition to which the protocol applies, and which patients can/cannot be included. Staff authorized to supply and administer medicines should be detailed, including their qualifications and measures of competence. The treatment to be given under protocol should be included, along with details of drugs involved (such as dose and methods of administration). The names of the professionals or professional advisory group involved in drawing up the protocol should also be given.

The Report recommended that protocols should be drawn up on a local basis by an interdisciplinary committee, including a doctor/pharmacist/ named representative of each profession likely to contribute care under protocol. The protocol would require approval of those professional managers using it, while all participants in care under the protocol would sign a copy. Group protocols were not only be used in the context of nurses, but should also cover persons not professionally trained but suitably trained and approved as competent in relation to the protocol. The Report emphasized the need for safety, and that in all situations group protocols should ensure that patient safety is not compromised or put at risk. Those using a protocol should be professionally trained, although in some situations those not so trained could be included if acting under the direction of those who are.

There are some potential problems with such protocols. For example, the localized nature of group protocols works against the policy *re* centralization and quality through the establishment of bodies such as NICE and CHI – although admittedly not the approach taken by local research ethics committees. Nurses also need to be aware that undertaking an enhanced role involves increased responsibilities, with the prospect of liability in negligence if a patient who is being treated under protocol suffers harm.

The second Report had a far broader scope, and has the effect of removing the dominance of the medical profession, sanctioning prescribing on a far broader basis. It was recommended that the legal authority in UK to prescribe should be extended. This should include those specific therapeutic areas related to particular competence and the expertise of the prescribing group. This may include prescription only medicines within the area. There would be independent prescribers, who were to be those responsible for the assessment of patients with undiagnosed conditions and for decisions regarding the clinical management required, including prescribing. Examples of such independent prescribers included:

- family planning nurses
- tissue viability nurses (who assess viability of patients' skin – particularly in their own homes)
- chiropodists and podiatrists (who undertake some forms of foot surgery)
- specialist physiotherapists.

There was also to be a category called 'dependent prescribers'. These would include groups such as: specialist diabetes nurses, who already give advice to patients and train them in the use of insulin and who, if they were dependent prescribers, could take over from doctors once the initial diagnosis of diabetes was established; specialist asthma nurses, who could vary diagnosis and prescribe further medication as was required; and specialist pallative care nurses, who could review and revise medication as necessary.

Certain groups of medicines would not be available for prescription by certain new groups of prescribers (para 6.53), e.g. controlled drugs (those subject to the Misuse of Drugs Act 1971) or drugs over which there is continuing professional concern (for instance drugs used to treat children and young people with mental health problems).

The dependent prescriber would be someone who was involved in the continuing care of patients who had been clinically assessed by an independent prescriber. This care could include prescribing, usually informed by clinical guidelines, and within designated treatment plans. Dependent prescribers would have the discretion to vary some aspects of repeat prescriptions, such as the dose/frequency/presentation/active ingredient group. There was provision for regular clinical review by the assessing clinician. The dependent prescriber would be different from the nurse administering drugs under group protocol, because:

1. the dependent prescriber would be working under a care plan drawn up for an individual patient following full assessment by the clinician
2. supply and administration in contrast was to be used in the case of patients who will not be individually identified by the clinician
3. dependent prescribers would have greater discretion over the choice of the treatment regime.

The report suggests that:

Administration or supply within a group protocol may be a suitable model where patients' clinical needs are broadly similar and individual prescriptions would be unwieldy or impracticable (as in mass vaccination campaigns), or where there is a need for urgent treatment (as in relief of acute asthma attacks by ambulance paramedics). Dependent or independent prescribing will be preferable where more detailed clinical assessment is needed and the range of treatment options required to meet the clinical needs of the patients is wider (as in family planning clinics).

The new scheme would be administered by a new Prescribing Authority, which would have the task of assessing existing prescribing rights for different groups of nurses and whether the training was of a sufficiently high standard. The body would be drawn from current prescribers, other relevant health care professions, professional regulatory bodies, education and training accrediting bodies, NHS commissioners and provider units, and patient groups.

The government is undertaking a consultation consequent upon the Crown review. It has already stated its support for the extension of nurse prescribing (DOH, 2000b, para 9.2). As with many expanded roles, the extension of prescribing powers has led to much controversy and debate. One important fact is that such an extension of powers may bring increased legal liability upon the nurse. Where nurses act as prescribers, they must ensure that they are acting within the powers given by statute. Crown noted the need for clear arrangements in relation to accountability (para 3.5):

It is essential, however, that the extension of professional roles is accompanied by clear arrangements for accountability. One professional should not be expected to take responsibility for clinical decisions that are actually taken by a colleague – for instance, if a district nurse has in fact decided on the appropriate clinical dressing for a particular patient, and the GP has not in any real sense reviewed this decision, it is wrong for the GP to take formal clinical responsibility for signing this prescription. This is not only professionally inappropriate for both parties, but it can lead to confusion which may prejudice patient safety and reduce confidence in the arrangements for care.

When prescribing drugs, the nurse will be judged by the standard of the experienced nurse undertaking such a role. If nurses are involved in prescribing drugs, then they must check the dose given; negligent prescription of an overdose may lead to an action in negligence (*Dwyer* v. *Roderick* (1983) 127 SJ 806), as may writing an illegible prescription (*Prendergast* v. *Sam and Dee; The Times* [1989] and 1 Med LR 36).

References

BMA (1996). Joint Consultants' Committee. *Protecting Patient Safety*. BMA.

Caine, N. (1993). Heart to heart. *Health Service J*, **103(5370)**, 22.

Carlisle, D. (1995). Nurse-led unity. *Nursing Times*, **91(47)**, 14.

Darley, M. and Rumsey, M. (1996). The scope of professional practice: work to date. *Nursing Times*, **11(4)**, 32.

Department of Health (1992). *The Extended Role of the Nurse. Scope of Professional Practice,* PL/CNO (92)4, DOH.

Department of Health (1996a). *Promoting Clinical Effectiveness: A Framework for Action in and Through the NHS*. DOH.

Department of Health (1996b). *Delivering the Future*. DOH.

Department of Health (1998). *Review of Prescribing, Supply and Administration of Medicines; a Report on the Supply and Administration of Medicines under Group Protocol (Crown Part I); Final Report*: March 1999 (*Crown Part II*). DOH.

Department of Health (1999a). *Making a Difference*. PL/CNO(99) (6), 29 September, DOH. See also www.doh.gov.uk/nurstrat.htm.

Department of Health (1999b). *Faster Access to Modern Treatment: How NICE Appraisal will Work*: *A Discussion Paper*. DOH.

Department of Health (2000a). Health Secretary lays out plans to liberate nurse talents. Press release, 2000/0209, February, DOH.

Department of Health (2000b). *The NHS Plan*. Command Paper 4818-1, The Stationery Office.

Dowling, S., Martin, R., Skidmore, P. *et al*. (1996). Nurses taking on junior doctor's work: a confusion of accountability. *Br. Med. J.*, **312**, 1211–14.

Doyal, L., Dowling, S. and Cameron, A. (1998). *Challenging Practice: An Evaluation of Four Innovatory Nursing Posts in the South West*. The Policy Press, University of Bristol.

Eaton, L. (1993). Vein hopes. *Nursing Times*, **89(36)**, 18.

Foster, C. (1998). Bolam: consolidation and clarification. *Health Care Risk Report*, **4(5)**, 5–7.

General Medical Council (1998). *Good Medical Practice*. GMC, pp. 12–13.

Giles, S. (1993). Passing the buck. *Nursing Times*, **89(28)**, 42.

Healey, P. (1996). Nurses doing junior doctor's work are safe claims unions. *Nursing Standard*, **10(34)**, 5.

Jones, M. (1999). *Nursing Prescribing*. Tindall.

Jowett, S., Peters, M., Wilson-Barnett, J. and Reynolds, H. (2000). *The Scope of Professional Practice – A Study of its Implementation*. UKCC.

Kerry, D. G. (1991). Lawyers comment, *Martin Wilsher* v. *Essex Area Health Authority* and causation. *AVMA Med. L. J.*, **12**, 12.

Kloss, D. K. (1988). Demarcation in medical practice: the extended role of the nurse. *Professional Negligence*, **4(2)**, 41.

Last, T., Seld, N., Kassat, J. and Rawan, A. (1992). Extended role of the nurse in ICU. *Br. J. Nursing*, **1(13)**, 675.

Mayor, S. (1997). Working to protocol. *Practice Nurse*, **13(4)**, 187.

Montgomery, J. (1992). Doctors' handmaidens: the legal contribution. In: *Law Health and Medical Regulation* (S. McVeigh and S. Whelar, eds). Dartmouth, Aldershot.

Naish, J. (1995). The extended role of the nurse: risk management implications. *Health Care Risk Report*, **1**, 22–4.

Naish, J. and Garbett, R. (1996). Don't administer drugs, says union. *Nursing Times*, **92(47)**, 5.

NICE (1999). *A Guide to Our Work*. National Institute for Clinical Excellence (NICE). See also www.nice.org.uk.

NICE (2000). NICE establishes guidelines advisory committee. Press release, 2000/015, 23 May, NICE.

Parker, S. and Wilson, C. (1992). *An Introduction to Medico-Legal Aspects of Practice Nursing*. MDU.

Peysner, J. (1995). The captain on the bridge. *Health Care Risk Report*, **1**, 8.

Shepherd, J. (1993). Nurses are changing, not extending their roles. *Br. J. Nursing*, **2(9)**, 447.

Standing Medical Advisory Committee and the Standing Nursing and Midwifery Advisory Committee Joint Working Party on Extended Role (1989). DHSS Professional Letter, PL/CMO, (89), 7.

Tingle, J. H. (1993). The extended role of the nurse; legal implications. *Care of the Critically Ill*, **9(1)**, 30–34.

Tingle, J. H. and Rodgers, M. E. (1999). Clinical Guidelines, NICE and the Court of Appeal. *Nottingham Law J.*, **8(2)**, 95–100.

UKCC (1992a). *The Scope of Professional Practice*. UKCC, (i) p. 7; (ii) p. 8.

UKCC (1992b). *Code of Professional Conduct*. UKCC.

UKCC (1992c). *Standards for the Administration of Medicines*. UKCC.

UKCC (1996). *Guidelines for Professional Practice*. UKCC.

UKCC (2000). Register, Spring 2000, No. 31. UKCC.

Waters, J. (1996) Horror stories warn of need for training. *Nursing Times*, **92(16)**, 9.

Chapter 5

Consent to treatment I: general principles

Jean McHale

One of the most fundamental principles of health care law and ethics is that treatment should be given only with the patient's consent. The nurse is frequently the person who has to obtain the patient's consent to treatment, whether on the wards or in the community. Even if the doctor has the task of obtaining the patient's consent, the patient may turn to the nurse for clarification or for further information regarding the proposed treatment. This chapter begins by considering the types of consent: express and implied, written and oral. Secondly, consideration is given to when a patient is legally capable of giving consent and the basis on which treatment may be given to an incompetent patient. Thirdly, liability in criminal and civil law is discussed, where treatment is given without consent.

Types of consent

Consent forms

Nurses are familiar with the consent forms given to patients to sign before they go in for an operation. The Department of Health (1992) has published model consent forms, which provide guidance to health professionals. In law, while a consent form may provide evidence that the patient has consented, the act of signing a form does not itself make the consent obtained legally valid. What is important is that the consent given is 'real' – that is to say, it has been obtained freely, without pressure being placed upon the patient, and that the patient understands the implications of what he or she is consenting to. There may be situations in which consent may be implied through the patient's actions, but considered consent is necessary in relation to all serious medical procedures, and failure to obtain that consent may leave a nurse in danger of being held liable in the criminal courts, or of being sued for damages in the civil courts.

Express and implied consent

Consent may be either express or implied. Consent may be expressly given in writing or orally. Alternatively, a patient may through actions signify consent – for example, by proffering a wrist to be bandaged. There are risks in assuming that a patient, in seeking treatment, is consenting to any medical procedure being undertaken. There has been much discussion as to whether, when blood is taken from a patient, it is necessary to obtain the patient's consent for undertaking tests on each individual sample. Particular difficulties have arisen where it is proposed to test one of the samples to determine a patient's HIV status. The simple fact that an HIV test has been undertaken may have considerable repercussions for the patient regarding employment and insurance. The UKCC has issued guidance, which states that if a nurse takes blood from a patient without that patient's consent, or co-operates in blood being removed without the patient's consent, the nurse may be reported to the UKCC for misconduct (UKCC, 1993i). They do, however, recognize that in certain 'rare and exceptional circumstances' blood may be tested without the patient's consent (UKCC, 1993ii). The guidance does not explain what these circumstances may be; they could possibly include the fact that in the future a cure may be found, and thus to test might facilitate diagnosis and treatment.

Capacity

Generally, patients are presumed capable of making their own treatment decisions. However, in some situations capacity may be called into question. A patient may not appear to understand what he or she has been told, or may appear confused, and the nurse may need to assess whether this patient is capable of making a particular treatment decision. This task may prove to be particularly difficult if a person has a learning disability or suffers from fluctuating mental capacity. In *Re C* the court upheld the right of a 68-year-old paranoid schizophrenic who had developed gangrene in his foot to prevent amputation in the future without his express written consent (*Re C* [1994] All ER 819). Thorpe J. suggested a three-part test to determine whether a patient possessed capacity:

1. Did the patient comprehend the information given?
2. Did the patient believe it?
3. Had the patient weighed up the information, balancing needs and risks, before reaching a decision?

At the hearing it was claimed that C was not competent because of his delusions that he was a doctor, and that whatever treatment was given to him was calculated to destroy his body. However, despite these claims Thorpe J. held that he was satisfied that C was capable of giving consent because he understood and had retained the relevant treatment information and believed it, and had arrived at a clear choice. One difficulty with the test laid down in *Re C* is that it makes capacity dependent upon the information the patient is actually given (Grubb, 1994). If the nurse provides a patient with a great deal of complex information, the patient may not understand it and so it may not fall within the definition of capacity set out in *Re C*, whereas had the patient been given a very simple basic explanation about the same treatment procedure, he or she may have possessed the necessary capacity to consent.

Some guidance to health care professionals as to how to approach the assessment of capacity is contained in a document produced by the British Medical Association in conjunction with the Law Society (the solicitors' professional organization), and this provides a useful source of reference for the nurse (BMA/Law Society, 1996). They suggest that a decision about capacity should be made on the basis of full information. The health professional should have access to all past medical/psychiatric records and, where appropriate, assessments should be obtained from a clinical psychologist, nurse or social worker. They note that information from relatives and carers is important, although this needs to be approached with caution. The guidelines state that views of relatives/carers:

> … may give clues as to whether current behaviour and thinking reflects an abnormal mental state. Aspects of a person's current thinking may derive not from a medical disability but from a normal personality, or from a particular cultural or ethical background, and this may be of great importance in determining capacity. It may even be necessary for the doctor to seek advice from others on such cultural issues, or to suggest that the patient be examined by a doctor of a cultural or ethical background similar to the person being assessed.

These are useful guidelines, and should provide a reference point for the nurse when involved in the consent process. Some very difficult and sensitive issues arise where treatment is refused on ethical or religious grounds. Certain ramifications of these issues are explored in the context of treatment refusal below.

The Law Commission, a body established by the government to examine areas of law and make recommendations for reform, undertook a study involving treatment of the mentally incompetent and published its recommendations in its report *Mental Incapacity* (Law Commission, 1995). It recommended that capacity to make decisions should be assessed on the balance of probabilities (Law Commission, 1995i). As with the test suggested by Thorpe J. in *Re C*, any test for capacity should be decision-specific; this emphasizes the fact that a person may be capable of making one decision while at the same time being incapable of making another. It proposed that legislation should provide that a person should be deemed to lack capacity if at the material time he or she is:

1. unable by reason of mental disability to make a decision on the matter in question, or

2. unable to communicate a decision on that matter because s/he is unconscious or for any other reason.

Mental disability was defined by the Law Commission (1995ii) as being:

... any disability or disorder of the mind or brain, whether permanent or temporary, which results in an impairment or disturbance of mental functioning.

The Law Commission (1995iii) recommended that a person should be unable to make a decision on the basis of mental disability:

... if the disability is such that, at the time when the decision needs to be made, he or she is unable to understand or to retain the information relevant to the decision, including information about the reasonably foreseeable consequences of failing to make that decision.

It suggested that a person who, while he or she understands the information given, is not able to absorb it, should be held to lack capacity. An example of such a situation is that of a person suffering from a compulsive disorder. The Law Commission (1995iv) recommended that the patient show a basic level of comprehension of the information given 'in broad terms and simple language'. There is a danger that a person is believed to lack capacity when in fact it is not that the person is unable to make a decision, but that there are problems both in communicating information and in receiving that information. The Law Commission noted this difficulty and suggested that, wherever possible, specialists in communication skills should be used. The Law Commission also recommended that the Secretary of State should prepare a code of practice for guidance in such decision making. The contents of any such code would be of vital importance in respecting patient autonomy.

The Law Commission's approach was followed in 1997 by the Court of Appeal in *Re MB*, a case discussed more fully in Chapter 9 in the context of enforced caesarean sections (see p. 197). In this case, the Court of Appeal adopted a version of the test of capacity stated in earlier cases. They held that a person is not capable of making a decision where:

(a) the person is unable to comprehend and retain the information which is material to the decision, especially as to the likely consequences of having or not having the treatment in question; and

(b) the patient is unable to use the information and weigh it in the balance as of the process of arriving at a decision.

In 1997 the government issued a document, *Who Decides* (Lord Chancellor's Department, 1997), followed in 1999 by the Green Paper *Making Decisions* (Lord Chancellor's Department, 1999), which announced their intention to enact certain provisions from the Law Commission's report, including placing the test for capacity upon a statutory basis.

Should capacity include the right to make an 'irrational' decision?

> If a patient refuses treatment on what the nurse treating him or her regards as an irrational basis, can treatment still be given?

As Brazier (1991) comments, an elderly woman with a diseased tooth may have sufficient capacity to understand the suggestion made to her that it should be removed, but she may nevertheless allow her fear of dentists and of the pain of treatment to overcome her wish to have the tooth extracted. One approach to problem patients such as this elderly lady would be to categorize her decision as 'irrational' and to override her decision. A variation on this approach, suggested by Kennedy (1991), is that an irrational decision should be respected where it derives from long-held beliefs and values on the basis of which a patient has run his or her life, but not if it is the result of a temporary delusion. Nevertheless, attempting to distinguish between different 'irrational' decisions may be difficult practically. Furthermore, there is also a real risk that those refusals that are found to be 'irrational' will be those of mentally handicapped and demented patients (Brazier, 1991).

In *Re MB* [1997] 2 FLR 426, in which MB refused a Caesarian section due to her needle phobia, the Court of Appeal discussed a number of cases in which a Caesarian section was authorized, noting that in all those cases, save *Re S,* the court had decided that the woman in question lacked capacity. After again stressing the right of the competent adult to consent or to refuse treatment, Butler Sloss L.J. commented that:

> A competent woman who has the capacity to decide may, for religious reasons, other reasons, for rational or irrational reasons or for no reason at all, choose not to have medical intervention, even though the consequence may be the death or serious handicap of the child she bears, or her own death. In that event the courts do not have the jurisdiction to declare medical intervention lawful and the question of her own best interests objectively considered, does not arise (at pages 436–7).

She went on to state that:

> Irrationality is here used to connote a decision which is so outrageous in its defiance of logic or of accepted moral standards that no sensible person who has applied his mind to the question to be decided could have arrived at it. ... Although it might be thought that irrationality sits uneasily with competence to decide, panic, indecisiveness and irrationality in themselves do not as such amount to incompetence, but they may be symptoms or evidence of incompetence. The graver the

consequences of the decision the commensurately greater the level of competence is required to take the decision.

The Court of Appeal noted that in *Re C*, Thorpe J. had suggested that a compulsive disorder/phobia may have the effect that the decision is not 'a true one'. Temporary incompetence, as the Court of Appeal commented, may erode capacity. This may be due to such factors, mentioned by Lord Donaldson in the earlier case of *Re T*, as 'confusion, shock, pain and drugs'.

Thus a patient has, as in *Re C* itself, the ability to make a decision that some may regard as being irrational, even though this may have serious consequences for their health, while in other situations a decision that may be irrational may be linked to a lack of competence. This is a fine line, and is a matter that is likely to come before the courts again in the future.

Fluctuating capacity

An elderly lady is cared for in a nursing home. She has good days and bad days. She can throw tantrums and yet later appear totally lucid. How far do the nurses caring for her need to respect her wishes?

Where a patient has a fluctuating mental state it may be acutely difficult to assess capacity, and this creates real difficulties for the nurses treating the patient. In such a situation it is tempting to say that she lacks capacity, because English law allows a mentally incompetent patient to be given such treatment as those treating her believe to be in her best interests (*Re F* [1990] 1 AC 1). In *Re T* ([1992] 4 All ER 649), the Court of Appeal held that the capacity of an adult patient is to be judged by reference to the particular decision to be made. This approach was at variance with an earlier Court of Appeal decision in which it was held that a child with fluctuating mental capacity was to be regarded as totally incapable (*Re R* [1991] 4 All ER 177). The approach in *Re T* is surely right, reinforced by the decision in *Re C*, which states that the test for capacity is decision-specific.

The BMA and the Law Society, in their guidelines (BMA/Law Society, 1996), provide a number of suggestions for dealing with patients with fluctuating capacity:

- Any treatable medical condition which affects capacity should be treated before a final assessment is made
- Incapacity may be temporary albeit for a prolonged period. For example, an older patient with an acute confusional state caused by infection may continue to improve for some time after successful treatment. If a person's condition is likely to improve, the assessment of capacity should, if possible, be delayed

- Some conditions, for example dementia, may give rise to fluctuating capacity. Thus, although a person with dementia may lack capacity at the time of one assessment, the result may be different if a second assessment is undertaken during a lucid interval. In cases of fluctuating capacity the medical report should detail the level of capacity during periods of maximal and minimal disability.

In assessing capacity, in practice much will depend upon the discretion of the individual practitioner. In making the decision, nurses should keep in mind clause 5 of the UKCC Code, which requires them to:

... work in an open and co-operative manner with patients, clients and their families, foster their independence and recognize and respect their involvement in the planning and delivery of care.

Good practice would suggest that, as far as possible, patients should be left to make their own decisions.

The mentally incompetent patient

Best interest test

Take a situation in which a nurse is asked to care for a patient who has profound mental handicap or severe brain damage: on what basis can the nurse lawfully treat that patient? Until 1990, the legal position as to treating mentally incompetent adult patients was uncertain. Prior to the Mental Health Act 1983, the court had had an 'inherent jurisdiction' to act for the benefit of incompetent adult patients, as they have today with regard to child patients (see Chapter 6). The basis for such treatment was discussed by the House of Lords in 1990. In *Re F* ([1990] AC 1), the court was asked to authorize the sterilization of a 36-year-old mentally handicapped woman. The House of Lords held that the operation could be undertaken. It held that the court had no power to authorize treatment of a mentally incompetent adult through the use of inherent jurisdiction as it had regarding a child patient (see Chapter 6). Prior to *Re F* it was common practice to get the relatives to sign the consent form, but in *Re F* the court said that such consent had no legal effect. No one had a legal right to give consent on behalf of a mentally incompetent adult. However, that did not mean that treatment could not be given; the House of Lords said treatment could be given on the grounds of necessity where this was in the patient's best interests.

'Best interests' is assessed by reference to what a responsible body of professional practice would regard as being in a particular patient's best interests (the *Bolam* test discussed in Chapter 2). The basis for the 'best interests' test in *Re F* has been criticized; for example, it has been suggested that the test raises questions of value and social policy, issues which are not the sole preserve of doctors (Kennedy and Grubb, 1994). The nurse acting as the patient's advocate may take the view that what a doctor believes to be medically expedient is not actually in that patient's best interests, and should be able to raise concerns and take the matter further should he or she believe that the patient's interests are being disregarded.

Which medical procedures can be authorized under the 'best interests' principle was left uncertain after *Re F*. While it appears that generally therapeutic procedures would clearly fall within 'best interests', the legality of many non-therapeutic procedures (such as non-therapeutic clinical trials) is questionable. This issue is returned to below.

The Law Commission proposed reform of the 'best interests' test (Law Commission, 1995v), recommending a set of criteria to be taken into account in determining 'best interests'. These are:

(1) ascertainable past and present wishes and feelings of the person concerned and the factors that a person would consider if unable to do so;

(2) the need to permit and encourage the person to participate or to improve his or her ability to participate as fully as possible in anything done for and any decision affecting him or her;

(3) the views of other people whom it is appropriate and practicable to consult about the person's wishes and feelings and what would be in his or her best interests;

(4) whether the purpose for which any action or decision is required can be as effectively achieved in a manner less restrictive of the person's freedom of action.

Such an approach could facilitate decision making. Nevertheless, there may be practical problems in the application of such a test. How would it operate, and how would the relevant criteria be weighed against each other? The Law Commission (1995vi) recommended that an appropriate approach would be the development of a code of practice to facilitate health professionals in ascertaining best interests.

In *Re F*, the court said that there was no legal duty to refer all cases concerning treatment of a mentally incompetent adult to the court for approval. Nevertheless, in certain situations (for example, before major surgery is performed) it believed that referral of the issue to the court would be desirable. This raises the question of whether it is appropriate to leave this assessment to the health professional at all. The Law Commission (1995) suggested in its report that the decision to undertake certain clinical procedures upon mentally incompetent adults should be referred to a decision maker outside those immediately caring for the patient. In some situations, the Law Commission suggested, the decision should be subject to a second opinion. Cases involving authorization of serious treatment may be referred to a new body, called a 'judicial forum', a court with specialist expertise in such treatment issues. The government has accepted the need for change in this area in their document *Making Decisions* (Lord Chancellor's Department, 1999), and it is also proposed that there will be a new specialist judicial forum.

Procedures ancillary to treatment

There are a number of practical difficulties in treating mentally incompetent adults. Treatment can be given regardless of consent if it can be shown to be in the patient's best interests. However, the patient cannot be confined to one particular place while treatment is provided unless certain statutory powers (such as those under the Mental Health Act 1983) apply. Frequently, confused elderly persons may be placed in beds that have cot sides to stop them from falling out. Is this justifiable? Is it part of treatment? It might be argued that to restrain patients in this situation might even constitute the tort of false imprisonment. The powers for treatment of such patients urgently require clarification. While the House of Lords has indicated that some detention of a compliant patient who is not sectioned under the Mental Health Act may be lawful, the precise boundaries of this power still remain to be determined (R v. *Bournewood Community and Mental Health NHS Trust ex parte L* [1998] 3 All ER 289 HC).

Criminal law liability

Bringing a criminal law prosecution against a nurse or doctor where a medical procedure has been undertaken without consent may seem only a remote possibility, but such a prosecution is not totally unforeseeable. In November 1992, a press report appeared concerning a 51-year-old journalist who woke up in hospital after a 'deep scrape' operation to find that during the operation her womb and ovaries had been removed (*Sunday Times*, November 1992). The surgeon had found a swelling in her abdomen, although it was not life-threatening condition, and had gone on to cut out her ovaries. He said that 'I thought at her age it was the wiser thing to remove them'. The woman took her case to the Director of Public Prosecutions, who considered prosecution.

Failure to obtain consent to treatment may amount to the crime of battery, a common law offence. Some types of battery cannot be consented to, such as prize fighting or beatings for sexual gratification (*R v. Donovan* [1934] QB 638 and *R v. Brown* [1994] 1 AC 212). However, it appears to be the case that reasonable surgical interference does not constitute an inherently unlawful action, and no crime will be committed as long as the patient has consented to the operation being undertaken (*AG Ref (No. 6 of 1980)* [1981] QB 715). There is the possibility that serious surgical procedures may also constitute an offence, under section 18 of the Offences Against the Person Act 1861. This section makes it an offence to cause grievous bodily harm 'unlawfully and maliciously' to a person with the intention of causing grievous bodily harm. A court is unlikely to find that an operation to improve the patient's health has been undertaken unlawfully.

Finally, there is the chance that an operation might be held to be unlawful, regardless of consent, because it constituted the crime of maim. This is an ancient crime, which makes it an offence to perform an operation or give an injury that has the effect of permanently disabling or weakening a man. Skegg (1984) suggests that such a prosecution is unlikely to be successful even if it were to be brought. First, most medical treatment does not have the effect of permanently disabling a man and rendering him less useful for fighting. Secondly, even if an operation did have that effect it may still be lawful if undertaken for therapeutic purposes. In a consultation paper which examines the scope of criminal liability in relation to consent to treatment, the Law Commission (1996) recommended reform of the law to recognize the legality of the performance of medical procedures such as surgical operations.

Civil law liability

Battery

While a criminal prosecution may be brought, it is far more likely that failure to obtain consent will lead to the patient suing for damages in the civil courts. This may be on the basis either that the treatment amounted to a battery or that the nurse or doctor was negligent in providing the patient with inadequate information. A battery refers to any unlawful touching, and consent is a defence to battery. But what amounts to consent? In *Chatterson* v. *Gerson* ([1981] QB 432), Bristow J. said:

> In my judgment once the patient is informed in broad terms of the nature of the procedure which is intended and has given her consent then that consent is real and the cause of action on which to base the claim is negligence not trespass.

It is sufficient that the patient understands the type of operation that is to be performed. The patient does not have to be informed of all the potential risks and implications of the clinical procedure.

Treating on the basis of temporary incompetence

Consent is not required if treatment is necessary in an emergency. The patient brought to Accident & Emergency bleeding and unconscious can be treated without consent. If it was later claimed that treatment was unlawful, then the nurse could claim the defence that the treatment was 'necessary'. If, during an operation, it is found that a patient is suffering from, for example, a life-threatening tumour, then this tumour may be removed if it is necessary to save the patient's life, even though the medical team does not have the patient's express consent to removal. However, while it is lawful to undertake treatment without consent where necessary to do so, how far does this principle extend? Guidance can be taken from two notable decisions in Canada. In *Marshall* v. *Curry* ([1933] 3 DLR 260), the plaintiff sought damages for battery against a surgeon. During a hernia operation the surgeon had removed a testicle. He claimed that the removal was necessary because otherwise the patient's life would have been in danger. The court held that the surgeon was correct to go ahead; it would have been unreasonable to have delayed removal by waiting to obtain the patient's consent and then undertaking a second operation.

However, 'reasonableness' is a question of degree, and is dependent upon the urgency with which the operation should be undertaken. This was illustrated in the later case of *Murray* v. *McMurchy* ([1942] 2 DLR 442). A woman underwent a Caesarean section. While operating, the doctor found that the woman's uterus was in such a state that it would have been exceedingly dangerous for her to undergo another pregnancy. He decided to sterilize her there and then, and tied her Fallopian tubes. On recovering from the operation and discovering what had happened, the woman brought an action for battery. The court upheld her claim. They were of the view that the doctor should have postponed the sterilization operation until after the patient's consent had been obtained.

In view of the uncertainty as to what constitutes necessary treatment, nurses should be exceedingly careful before proceeding with treatment in the absence of consent, save in an emergency situation where it is required to preserve the patient's life.

The patient who refuses treatment

A woman who is lying in Accident and Emergency critically ill after a car accident refuses treatment because she says that she is opposed to conventional medical therapies and in particular will not receive blood products. Can she be treated?

If the nurse goes ahead and gives treatment against the patient's wishes, this may well amount to a battery. Take, for example, the Canadian case of *Malette* v. *Schumann* ([1990] 67 DLR (4th) 321). The plaintiff was brought into hospital after a road accident. A nurse found a card in her pocket identifying her as a Jehovah's Witness and requesting that she never be given a blood transfusion. Despite this, the doctor went ahead and administered the transfusion. On recovering her health, the patient brought an action for battery and was awarded some $20 000 damages.

While this is the general rule, the English courts have indicated there may be situations in which treating a patient against his or her express wishes may be lawful. In *Re T* ([1992] 4 All ER 649), T, a woman 34 weeks pregnant was taken to hospital after she had been involved in a road accident. She developed pneumonia and her condition deteriorated. While in hospital she was visited by her mother. Although T was not a Jehovah's Witness, her mother was. There was some discussion between T and the medical team treating her as to whether she should be given a Caesarean section. After some time alone with her mother, T stated clearly that she did not want a blood transfusion. T then gave birth to a stillborn child, and her condition subsequently deteriorated. The hospital went to the court and asked for a declaration stating whether it would be lawful for T to be given a transfusion should it prove necessary. The court granted the declaration.

The Master of the Rolls, Sir John Donaldson, stressed that a patient's refusal to consent should lead those treating the patient to ask, was the patient capable of refusing consent to that treatment? He emphasized that refusals varied in the degree of seriousness, and the scope of the refusal must be considered: Did it apply to all situations? Was it based upon assumptions that had not been realized? He recommended that consent forms should be redesigned so that the consequences of refusal were brought forcibly to the patient's attention. This is a very controversial judgment. Were it to be followed, nurses and other members of the health care team would have to scrutinize very carefully any decision to refuse treatment. The other judges in this case did not go so far as Lord Donaldson, preferring to base their decision upon the fact that T had made her decision under pressure from her mother. Where there is doubt as to the patient's capacity to refuse treatment, Lord Donaldson stressed that the health care team should seek a declaration from the court.

In a case decided not long after that of *Re T*, *Re S* ([1992] 4 All ER 671), a medical team was again able to override a patient's decision to refuse treatment. S was 6 days overdue giving birth. The team treating her believed that there was a very grave risk of a rupture to the uterus were the pregnancy to continue in the normal way. Essentially, the life of both the woman and the fetus were at stake if the Caesarean did not go ahead. S, a born-again Christian, refused the procedure on the basis that the operation was against her religious beliefs. The hospital sought a declaration from the court. Sir Stephen Brown granted the declaration, though in a short expedited judgment. Subsequent to *Re S* in *Re MB* [1997] FLR 426 the court has confirmed the right of the competent patient to refuse treatment and, in particular, the right of the competent woman to refuse a caesarean section. If there is real doubt as to whether to proceed against the patient's wishes and the patient's life is in danger, advice should be sought from the court as to the legality of proceeding with treatment.

Using compulsion in health care – public health powers

Generally speaking, in order for clinical procedures to be lawful a patient must give consent freely. However, in some situations compulsion may be sought. In Chapter 6, the operation of the Mental Health Act 1983 is examined. In addition, there are a number of powers relating to compulsory care in the context of public health. If a patient is suffering from a notifiable disease, then the Public Health (Control of Disease) Act 1984 s37 allows such a patient to be forcibly removed to hospital. The order must be made by a magistrate. The statute applies only to those persons suffering from notifiable diseases, such as cholera or typhoid. While HIV or AIDS are not notifiable conditions, special regulations have extended the power to make an order to persons who are HIV-positive or who have AIDS (Public Health (Control of Infectious Diseases) Act 1984). There are also provisions under the National Assistance Act 1948 (section 48) that allow the removal of persons who are aged, infirm, suffering from chronic disease or who are incapacitated from their homes to hospital. Removal can only be undertaken after a magistrate's order has been obtained, and this order allows removal for a period of up to 3 months. There is also a special provision allowing a person to be removed in an emergency for a period of up to 3 weeks (National Assistance (Amendment) Act 1951 s1(1)). This may be undertaken on the recommendation of the community physician if supported by another practitioner.

Negligence

Once the patient has been told in general terms what is involved in medical procedures, then there will no longer be liability in battery. However, the patient may claim that while a general explanation has been given, he or she has not been told of the risks of the treatment and that this amounts to negligence. In establishing negligence for failure to inform, the legal principles are the same as in any other negligence claim (see Chapter 2). The plaintiff must show that he or she was owed a duty, that there was a breach of duty, and that damage resulted from that breach.

In English law there is no doctrine of 'informed consent'; no requirement to inform the patient of all risks. This was made clear by the courts in the case of *Sidaway* v. *Bethlem Royal Hospital Governors* ([1985] 1 All ER 643). Mrs Sidaway underwent an operation after having suffered for some time from a recurring pain in her neck, right shoulder and arm. The operation was performed by a senior neurosurgeon at the Bethlem Royal Hospital. Even if carried out with all due care and skill there was a 1–2 per cent risk of damage to the nerve root and spinal column. While the risk of damage to the spinal column was less than to the nerve root, the consequences were more severe.

The plaintiff was left severely disabled after the operation. She claimed that she had not been given adequate warning as to the risks of the operation, and she sought damages for negligence. During the proceedings it was found that, while the surgeon had told the patient of the risks of damage to the nerve root, he had not told her of the risks of damage to the spinal column. In doing this, he had conformed with what in 1974 would have been accepted as standard medical practice by a responsible and skilled body of neurosurgeons. The House of Lords rejected the claim that the surgeon had acted negligently. The majority held that the test the courts should use in deciding whether the advice given was negligent was the same as that used in deciding whether medical treatment was negligent – the *Bolam* test. This test provides that a doctor:

> ... is not guilty of negligence if he has acted in accordance with a practice accepted as proper by a responsible body of medical men.

That does not mean, however, that the court will always accept the word of the health care professional as to which risks should and which should not be disclosed. Only one member of the court in *Sidaway*, Lord Diplock, unreservedly accepted the *Bolam* test. Lord Bridge said that a judge could disagree with the evidence given to him:

> I am of the opinion that the judge might in certain circumstances come to the conclusion that disclosure of a particular risk was so obviously necessary to an informed choice on the part of the patient that no reasonably prudent medical man would fail to make it.

Lord Templeman stressed that it was for the court to decide whether the doctor had acted negligently or not.

The requirement that the standard of disclosure should be that which would be recognized by a competent body of health care professionals can be contrasted with the approach taken in certain other countries that have recognized the doctrine of 'informed consent'. In the case of *Canterbury* v. *Spence* ([1972] 464 F 2d 772), in the USA, the court declared that:

> ... respect for the patient's right of self-determination on particular therapy demands a standard set by law for the physician rather than one which physicians may or may not impose on themselves.

Several states adopted a standard of disclosure based upon the information a 'prudent patient' would expect to receive. In *Sidaway*, one member of the House of Lords, Lord Scarman, favoured the informed consent approach, but he was very much in the minority. Whether such a test would make a radical difference to the amount of information a patient receives is open to question. It is interesting to note that, in the USA, some courts have used the notion of therapeutic privilege to restrict the requirement to disclose (see also the discussion of therapeutic privilege on p. 105). A broader duty of disclosure has also been recognized in the Australian case of *Rogers* v. *Whittaker* ([1993] 4 Med LR 79).

Overriding the responsible body of professional practice

While the court has the ultimate power to overrule the view of the responsible body of professional practice as to what risks should be disclosed, the courts have been traditionally unwilling to do so. In *Maynard* v. *West Midlands Health Authority* ([1984] 1 WLR 643), for example, the trial judge preferred one body of professional medical opinion to another and was held to have been wrong to do so. Even if the body of professional practice is very small in number, four or five out of 250 specialists, for example, the court will still be prepared to accept its opinion (*De Freitas* v. *O'Brien* [1995] 6 Med LR 108).

Nonetheless, the fact that a responsible body of medical practice does support the actions of the clinician is not by itself necessarily conclusive. In *Smith* v. *Tunbridge Wells Health Authority* ([1994] 5 Med LR 334), the failure to warn a 28-year-old man of the risks of impotence subsequent to surgery upon a rectal prolapse was found to constitute negligence. It was held that while some surgeons were not providing warnings of that risk at that time, nonetheless the omission to inform in this particular case was 'neither reasonable nor responsible'.

The House of Lords, in *Bolitho*, subsequently illustrated the fact that there is greater judicial willingness to scrutinize the opinion expressed by the body of professional practice (*Bolitho* v. *City and Hackney Health Authority* [1998] AC 232). Lord Browne Wilkinson stated that:

> In particular where there are questions of assessment of the relative risks and benefits of adopting a particular medical practice, a reasonable view necessarily presupposes that the relative risks and benefits have been weighed by the experts in forming their opinions. But if in a rare case, it can be demonstrated that the professional opinion is not capable of withstanding logical analysis, the judge is entitled to hold that the body of opinion is not reasonable or responsible. I emphasise that in my view it will be very seldom right for a judge to reach the conclusion that views genuinely held by a competent medical expert are unreasonable.

In this case, Lord Brown Wilkinson excluded from his discussion the issue of disclosure of risk. He stated that (p. 243):

> ... in cases of diagnosis and treatment there are cases where, despite a body of professional opinion sanctioning the defendant's conduct, the defendant can be properly held liable in negligence (I am not here considering questions of disclosure of risk).

However, the application of *Bolitho* to diagnosis and treatment was considered recently in the decision of *Pearce* v. *United Bristol NHS Trust* ([1999] PIQR) P53.(CA)). Here, the Court of Appeal looked at both the decisions in *Bolitho* and the earlier House of Lords judgment in *Sidaway*. Lord Woolf held that:

> ... if there is a significant risk which would affect the judgment of a

reasonable patient then in the normal course it is the responsibility of a doctor to inform the patient of that significant risk, if the information is needed so that the patient can determine for him or herself as to what course he or she should adopt.

On the facts of that particular case the plaintiff failed to establish negligence, in that had the risk of the stillbirth been disclosed the evidence suggested that she would still have gone ahead with a natural delivery. Nonetheless, the approach taken by the Court of Appeal in this case indicates that this decision may again be regarded as a further step towards a broader duty of disclosure upon clinicians (Grubb, 1999). Jones (1999) has argued that the effect of the judgments is that of a combination of the 'prudent patient' standard with the reasonable doctor standard, and that in the light of this case it could be argued that 'no reasonable doctor would fail to disclose a risk regarded as significant by a reasonable patient'. Moreover, it appears to be the case that the risk does not necessarily have to be such that patients would have changed their mind had they known about this particular risk, but rather that it could be sufficient if this risk is one that is *relevant* alongside other factors in reaching a decision.

The implications of the judgments in *Bolitho* and *Pearce* are yet to be explored by the courts. However, the prospect of such enhanced judicial scrutiny may suggest that in the future it will become increasingly difficult to justify withholding information regarding the risks of treatment from patients. This may be particularly the case in the light of the fact that the Human Rights Act 1998 came into force in October 2000. It may also be reflective of the fact that there is a tendency today towards enhanced disclosure on a routine basis in health care, and that in many cases the responsible body of professional practice is likely to favour broader disclosure. The duty of disclosure required under the *Sidaway* test is not fixed; it changes as the approach taken in professional practice changes. The recent guidelines of the GMC, *Seeking Patients' Consent; The Ethical Considerations* (GMC, 2000), are illustrative of the changing approach in health care practice. This document, giving guidance to doctors regarding the provision of information, states that:

6. When providing information you must do your best to find out about patients' individual needs and priorities. For example, patients' beliefs, culture, occupation or other factors may have a bearing on the information they need in order to reach a decision. You should not make assumptions about patients' views, but discuss these matters with them, and ask them whether they have any concerns about the treatment or the risks it may involve. You should provide patients with appropriate information, which should include an explanation of any risks to which they may attach particular significance. Ask patients whether they have understood the information and whether they would like more before making a decision.

As patient expectations change regarding their involvement in decisions concerning their treatment, so the levels of disclosure required of practitioners are likely to change.

This is a very patient-based test, and if followed may have the effect that the nature of the *Sidaway* test over time changes fundamentally in character. Furthermore, the information required to be provided may be affected by external factors. For instance, a directive from Europe now requires that explanatory leaflets be enclosed in certain pharmaceutical products, and this may affect the duty of disclosure in the future (Dir. 92/27/EEC (L113/8)). In addition, the Clinical Negligence Scheme for Trusts (CNST) (2000) requires in Risk Management Standard No. 5 that patients should be provided with appropriate information of risks and benefits before a patient signs a consent form.

Therapeutic privilege

There may be some situations in which it is thought that the patient would be unable to cope if told all the details of the prognosis. In *Sidaway*, Lord Scarman indicated that in such a situation information may be withheld on therapeutic grounds – the so-called 'therapeutic privilege'. This approach is reflected by the UKCC (1996i) in the document *Guidelines for Professional Practice*:

> If patients or clients do not want to know the truth it should not be forced upon them. You must be sensitive to their needs and must make sure that your communication is effective. The patient or client must be given a choice in the matter. To deny them that choice is to deny their rights and so reduce dignity and independence.

Therapeutic privilege must of course be exercised sensitively. Generally nurses should be cautious about withholding information from patients, particularly in the light of the trend towards greater information disclosure.

The questioning patient

A patient is provided with information about the proposed treatment, but then asks questions as to the risks of the treatment and any complications that may arise. To what extent is the nurse obliged to give a full answer?

In *Sidaway*, it was suggested that there might be a duty to respond fully if the patient asked specific questions. For example, Lord Bridge said that:

... when questioned specifically by a patient of apparently sound mind about the risks involved in a particular procedure proposed, the doctor's duty must, in my opinion, be to answer both truthfully and as fully as the questioner requires.

However, the statements made were only judicial opinions, which did not relate to the decision in that case, and so were *obiter* not binding on later courts.

In the later case of *Blyth* v. *Bloomsbury AHA* ([1987] (1993) 4 Med LR 151 CA), the court indicated that the *Bolam* test should also apply to this situation. The plaintiff, Mrs Blyth, was a qualified nurse. She went into hospital to give birth, and after the birth she was given a vaccination against rubella and an injection of the contraceptive Depo-Provera®. Mrs Blyth said that she did not want to be given Depo-Provera until she had been told about the side effects. At the trial, her claims as to what information she had been given were disputed. Expert evidence put forward at the trial indicated that at that time it was the practice to inform the patient that Depo-Provera led to irregular bleeding, but not to inform about the other side effects. Kerr L.J. said that there was no obligation to disclose all information when a question was asked; it was sufficient if the information given was that which would be given by a responsible body of clinical practitioners (the *Bolam* test). In responding to questions, he stressed that the answer given should depend upon the circumstances, the nature of the information, its reliability and relevance, the condition of the patient, etc. In deciding what information should be given initially, the nurse would need to examine the patient to see if he or she were capable of comprehending the information. Nevertheless, questioning patients must be treated with respect and their questions given a serious response.

While the general obligation regarding disclosure of information relates to the standard of the responsible body of clinical practice, should that standard apply to all types of medical procedure? This question came before the courts in the case of *Gold* v. *Haringey Health Authority* ([1987] 2 All ER 888). Mrs Gold underwent a sterilization operation, and the operation was unsuccessful. She brought an action claiming that the surgeon was negligent because she was not told of the risk that the sterilization operation might be reversed naturally, nor of the fact that a vasectomy operation upon her husband would have carried less risk of reversal. At the time she underwent her operation there was a body of medical opinion that supported giving further information, but also a body of medical opinion that supported what her surgeon had done.

At first instance, Schiemmann J. drew a distinction between the level of information that had to be given in cases involving therapeutic as opposed to non-therapeutic treatment. He said that a sterilization operation was non-therapeutic treatment, and as such the approach taken in *Sidaway* was not applicable. It was for the court to decide whether or not the person giving advice should mention the chance that the operation would not achieve the desired result. However, on appeal this approach was rejected. In the Court of Appeal, Lloyd L.J. said that the *Bolam* test applied. He saw problems in trying to draw a line between advice given in relation to therapeutic treatment and non-therapeutic treatment. For example, a plastic surgeon carrying out a skin graft may be acting therapeutically, but he may not be if he were carrying out a facelift or some other cosmetic operation.

Causation

As with any negligence claim, if the patient can show that inadequate information was given by the nurse providing treatment, the patient must still go on to show that the failure to provide such information as to the risks of a particular clinical procedures caused the harm suffered. The court will ask, 'If this patient had been given the information which she should have been given, then would she have decided to go ahead with the treatment?' (*Chatterson* v. *Gerson* [1981] QB 432).

Providing information: professional conflicts over disclosure

In some situations the nurse may be of the view that a doctor or another nurse treating the patient has not provided the patient with adequate information, or that the patient has not understood the information given. What should the nurse do?

In the document *Guidelines for Professional Practice*, the UKCC (1996ii) states that:

> Sometimes you may not be responsible for obtaining the patient's or client's consent as, although you are caring for the patient or client, you would not actually be carrying out the procedure. However, you are often best placed to know about the emotions, concerns and views of the patient or client and may be best able to judge what information is needed so that it is understood. With this in mind you should tell the other members of the health care team if you are concerned about the patient's or client's understanding of the procedure or treatment, for example, due to language difficulties.

What if the nurse draws the doctor's/other nurse's attention to the perceived problem but they disagree with her? What should she do? The UKCC (1996iii) states that:

> There is potential for disagreement or even conflict between different professionals and relatives over giving information to a patient or client. When discussing these matters with colleagues or relatives, you must stress that your personal accountability is firstly to the patient and

client. Any patient or client can feel relatively powerless when they do not have full knowledge about their care or treatment. Giving patients and clients information helps to empower them. For this reason, the importance of telling the truth cannot be over-estimated.

The standard of disclosure laid down by the courts is that of the responsible body of professional clinical practice. If, for example, a doctor had given a patient the amount of information that a body of professional opinion would believe was sufficient, then he would have acted lawfully even though the nurse may disagree with the amount of information given. It is very unlikely that the court would go against the approach the doctor had taken.

Should the nurse inform the patient personally? If he or she does so, then there may be the risk of being disciplined for overstepping authority and disobeying the doctor. It is also possible that the doctor may be withholding the information for a specific reason, such as on therapeutic grounds, and the patient may not be able to cope with the information once given and may actually suffer harm. In such a situation, the nurse is at risk of an action subsequently being brought against him or her in negligence. The court would examine the nurse's actions and determine whether his or her conduct was such as would be supported by a responsible body of professional nursing practice.

If the nurse fails to act and the patient suffers harm, then the nurse may also be at risk of legal proceedings. However, were proceedings to be brought against the nurse, he or she could claim to be simply following the doctor's orders. In earlier cases the courts have been willing to find that a nurse was not negligent because he or she had been following the orders of the doctor (*Gold* v. *Essex CC* [1942] 2 All ER 237). Nonetheless, with the increasing autonomy of the nurse and the growth of professional practice, whether this approach would be given unreserved acceptance may be questioned.

In practice, should this situation arise, it is suggested that the nurse should not go ahead and disclose immediately but should ask the doctor why more information is not being given. If the doctor gives what the nurse regards to be an inadequate reason, then the matter should be referred to the nurse's line manager.

Concluding comments

The principles of consent to treatment outlined in this chapter underpin much of health care law. Matters of consent are considered further in the chapters on reproductive choice, medical research and end of life. In Chapter 6, consent in relation to two particular groups of patient, child patients and the mentally ill, is considered.

References

BMA/Law Society (1996). *Assessment of Mental Capacity: Guidance for Doctors and Lawyers: A report of the British Medical Association and the Law Society*. BMA.

Brazier, M. (1991). Competence, consent and proxy consents. In: *Protecting the Vulnerable* (M. Brazier and M. Lobjoit, eds). Routledge.

Clinical Negligence Scheme for Trusts (2000*). Risk Management Standards and Procedures, Manual of Guidance*. CNST.

Department of Health (1992). *Patient Consent to Examination or Treatment*, Appendix A(1). NHS Management Executive, HSG 92(32). DOH.

General Medical Council (2000). *Seeking Patients' Consent; The Ethical Considerations*. GMC.

Grubb, A. (1994). Treatment without consent: adult. *Med. Law Rev.*, **2**, 92.

Grubb, A. (1999). *Med. Law Rev.*, **7**, 61.

Jones, M. (1999). Informed consent and other fairy stories. *Med. Law Rev.*, **7**, 103.

Kennedy, I. (1991). Consent to treatment. In: *Doctors, Patients and the Law* (C. Dyer, ed.). Blackwell Scientific.

Kennedy, I. and Grubb, A. (1994). *Medical Law: Text and Materials*, 2nd edn. Butterworths.

Law Commission (1995). *Mental Incapacity*. Law Comm Report No. 231. HMSO, (i) para 3.2; (ii) para 3.12; (iii) para 3.16; (iv) para 3.18; (v) para 3.28; (vi) para 4.37.

Law Commission (1996). *Consent in the Criminal Law: A Consultation Paper*. No. 139. HMSO.

Lord Chancellor's Department (1997). *Who Decides*. LCD.

Lord Chancellor's Department (1999). *Making Decisions*. LCD.

Skegg, P. D. G. (1984). *Law, Medicine and Ethics*. Oxford University Press.

UKCC (1993). *AIDS and HIV Infection: A UKCC Statement* (Registrar's letter, 6 April). UKCC, (i) para 25; (ii) para 29.

UKCC (1996). *Guidelines for Professional Practice*. UKCC, (i) para 29, (ii) para 29, (iii) para 25.

Chapter 6

Consent to treatment II: children and the mentally ill

Jean McHale

In Chapter 5, the basic principles of the law as it relates to consent to treatment were examined. This chapter focuses on the treatment of two particular groups of patients: children and the mentally ill. The basis on which treatment may be given and from whom consent to treatment should be obtained is examined in relation to the child patient. Particular difficult treatment issues arise with the child patient, as with the adult counterpart, in the context of treatment refusal. These issues are further complicated in the context of the child patient in a situation in which conflicts arise between child and parent. The second part of the chapter considers legal regulation of treatment of the mentally ill patient in hospital and the community. Here a statutory regime exists, which regulates treatment procedures, in the form of the Mental Health Act 1983.

Treating the child patient

Where the nurse is treating a child patient, he or she must take care to ensure that the appropriate consent has been obtained. Where a child is very young, consent must be obtained from the person with 'parental responsibility'. This may be the child's mother, married father and unmarried father (s2 and s4 Children's Act 1989) (with agreement with the mother or where a court order has been made giving him that power), a person holding a residence order (s12), or a local authority (s33). However, there may be situations where is not sufficient time to consult a person with parental responsibility – for example, a child on her way to school who is injured by a hit and run driver and is taken to hospital bleeding profusely, in a critical condition. In an emergency, such treatment may be given as is immediately necessary without parental consent being obtained. In addition, a child minder or a teacher has the right to do what is 'reasonable in all the circumstances' of the case for the purpose of safeguarding or promoting the child's welfare. This would include authorizing medical treatment (s3(5) Children's Act 1989). The Family Law Reform Act 1969 gives children who are 16 years and over the right to give consent themselves to surgical, medical or dental treatment (s8 Family Law Reform Act 1969).

Many uncertainties remain, however, as to what exactly constitutes 'treatment' for these purposes. It is obvious that the plaster on the wound and the surgery on the car accident victim are covered. What is less clear is the extent to which procedures ancillary to treatment are lawful. A difficult issue concerns the use of constraints upon young children – for example, holding down a child to give treatment. It is submitted that wherever possible treatment should be given with the co-operation of the child, and that the use of compulsion should be contemplated only in highly exceptional circumstances. Generally the performance of non-therapeutic procedures on a child creates difficulties because often they cannot be said to be in the child's best interests. One approach is to say that certain procedures are justifiable as long as they are not *against* the child's best interests (*S* v. *McC*, *W* v. *W* [1972] AC 24). Whether parents can consent to involvement in certain non-therapeutic procedures such as organ donation or involvement in clinical research is discussed further in later chapters.

The parental power of consent does not cover whatever treatment they believe to be in the child's best interests. Any treatment given is ultimately dependent upon the health professional's assessment of whether that treatment is appropriate for the child. Certain procedures are also unlawful *per se* – for example, a mother cannot consent to her daughter being circumcised, because this practice was made illegal by the Prohibition of Female Circumcision Act 1985.

When is the child competent to consent to medical treatment?

A young girl approaches a school nurse and wants advice because she intends obtaining the contraceptive pill. What is the legal position? Can such a girl be given such medication without parental consent?

As stated above, there is a statutory right for children aged 16 years and over to consent to medical or dental treatment. However, some children reach maturity earlier than others – 16 years is an arbitrary point. In *Gillick* v. *West Norfolk and Wisbech AHA* ([1985] 3 All ER 402), the House of Lords clearly stated that even if a child is under 16 years of age he or she may be able to give consent to medical treatment. In this case, Mrs Victoria Gillick sought a declaration that the DHSS had been wrong to issue a direction indicating that a doctor might give contraceptive advice/treatment to a child under 16 years without parental consent. The House of Lords, by a narrow majority, dismissed her claim. Lord Fraser held that a doctor would be justified in giving a girl contraceptive advice without her parent's knowledge and/or consent. He suggested a number of factors to be taken into account in making such an assessment. These included that: the doctor is satisfied that the girl would understand his advice; he has been unable to persuade her to tell her parents or to let him tell her parents; the girl is likely to begin having intercourse with/without contraceptive treatment; without contraceptive advice/treatment her physical or mental health could suffer; and that it would be in the girl's best interests to receive contraceptive assistance without a parent's consent.

Another member of the House of Lords, Lord Scarman, saw the issue in terms of the rights of the child (p. 423):

> ... as a matter of law the parental right to determine whether or not a minor child below the age of 16 will have medical treatment terminates if and when the child achieves a sufficient understanding and intelligence to enable him to understand fully what is proposed. It will be a question of fact whether a child seeking advice has sufficient understanding of what is involved to give a consent valid in law.

Two members of the House of Lords, Lords Brandon and Templeman, dissented. Lord Templeman said that there are many things that a girl under 16 years of age needs to practise, but sex is not one of them.

After the *Gillick* decision, it is clear that a child under 16 years of age may consent to medical treatment if he or she is judged to be competent to give that consent. The difficulty with the test laid down in *Gillick* is that it means that a nurse treating a child patient has the task of assessing whether this particular child is competent to consent to this particular treatment. A child may have sufficient maturity to consent to one type of treatment, such as treatment for cuts and bruises, while at the same time not being competent to decide about another type of treatment, such as an operation. It must be emphasized that even if a child is under 16 years of age, good practice would dictate that, wherever possible, an effort should be made to involve the child in any decisions regarding care and treatment.

Court orders

The vast majority of treatment decisions are straightforward and will present no legal difficulties as long as the nurse complies with the general legal principles in relation to disclosure of information set out in the previous chapter, and if she obtains consent from the appropriate person. There are, however, some situations in which difficult dilemmas arise. The health care professionals may be uncertain as to what action to take. There are three main routes through which an application may be made to the court:

1. The case may be referred under what is known as the court's 'inherent jurisdiction'; the court has a power to make orders regarding medical treatment.

2. The child may be made a ward of court. This power was limited by the Children's Act 1989 and today a local authority cannot apply for wardship, although other interested bodies such as a health authority may do so. In addition, wardship cannot be sought if the child is in local authority care.

3. The third option is to ask the court to make one of two orders created by the Children's Act 1989, section 8. The first of these is a 'prohibited steps' order; this has the effect of stopping a parent exercising his or her parental responsibility without the consent of the court. Secondly, an application could be made for a 'specific issue order'. This involves asking the court to give directions on a specific question before it, for example, giving consent to treatment. In making an order the court considers whether the child's welfare dictates that the treatment be undertaken.

Refusal of treatment by those with parental responsibility

What if a course of treatment is proposed for a critically ill child but the parents refuse to give their consent? Can treatment be given? The parents may be refusing treatment for a particular reason, such as their own ethical or religious beliefs. In such circumstances, health care professionals should hesitate before treating. The impact upon the child, were treatment to be authorized in the face of parental opposition, requires some consideration; if treatment were to be given in such a situation, this may have the effect that the child is alienated from his or her own family. The action taken is likely to relate to the urgency with which treatment is required. If a child is literally bleeding to death, then it is suggested that it is justifiable to treat, even in the face of parental opposition.

If, however, although a child's life is in grave danger death is not imminent, then the matter may be referred to the court by the hospital or by the local authority under the court's inherent jurisdiction, or through a specific issue order asking for clarification of their legal position in undertaking treatment.

Such an issue came before the courts in the case of *Re S (a minor)* ([1993] 1 FLR 376). A 4½-year-old child was suffering from T-cell leukaemia, with a high risk that death would occur. Chemotherapy was offered, but this required a blood transfusion. S's parents, who were dedicated Jehovah's Witnesses, refused to consent to the treatment. The local authority went to court and asked for an order under its inherent jurisdiction, and the parents asked for a prohibited steps order. In authorizing treatment, Thorpe J. noted that the parents' refusal of treatment would deny their son the 50 per cent chance of survival that was offered by the therapy. It had been suggested that one reason why treatment should not be given was that the child would have to live for years to come with parents who 'believed that his life was prolonged through an ungodly act'. Thorpe J. recognized that by providing the child with a transfusion there was a further risk of conflict between child and parent; however, as the judge said:

> The reality seems to me that family reactions will recognize that the responsibility of consent was taken from them, and as a judicial act, absolved their conscience of responsibility.

In the case of *Re O (a minor) (Medical Treatment)* ([1993] 2 FLR 149), a baby was born prematurely. The child suffered from a respiratory distress syndrome, which meant that she would require a blood transfusion. The parents were Jehovah's Witnesses and were opposed to the transfusion. Other options were tried, but it was realized that a blood transfusion was inevitable. The inherent jurisdiction of the High Court was invoked, and Johnson J. gave directions to the effect that if medical advice deemed it necessary the child should be given a blood transfusion.

A more recent and contrasting case provides an illustration of judicial willingness to support a parent's decision to refuse treatment. In *Re T* ([1997] 1WLR 242), a child was born with a liver defect which was life threatening. An operation had initially been carried out on the child at the age of 3½ weeks, which had been unsuccessful and had resulted in the child suffering a great deal of pain. The child then needed a liver transplant. At the time of the hearing, both child and parents were in a foreign country. The parents, who were health care professionals, were opposed to the treatment being undertaken because the mother did not want the child to undergo the suffering that this procedure would involve. The operation was not available in the Commonwealth country where the treatment was being given, and had an order been made the parents would have had to bring the child back to this country for treatment.

At first instance, the judge held that leave should be given to the health professionals to perform the operation despite parental opposition. In the Court of Appeal, this order was reversed. Butler Sloss L.J. examined a number of cases involving the decision to treat the incompetent minor. She noted the exceptional nature of this case, and stated that:

> This mother and child are one for the purpose of this unusual case and the decision of the court to consent to the operation jointly affects the mother and son and it also affects the father. The welfare of this child depends upon his mother.

The decision of the Court of Appeal in *Re T* has proved controversial. The court placed great weight on the views of the parents. This case may appear to run contrary to a number of cases concerning refusal of treatment by parents on religious grounds, where the views of the parents have been overridden by the courts. Emphasis was placed upon the fact that the parents were health professionals. Does this place the opinions of such parents in a special category apart from those of parents generally – even where the parents possess deep religious convictions? While the decision of the Court of Appeal in *Re T* has attracted considerable public attention, its wider implications remain to be assessed. In *Re T* the court stressed the unusual nature of this case and the close emotional attachment which existed between the mother and baby. It may be speculated as to whether the location of the parties may have had some influence on the ultimate decision reached, as the parents were abroad at the time. There are a number of cases in which the court has granted orders allowing active treatment to be withheld from newly born infants, and these cases are explored in Chapter 10.

An illustration of some of the difficult issues that may arise in the context of parental treatment refusal was provided by the case of *Re C (HIV Test)* ([1999] 2 FLR 1004). Here the parents of a 4-month-old child refused to have the child tested for HIV. The mother was HIV-positive, although the father had tested negative. The parents were opposed to the testing; they said that the child was healthy and they wanted to decide what was in her best interests. They were both alternative health practitioners, and were sceptical regarding conventional medical treatment. The mother was breast-feeding the baby. The judge held that he was prepared to sanction the test', and that here there was an 'overwhelming case for the baby to be tested'. The order applied only to testing, and the Council would be required to return for a further order in relation to treatment. The Council had not sought an order preventing the mother from breast-feeding. Mr Justice Wilson was of the view that had such an order been sought it would have been unenforceable. As he stated: 'My belief is that the law cannot come between the baby and the breast'. The parents sought leave to appeal, but their application was dismissed. They had argued that the judge should have evaluated why they were critical of the use of orthodox clinical approaches to HIV, that parents in a developing area of medicine such as this should be given certain clinical autonomy and that the court should not intervene with this. The Court of Appeal rejected the appeal. They held that there was strong medical evidence that the child was at risk of harm unless the test was undertaken. Moreover, the court could overrule the decision of a parent even though this decision may be reasonable. It may be the case that there will be litigation regarding the application of Article 8 of the Human Rights Act 1998, which came into force in October 2000. This Article concerns the right to privacy of home and family life. The extent to which this provision will be successfully used to alter the judicial approach in cases such as *Re C (HIV Test)* may be questioned (Grubb, 2000). Grubb has suggested that:

> It would, however, require a substantial 'u-turn' in judicial behaviour and inclination and would contradict the philosophy of the Children's Act which sees the child's welfare as paramount.

It is submitted that this is the better view and that unless there is a radical reconception of the role of parent's rights in treatment decision making, successful use of Article 8 is somewhat unlikely.

When can treatment be given in the face of a child's refusal?

> Parents bring their son to be vaccinated. The boy goes into the treatment room but then begins to scream and refuses to let the nurse touch him. Can he be compelled to have the injection?

In the case of a very young child, while actually giving this injection may not be very easy, in strict law the parent may consent to treatment despite the child's refusal. However, in practice the nurse may suggest to the parents that the vaccination does not go ahead at that time, but that they bring the child back another day. Difficult issues arise in relation to older children who are assessed as *Gillick* competent. Such a child may be able to consent to medical treatment, but what if he or she refuses? Can treatment be given, and if so on what basis? In the professional role as patient advocate, the nurse is required to respect the autonomy of the patient, which includes providing support for a patient who decides to refuse treatment or that treatment should be withdrawn (UKCC, 1996). Nonetheless, it has been noted that in law the power of the adult patient to refuse treatment is not unlimited (see Chapter 5). As far as the child patient is concerned, it is clearly the case that the right to refuse treatment is again not absolute. It is also likely that where a child refuses treatment this will mean that, as with the adult patient, a more rigorous assessment is made of that child's competence.

The Court of Appeal has indicated that if a competent child refuses treatment, his or her parents may override this refusal. In *Re R* ([1991] 4 All ER 177 CA), Lord Donaldson said that the fact that a child was competent to consent to treatment did not mean that all parental rights were removed. Once a child reaches maturity, he or she receives a key to the door of treatment. However, the child's parents have keys, and they also keep the keys once the child gains maturity. A parent can authorize treatment even though the child refuses. Lord Donaldson's words in that case were *obiter* and the other members of the Court of Appeal did not agree with his approach.

However, in the later case of *Re W* ([1992] 3 WLR 758), the Court of Appeal confirmed that the parents could lawfully override the refusal of a competent child. This case concerned an anorexic 16-year-old girl who opposed removal to a treatment centre where it was likely that an active treatment regime might be imposed. The court held that although she was competent to consent to treatment, her refusal could be overridden. Lord Donaldson moved away from the keyholder analogy, and instead said that a doctor acquires a legal 'flak jacket' as protection against being sued when he receives consent from a child over 16, a *Gillick* competent child or from a person with parental responsibility. He went on to say:

No minor of whatever age has power by refusing consent to treatment to override a consent to treatment by someone who has parental responsibility for the minor. Nevertheless such a refusal was a very important consideration in making clinical judgments and for parents and the court in deciding themselves whether to give consent.

The judgment in this case was contrary to general opinion as to the interpretation of the *Gillick* case and the Family Law Reform Act 1969. However, at present, even if a *Gillick* competent child refuses medical treatment it appears that his or her parents may override the refusal. Even so, the court in *Re W* suggested that before a major surgical procedure is undertaken on a child against the child's will, it is desirable for the issue to be referred to the court. The court will then determine what is in the child's best interests, taking into account the child's expressed wishes and the strength of the child's beliefs. It may be, for example, that while a child has strong convictions at present, this may be only a passing phase. The urgency of the treatment is also a relevant factor.

In *Re W*, Nolan L.J. suggested that the court could intervene where the child's welfare was 'threatened by serious and imminent risk that the child will suffer grave and irreversible mental or physical harm', while Balcombe L.J. stated that the court should only intervene where refusal would lead to the child's death.

Children were given certain statutory rights to refuse court-ordered assessment and treatment under the Children's Act 1989. This may seem rather at odds with the approach of the courts in *Re R* and *Re W*. However, in the case of *South Glamorgan CC* v. *W and B* ([1993] 1 FLR 574), the court confirmed that a court still possessed certain residual powers under its inherent jurisdiction to override a child's refusal. The decision in this case has been criticized on the basis that it goes against clear words of statute.

Authorization of treatment in the face of a child's opposition may also give rise to problems as to the relationship between the powers to treat compulsorily under the Mental Health Act 1983 (which will be considered later) and the powers at common law. In *Re K, W and H (minors) (Medical Treatment)* ([1993] FLR 584), advance parental consent was required before children were admitted for treatment in a specialist psychiatric institution. Three children were admitted. They later complained regarding their treatment, including the administration of emergency medication. An action was brought before the court under section 8 of the Children's Act 1989 to clarify the legality of the treatment of these three children. Two were 15 years old and were suffering from unsocialized adolescent conduct disorder; the other child, who was almost 15 years of age, was suffering from bipolar affective disorder. Thorpe J. said that none of the children was *Gillick* competent, but that even if they were, the doctor had received parental authorization of treatment in the form of the advance consents before they had entered the psychiatric institution, and thus was justified in law in going ahead and providing treatment. He commented that a specific issue order to authorize treatment under section 8 of the Children's Act 1989 was not required where parental consent existed. The difficulty with such an approach is that it denies children the safeguards in the form of the statutory provisions limiting provision of treatment contained in the Mental Health Act 1983 (Bate, 1995).

In *Re M* ([1999] 2 FLR 1097), a 15-year-old girl required a heart transplant without which she was likely to die within the week. M refused consent and claimed that she did not want to follow the long post-operative course of therapy with a daily course of tablets for the rest of her life, and that she would rather die than live on with the heart of another person inside her. Johnson J. in the Family Division held that M was in effect incompetent. He commented: '... events have overtaken M so swiftly that she has not been able to come to terms with her situation'. While there were consequent risks in the heart transplant operation itself being undertaken, as Johnson J. noted, these were overridden by what was otherwise the certainty that in this situation M would die.

While certain powers are given to courts and parents to override the decisions of competent children, these powers should be used only in exceptional circumstances. Generally it is not clinically beneficial to treat a child where he or she is objecting, particularly where this involves detention against a child's will.

Refusal of treatment by both children and parents

What if both parents and child patient are in agreement in their opposition to treatment and emphasize that this is on religious grounds? In such a situation the consequences of refusal of treatment should be clearly explained to the child. Dilemmas may arise, however, where that refusal is likely to result in the patient's death. It may be the case that the child's will is being overborne, but equally the child may have a fundamental religious belief and have reached his or her own decision to refuse treatment based on that belief. In such a situation where refusal of treatment would have the consequence that death would result, an application to the court would be appropriate, to ask for the authorization of treatment.

This issue came before the courts in the case of *Re E (minor) (Wardship: Medical Treatment)* ([1993] 1 FLR 386). A was 15 years and 9 months, and was suffering from leukaemia. A's parents were devout Jehovah's Witnesses, and both A and his parents were opposed to a blood transfusion. Consent was given to therapy which avoided a blood transfusion but had a 40–50 per cent chance of full remission, as opposed to 80–90 per cent with treatment involving a blood transfusion. The health authority made an application to the court when it became apparent that within a matter of hours blood platelet levels would fall to unacceptable levels and A was at risk of a stroke or heart attack. The judge, Ward J., stated that although A was a calm and intelligent person, in his view he did not really understand the implications of his decision:

I am quite satisfied that A does not have any sufficient comprehension of the pain he has yet to suffer, of the fear that he will be undergoing, of the distress not only occasioned by that fear but also – and more importantly – the distress he will inevitably suffer as he, a loving son, helplessly watches his parents' and his family's distress. They are a close family and a brave family, but I find that he has no realization of the full implications that lie before him as to the process of dying.

While noting A's religious convictions, he stated:

I respect this boy's profession of faith but I cannot discount at least the possibility that he may in later years suffer some diminution in his convictions. There is no settled certainty about matters of this kind.

In *Re L (Medical Treatment: Gillick Competency)* ([1998] 2 FLR 810), L was a Jehovah's witness who was 14 years of age. She refused a blood transfusion orally, and had also executed a blood transfusion card. L fell into a bath of hot water and suffered severe scalds; 54 per cent of the body surface was covered with severe burns, and 40 per cent were third-degree burns. Surgery was necessary to save her life, and she required a blood transfusion. The hospital authority obtained an application under the inherent jurisdiction to administer blood and blood products as necessary during treatment without L's consent. Sir Stephen Brown stated that L lacked *Gillick* competence. She had not been informed by her family or by the doctors as to the distressing nature of her death. He held that here:

It may be that because of her belief she is willing to say, and to mean it, 'I am willing to accept death rather than to have a blood transfusion', but it is clear that she has not been able to be given all the details which it would be right and appropriate to have in mind when making a decision.

This type of case poses difficult questions. In *Re L* the patient had not been appraised of all the circumstances when making her decision, and the court's decision in that case reflects that fact. It is also the case that the patient's perception of the situation may alter consequent upon treatment. However, while the patient's views may very well change, equally they may not. The minor in *Re E* subsequently died when, on reaching the age of 18 years, he refused treatment.

Seeking treatment and care when a child is being neglected or put at risk

If a health visitor believes that a child is being neglected by his or her parents or that he or she is being abused, what can the health visitor do? The actions of the health visitor will obviously depend upon the gravity of the situation and the child's need for immediate care. If a child is suffering from a particular medical condition and it is believed that the child still needs care, what can be done? In this situation, the matter should be referred to the line manager who may decide to refer the matter to Social Services. All local authorities and county councils have child protection policies, which should be consulted by health care professionals. The local authority may decide to instigate an investigation. The health visitor would be consulted while any investigation was being undertaken. Measures may be taken to bring the child under the care or supervision of the local authority. These are matters that go beyond the scope of this book, and readers are referred to specialist texts on the subject.

Treating the mentally ill patient

In Chapter 5, the question of treatment of mentally incompetent patients was examined. Here, the question of treatment of the mentally ill patient is considered. Mental illness and mental incompetence should not be equated. A mentally ill person may be perfectly competent to consent to involvement in some clinical procedures – for example, involvement in clinical research – even though he or she has diminished competence in relation to other matters.

It is important for the nurse to be aware of the operation of the Mental Health Act 1983, not only if he or she intends to specialize in mental health nursing, but also because issues involving treatment of the mentally ill arise in a wide variety of nursing situations. The nurse should also be aware of the Mental Health Act Code of Practice. This is not legally binding, but provides an indication of good practice. For fuller discussion of this area, the nurse is referred to specialist texts dealing with mental health law (Gostin, 1985; Dimond and Barker, 1996; Hoggett, 1996; Bartlett and Sandland, 2000). Here, the focus is on treatment given after detention under civil law power. Powers of detention are also available in the context of the criminal law.

Admission into hospital for treatment

A mentally disordered patient may be informally admitted to a hospital for psychiatric treatment. Such a patient may refuse any treatment, and may leave hospital freely at any time (s131 Mental Health Act 1983). Any attempt to detain the patient may lead to a civil law claim for damages for false imprisonment being brought. It appears that the use of 'constraints' such as special locks on doors to prevent patients wandering out onto the street is lawful (Hoggett, 1996). However, as Hoggett notes (p. 143), 'consideration should be given to "sectioning" people who persistently and purposefully try to leave'.

The Mental Health Act Code of Practice (1998) indicates that, wherever possible, preference should be given to informal admission. However, in some situations it is necessary compulsorily to admit a patient. Considered below are first, the basis on which a patient can be brought from the community into hospital and given treatment, and second, the grounds for detaining a patient who is presently in a hospital on an informal basis.

Emergency removal under the Mental Health Act 1983

The Mental Health Act 1983 contains emergency powers enabling a person to be removed to hospital for treatment. Section 135 of the Act provides that a magistrate may authorize a warrant allowing a police officer to gain entry to premises and remove a person to a 'place of safety'. The warrant will be granted if a magistrate is satisfied that the person is suffering from mental disorder and 'has been or is being ill-treated, neglected or kept otherwise than under proper control, or is living alone and is unable to care for themselves'. When entering premises, the Act requires a police officer to be accompanied by an approved social worker and a doctor. A person may only be detained under section 135 for up to 72 hours. After this point, any continued detention must be authorized under one of the other powers contained in the Mental Health Act 1983.

Power of police to remove a person found in a public place

If a man is found wandering in the street showing clear signs of mental disorder and a policeman believes that the man is in immediate need of care or control, he may remove him to a 'place of safety', such as a hospital, for up to 72 hours (s136 Mental Health Act 1983). The powers under section 136 apply to 'any place to which the public has access'. They enable an individual to be examined by a doctor and interviewed by an approved social worker as a preliminary to providing care or admission to hospital for treatment under the Mental Health Act 1983. The operation of this section has come under considerable criticism, with claims that the section has been inadequately supervised and details of patients admitted under the section inadequately recorded.

At present, if a person opposes removal from his or her home and treatment is needed, there is no alternative but forcible removal to hospital under the Mental Health Act 1983. The Law Commission has proposed a new power to allow the removal of a vulnerable person 'at risk' from his or her home (Law Commission, 1995). This would be for the purpose of an assessment order or a temporary protection order being made, enabling removal to protective accommodation for a period of up to 10 days.

Admission for assessment

Section 2 of the Mental Health Act 1983 allows a patient to be admitted for 'assessment'. Section 2 applies to patients suffering from a mental disorder justifying detention in hospital at least for a limited period. It must also be shown that detention is needed in the interests of the patient's own health and safety, or to protect others. The application must be made by the patient's 'nearest relative' or by an approved social worker. The approved social worker should inform the nearest relative that an application is being made (s11(3)). The application must be supported by two doctors, one of whom must have been approved by the Secretary of State as having special experience in the treatment of mental disorders. The 'nearest relative' is defined in the Act as being the relative who usually lives with that patient, or the person with the closest connection as determined in relation to a long list of relatives – in order of priority. The approved social worker is a social worker appointed to work under the Mental Health Act. Section 2 is intended to provide a short-term detention, with the limited purpose of determining suitability for continued assessment (*R* v. *Wilson and Williamson* [1995] *The Independent*, 19 April). Admission under this section is for a <u>period of up to 28 days.</u> This is a one-off admission, as the period cannot be renewed.

'Mental disorder' under this section is defined as 'mental illness, arrested or incomplete development of mind, psychopathic disorder and any other disability of mind' (s1(2)). The Act does not define mental illness, but the courts have indicated that it should be given its ordinary meaning (*W* v. *L* [1974] QB 711). This is commonly known as the 'man must be mad' test (Hoggett, 1996). The definition of mental disorder expressly excludes sexual deviations and alcoholism (s1(3) Mental Health Act 1983). Psychopathic disorder refers to a disorder or disability of mind (whether or not including significant impairment of intelligence) resulting in abnormally aggressive or seriously irresponsible conduct.

Admission for treatment

A person may be admitted for treatment for longer periods under section 3 of the Mental Health Act 1983. Application for admission under this section may be made by the same persons as under section 2. It must be shown that the patient is suffering from 'mental illness, severe mental impairment, psychopathic disorder or mental impairment' (s 3(2)). Mental impairment refers to arrested/incomplete mental development, including significant impairment of intelligence/social functioning, associated with abnormally aggressive/seriously irresponsible conduct. The condition must be of a nature such that it is appropriate for the patient to receive treatment in a hospital.

Where treatment is sought for psychopathic disorder or mental impairment it must be shown that the treatment is likely to alleviate or prevent deterioration in the patient's condition, although it is not necessary to show that it would provide a guaranteed cure. Treatment may include nursing and rehabilitation, including group therapy, which could result in the patient being rendered more co-operative (R v. *Canons Park Mental Health Review Tribunal Ex parte A* [1994] 1 All ER 481). Finally, it must be shown that admission is necessary for the patient's health and safety or for the protection of other persons, and that necessary treatment cannot be given unless the patient is detained under this section. Admission under section 3 allows the patient to be detained for up to 6 months. This period can be renewed, initially for 6 months and then on an annual basis.

Emergency power – section 4

In an emergency, a patient can be admitted under section 4 of the Mental Health Act 1983 if one doctor certifies that he or she is suffering from 'mental disorder'. The doctor should, if possible, already know the patient. A doctor who certifies admission under section 4 does not have to be a specialist in mental illness. The person making the application should have examined the patient in the previous 24 hours. Section 4 allows detention for up to a maximum of 72 hours, and this period can be extended by conversion into 'admission for assessment' under section 2.

Detaining a patient in hospital

In some situations it becomes obvious that a patient receiving care in hospital on a voluntary basis requires compulsory detention. The Mental Health Act 1983 contains powers to allow a patient to be detained to enable assessment of whether prolonged detention is necessary. One of these powers applies expressly to nurses. Section 5(4) of the Mental Health Act 1983 gives the nurse power to detain an inpatient, if the nurse is of the view that the patient is suffering from a mental disorder to such a degree that it is necessary for the patient to be immediately restrained from leaving hospital, and a doctor is unable to examine the patient at that time.

The power applies to nurses on part 3 or part 5 or parts 13 or 14 of the statutory Register (part 3 includes first level nurses trained in nursing people suffering from mental illness; part 5, first level nurses trained in nursing those with learning disabilities; part 13, nurses who have obtained qualifications after following a course of mental health nursing; and part 14, those qualified from a course of learning disabilities nursing). If the nurse decides to exercise this power, he or she must record this fact in writing. Detention under section 5(4) is limited to 6 hours, or to the point at which the doctor can see the patient. This is an important power, and one the nurse should use with discretion. There is a danger in these cases that, as Unsworth notes, the nurse may be seen as 'gaoler' rather than a carer (Unsworth, 1987).

The Mental Health Act Code of Practice sets out a number of criteria that a nurse should take into account before exercising power under section 5(4) (para 9.2).

Under the Mental Health Act Code of Practice, the nurse should consider the following criteria before exercising power under section 5(4) (para 9.2):

a. the likely arrival time of the doctor as against the likely intention of the patient to leave. Most patients who express a wish to leave hospital can be persuaded to wait until a doctor arrives to discuss it further. Where this is not possible, the nurse must try to predict the impact of any delay upon the patient.

b. the consequences of a patient leaving hospital immediately – the harm that might occur to the patient or others – taking into account:
   - the patient's expressed intentions including the likelihood of the patient committing self-harm or suicide
   - any evidence of disordered thinking
   - the patient's current behaviour and in particular any changes in usual behaviour
   - the likelihood of the patient behaving in a violent manner
   - any recently received messages from relatives or friends
   - any recent disturbance on the ward
   - any relevant involvement of other patients.

c. the patient's known unpredictability and any other relevant information from other members of the multi-disciplinary team.

The wording of section 5(4) appears to assume that a nurse should complete the forms before detaining the patient. Does this mean that the patient cannot be detained until the forms have been completed? The question is not expressly dealt with in the 1983 Act. At common law there were powers allowing the insane to be arrested, but it is uncertain how far these powers still exist; in one view sufficient common law powers do exist justifying such detention (*Black* v. *Forsey* (1988) *The Times*, 21 May). Nonetheless, the House of Lords in *R* v. *Bournewood NHS Trust ex parte L* ([1998] 3 All ER 289) did confirm that informal powers of detention may be used. An informal patient may be in hospital and being treated without formal detention powers being used. Of course the scope of such informal detention needs to be exceedingly carefully monitored to ensure that the provisions of the Mental Health legislation are not being undermined, with care and treatment being justified because detention has been authorized through informal means.

The section requires that detention must be authorized by suitably qualified nurses – RMNs or RNMHs. But what if there are no suitably qualified nurses on the ward? The Code of Practice provides that if it is likely that section 5(4) might be used, then:

... they should ensure that suitable arrangements are in place for a suitably qualified nurse to be available should the power need to be invoked.

The holding power under section 5(4) applies for a maximum of 6 hours.

Detention may be authorized under section 5(2) by a doctor. The doctor must provide the hospital managers with a report as to why he or she believes that the patient's detention is required, and once the managers have obtained a copy of the report then detention can be authorized for a period of up to 72 hours. It should be noted that this power applies to inpatients as opposed to patients simply visiting the hospital for treatment. It should be noted that while section 5(2) powers can be applied to any inpatient as long as the relevant criteria are satisfied, section 5(4) can be used by a nurse only in relation to a patient receiving treatment for a mental disorder as an in-patient.

It should be emphasized that sections 5(4) and 5(2) are holding powers to allow detention and assessment prior to possible authorization of longer detention under one of the other provisions of the 1983 Act.

Providing the patient with information

A detained patient must be given information enabling him or her to understand the grounds for and conditions for detention (s132 Mental Health Act 1983). This duty is one that is likely to be delegated to the nurse. The patient must be informed of what provisions of the Mental Health Act 1983 he or she is being detained under, the right to apply to a mental health tribunal for discharge, and how certain provisions of the Mental Health Act 1983 (such as those relating to consent to treatment) affect him or her (s132 Mental Health Act 1983). This information must be given as soon as reasonably practicable after detention has begun. Good practice dictates that the information should be given orally and in writing. There should be a procedure in existence stating who should give the information to the patient.

Treatment of the detained patient

The Mental Health Act 1983 only regulates treatment given for the patient's mental disorder (s63); a mentally disordered person may still have capacity to give consent or refusal to other types of treatment. 'Treatment' includes medication and nursing care, but may also extend to, for instance, feeding, if the patient's mental illness leads to the refusal of food (*B* v. *Croyden HA* [1995] 1 All ER 683). It has been suggested that the definition of mental illness includes anorexia nervosa (Mental Health Act Commission Fourth Biennial Report and *Riverside Mental Health Trust* v. *Fox* [1994] 2 *Med Law Review* 95). There has been recent judicial criticism of the use of this section in relation to the authorization of a Caesarean section upon a protesting patient (*St Georges NHS Trust v. S*; see also below). It should be noted that even where a patient may be compelled to receive medication within 3 months under section 63, every attempt must be made to obtain the consent of the patient.

Psychosurgery/surgical implantation of hormones

Section 57 sets out a special procedure for psychosurgery and for other procedures governed by regulations, including the surgical implantation of hormones. The patient must consent to the administration of this treatment.

In addition, a second opinion approved doctor appointed by the Secretary of State and two other persons appointed by the Mental Health Act Commission must have (s57(2)(a)):

> ... certified in writing that the patient is capable of understanding the nature, purpose and likely effects of the treatment in question and has consented to it.

One of these persons must be a nurse, and the other should be neither a nurse nor a doctor.

The second opinion approved doctor is appointed for these purposes by the body that regulates the conduct of the Mental Health Act, the Mental Health Commission. The doctor must also certify that (s57(2)(b)):

> ... having regard to the likelihood of the treatment alleviating or preventing a deterioration of the patient's condition the treatment should be given.

These safeguards apply both to patients detained under the Mental Health Act 1983 and to informal patients.

Electroconvulsive therapy and administration of medicines after 3 months

The administration of medicines and electroconvulsive therapy (ECT) is governed by section 58 of the 1983 Act. ECT may be appropriate, for instance, if a patient suffers from severe depression. As far as the administration of medicines is concerned, once 3 months have passed from the point when the patient was first admitted and given treatment for his or her mental disorder, special authorization is required before the nurse may continue to administer any medicines. Before ECT is given or medicines are administered after 3 months, one of two additional criteria must be satisfied. Either the patient must consent, with this consent being verified by the practitioner treating the patient, or, if the patient refuses consent, treatment may still be given if authorized by a second opinion approved doctor.

The doctor must state either that the patient is not competent because he or she cannot understand the nature, purpose or likely effects of treatment, or that, although the patient is competent and is refusing treatment, in view of the likelihood of it alleviating or preventing a deterioration in the patient's condition, treatment should be given (s58(3)(b)). In forming his or her opinion, the second opinion approved doctor should also consult two other persons professionally involved in that person's care.

The statute requires that at least one of these persons is a nurse (s58(4)). The grade of nurse is not specified. Again, the other person must be neither nurse nor doctor (s58(4)).

Treatment under sections 57 and 58 should be the subject of regular review. It should be noted that consents here are not always required on each separate occasion; it is sufficient that the consents relate to the overall plan of care (s59).

Treating in an emergency

In an emergency, the safeguards contained in section 57 and section 58 may be bypassed under section 62 of the Act. First, treatment may be given if it is immediately necessary to save the patient's life. Secondly, treatment that is not irreversible may be given to alleviate serious suffering by the patient. Thirdly, treatment which is immediately necessary and represents the minimum interference necessary to prevent the patient from behaving violently or being a danger to him- or herself or others may be given if it is not irreversible or hazardous in nature. 'Irreversible' is defined as treatment entailing unfavourable physical or psychological consequences; 'hazardous' refers to treatment that entails significant physical hazard. Gunn (1995) has suggested that those situations in which treatment may be given lawfully under this section are likely to be exceedingly limited. It is difficult to see how the performance of psychosurgery or surgical implantation of hormones can be justified in an emergency. Medication can, in any case, be given in the absence of the patient's consent within 3 months of a person first receiving medication for mental disorder during any continuous period of detention within 3 months of a person being sectioned. The only situation in which Gunn (1995) envisages use of section 62 is in an emergency to give ECT to a patient who is in a catatonic stupor and who might otherwise die.

It has been claimed that in some instances treatment given under section 62 has extended beyond what is justifiable within the provisions of the section. For example, there were three reported cases in Broadmoor Special Hospital where patients have died following doses of antipsychotic medication in excess of the those in the guide produced jointly by the BMA and the Royal Pharmaceutical Society of Great Britain (Fennell, 1994). A nurse who believes that the criteria laid down in the Mental Health Act 1983 are not being followed should make her or his concerns known to those who authorized this treatment. If necessary, the nurse should inform the line manager. Where an abuse has occurred, the line manager should inform the hospital authorities and make the Mental Health Act Commission aware of the situation. (See also the discussion on whistleblowing in Chapter 7, p. 150).

Use of seclusion

The use of seclusion in mental hospitals came under scrutiny in the report into the abuses of mentally ill patients at Ashworth Special Hospital. Seclusion is defined in the Mental Health Code of Practice (para 19.16) as: 'the supervised confinement of a patient in a room which may be locked for the protection of others from significant harm'. The Code of Practice emphasizes that it must be used as a last resort and for the shortest time possible. It should also not be used as a punishment/threat, as part of a treatment programme, as a measure because of staff shortages, or where there is any risk of suicide or of self-harm.

The precise legality of seclusion is unclear. It may be lawful because it is the application of reasonable force, which amounts to self-defence.

The Code of Practice provides that the nurse in charge of the ward may impose seclusion on a patient, but where this is done a doctor should be called immediately. A number of criteria must be fulfilled. First, a nurse should be within sight and sound of the place where the patient is being held and should be present if the patient has been sedated (para 19.19). Secondly, the patient should be observed and a documented report should be made every 15 minutes as to whether seclusion is necessary (para 19.20). Thirdly, if seclusion is continued, then two nurses in the seclusion room should undertake a review every 2 hours and a doctor should review every 4 hours. Where the seclusion has continued for more than 8 hours consecutively or for more than 12 hours intermittently over 48 hours, an independent review is required. This should be undertaken by a consultant 'or other doctor of suitable seniority' and a team of nurses and other health professionals, none of whom were involved in the care of the patient when the original seclusion was undertaken (para 19.22).

The Mental Health Act Commission commented in their Eighth Biennial Report that nearly 5000 episodes of seclusion were used in 1997–1998 in relation to slightly under 2000 patients. The Report also noted (para 10.18) that: 'there is a considerable number of units where policies are either inadequate or out of date and the guidance in the Code is not followed'.

Transfer

A patient detained under the Mental Health Act 1983 may be transferred to another unit managed by a different NHS trust, or to a registered mental nursing home registered to take detained patients.

Discharging the patient

The period of detention may come to an end or the patient may leave as a result of being discharged. A trust or authority can discharge any patient who has been admitted for assessment or treatment at any time (s23). The decision to discharge is to be taken by a committee of three persons (s24(4)(5)). The nearest relative may also apply to the hospital for the patient's discharge (s23(2)(a)), and must give notice in writing (s25). The patient has the right to apply for discharge to a mental health review tribunal (s66). In addition, an automatic reference will be made to a tribunal if the patient has not exercised the right to apply during the first 6 months of detention. Under section 68, automatic referral must be made if the patient has not been before the tribunal for 3 years. A Mental Health Review Tribunal (of which there are eight nationally) is a body comprised of three members; one legal, one medical and one lay. It is required to discharge patients if they are no longer suffering from mental disorder/illness, or if further detention is not required for the purposes of the patient's health or safety or to protect other persons. It may also exercise discretion to discharge even if these criteria have not been satisfied.

Detaining informal patients

One of the most debated issues has been that of the detention of informal patients in a situation in which statute itself does not legitimize the detention. In *R* v. *Bournewood NHS Trust, ex parte L* ([1998] 3 All ER 289), the House of Lords confirmed that where a patient was incompetent but compliant, he or she could be detained in hospital other than through the formal sectioning process. Regarding detention through the use of locked doors, in such a situation the Code of Practice 1999 (para 19.27) provides that:

> combination locks and double-handed doors should be used only where there is a regular and significant risk of patients wandering off accidentally and being at risk of harm and there should be clear policies on such use.

The precise legal scope of such restrictions may be debatable (Gunn and Rodgers, 2001), and the issue as to whether this may constitute false imprisonment remains to be determined. However, as Gunn and Rodgers (2001) note, compliance with the Code of Practice may provide a defence in that this constitutes good practice in the case of subsequent litigation.

Liability of the nurse under the Mental Health Act 1983

As long as a nurse acts in accordance with her or his statutory powers under the Mental Health Act 1983, then section 139 provides that:

> No person shall be liable ... to any civil or criminal proceedings ... in respect of any act purporting to be done in pursuance of this Act ... unless the act was done in bad faith or without reasonable care.

This limits the possibility of a civil action against the nurse (*Poutney* v. *Griffiths* [1975] 2 All ER 881). A patient may still bring an action challenging his or her detention under judicial review on the basis that the health care professionals have acted outside their powers.

Treating mentally incapacitated persons in the community

Some patients suffering from a mental disorder may benefit from treatment in the community rather than in hospital. The 1983 Act allows such patients to be made the subject of what are known as 'guardianship' orders (s7(2) Mental Health Act 1983). A person aged 16 years or over may be received into guardianship if he or she is suffering from mental disorder, i.e. mental illness, severe mental impairment, psychopathic disorder or mental impairment, and the disorder is of a nature or degree warranting the use of guardianship, and it is in the interests of the patient or for the protection of others that guardianship powers be used. The guardian may be the local social services authority or other named person. An application for admission to guardianship may be made by an approved social worker or by the patient's nearest relative (s11(1)), and must contain the recommendation of two doctors. A clinical description of the patient's mental condition must be given, and it must be explained why the patient cannot be appropriately cared for without the powers of guardianship.

One criticism made of the powers of guardianship has been that they are limited in scope. A patient may be required to live at a place specified by the guardian, and required to attend for treatment, occupation, education or training (s8). In addition, the order may require that a doctor or approved social worker be given access to the patient at his or her residence (s8). However, a patient cannot be compelled to receive treatment. It appears that in practice these powers are rarely used (Gunn, 1986).

If a patient detained under section 3 is then released into the community, he or she may be required, as a condition of discharge, to continue taking medication. However, section 3 cannot be used to admit a patient with the aim of requiring that patient to receive medication and then releasing him or her into the community (*R* v. *Hallstrom exp W* [1986] QB 1090).

Some have argued that patients were being released into the community but there were inadequate powers for regulating their care, and thus patients entered into a cycle of admission, treatment and discharge followed by readmission. Concern regarding this 'revolving door' led to the issue being considered by a House of Lords Select Committee in their 5th report (1992–1993), and this was followed by a Department of Health Inquiry (DOH, 1993a). The results of many of the recommendations for reform are to be found in the Mental Health (Patients in the Community) Act 1995. This legislation provides a new regime for supervision in the community of persons who have been released from detention (Mental Health Act 1983 s25A–H). The patient's responsible medical officer (RMO) makes an application for supervision to the health authority which is to have responsibility for providing the patient with aftercare facilities (s25(A)s). The RMO must be satisfied that supervision is justified on the basis of risk of harm to the patient or risk to the safety of others. In making this assessment, the RMO should take into account the patient's views and those of persons who will be professionally concerned with the after care, and others such as relatives who may be caring for the patient in the community (s25B). Once in the community, the patient is under the care of a supervisor. As with guardianship, the patient can be required to live in a particular place and can be compelled to attend for treatment, but cannot be compelled to receive treatment (s25D). However, unlike guardianship, if the patient refuses treatment this may lead to his or her condition being reviewed to see whether readmission is necessary. Supervision under this power is for an initial period of 6 months, with the possibility of renewal for a further 6 months. It may be ended at any time by the responsible medical officer after undertaking consultation (s25H(1)–(3)). This measure considerably strengthens the power to treat in the community.

Monitoring care – the role of the Mental Health Act Commission

The Mental Health Act Commission was established under the Mental Health Act 1983 (s120(1)) (Bingley, 1995). The Commissioners are drawn from medical practitioners and others such as social workers, academics, psychologists and lawyers. The Commission has the task of monitoring care given under the Act. The Commission monitors the implementation of the Mental Health Act Code of Practice. The special hospitals are visited by the Commissioners on a regular basis. They also visit other NHS hospitals and mental nursing homes that are registered to receive detained patients. They undertake periodic reviews of situations in which treatments have been authorized by the second opinion approved doctor. Where a nurse becomes concerned as to the regime at a mental health hospital and believes that her or his concerns have not been adequately addressed within the complaints structure available for hospital staff, then the Mental Health Act Commissioners provide one avenue through which he or she can address concerns as to standards of patient care (DOH, 1993b). They can also investigate complaints from patients (s120(1)(b) Mental Health Act 1983). They have the power to visit and interview detained patients, and can require the production of and inspection of records relating to detained patients.

The Commissioners may also make visits without giving advance warning if there is particular concern regarding patients. An example of this was a 'dawn raid' undertaken on 21 November 1996 on 31 acute psychiatric hospitals in England and Wales by the Mental Health Act Commission and the Sainsbury Centre for Mental Health. These raids led to a report that noted difficulties facing staff nursing and the mentally ill, and the fact that staff appeared to be demotivated and there were breakdowns in communication between staff and patients. The report noted that there were on average 80 patients for every 100 beds, which left little room for manoeuvre.

The Commission publishes a biennial report, which is laid before Parliament. It also publishes Practice Notes. Other functions include the appointment of second opinion doctors. The Mental Health Act Commission is itself accountable to the Secretary of State and to Parliament as a Special Health Authority.

Reforming the system

The system of care and treatment of those with mental illness and mental incapacity is under review in a number of areas. Concerns as to the operation of care regimes in particular institutions, such as that of Ashworth Hospital, have led to major inquiries being undertaken. In the previous chapter, the Law Commission's proposals on mental incapacity were discussed. In addition, proposals have been advanced for the care of those with dangerous serious personality disorders and for reform of the Mental Health Act 1983.

Proposals in relation to dangerous severely personality disordered people

There has been much debate regarding the appropriate measures to take in relation to those persons with dangerous severe personality disorders where the condition is not amenable to treatment. Such persons cannot be treated under the provisions of the Mental Health Act. The perception was that this group may present a considerable risk of harm to members of the community. The government responded to these concerns with a consultation paper (DOH/HO, 1999), in which the major proposals were:

- The provision of arrangements for identification of dangerous severely personality disordered people and assessment of risk based on agreed national protocols
- A case management system for those who have been assessed
- Conditions for managing people in detention that protect the public and are safe for staff and those who are subject to detention; programmes for the management of dangerous severely personality disordered people, in detention and following discharge from detention, based on best practice including risk assessment.

Persons are regarded as falling within the category if they have antisocial and self-damaging behaviour which is, at least in part, a product of abiding character traits such as impulsivity and suspiciousness, combined with abnormalities of mental state, including instability of mood and dissociative symptoms. There has been criticism of the government's proposals in that they could have the effect of criminalizing those persons in need of treatment rather than punishment. There is also a risk that certain persons may be labelled indefinitely as dangerous. While the Home Affairs Select Committee supported the concept of a system separate, although linked to, hospitals and prisons, they commented that there was a need for considerable expenditure of resources. They indicated that stringent safeguards were necessary to ensure that the plans complied with the European Convention on Human Rights – particularly important in view of the fact that the Human Rights Act 1998 came into force in October 2000 (Home Affairs Select Committee, 2000). A private members' bill, the Dangerous People with Severe Personality Disorder Bill, was introduced into Parliament; however this Bill did not obtain further parliamentary time.

Reforming the Mental Health Act

A major report into the system of treatment and care for the mentally ill was published in 1999 (DOH, 1999a). Chaired by Professor Genevra Richardson, the committee recommended a total reform of the 1983 Act. In their consultation document responding to the Richardson review, the government, while accepting some of the proposals, were by no means sympathetic to the whole report (DOH, 1996b). The report set out a series of principles that would underpin the proposed legislation. In their response to Richardson, the government endorsed this approach and proposed a series of principles:

1. informal care and treatment should always be considered before recourse to compulsory powers
2. patients should be involved as far as possible in the process of developing and reviewing their own care and treatment plans
3. the safety of both the individual patient and the public are of key importance in determining the question of whether compulsory powers should be imposed
4. where compulsory powers are used, care and treatment should be located in the least restrictive setting consistent with the patient's best interests and safety and the safety of the public.

This is more restrictive than the list of principles contained in the Richardson review, such as patient autonomy, consensual care, reciprocity, respect for diversity, equality, respect for carers, effective communication and provision of information, and a principle of evidence-based practice. While the government acknowledged their importance, it was of the view that these should be enshrined in a Code of Practice because some of these principles were already covered by primary legislation while others, such as clinical governance, were contained in existing government strategies. The government was concerned that the balance of rights and interests could be upset if these principles were given statutory force.

The committee proposed that the new legislation should apply to those with a 'mental disorder', and that this should refer to 'any disability or disorder of mind or brain, whether permanent or temporary, which results in an impairment or disturbance of mental functioning'. This definition is in line with that proposed by the Law Commission (1995) in their report, *Mental Incapacity*. The review proposed that certain disorders should be

excluded from the general definition – namely disorders of sexual preference (such as paedophilia), and misuse of alcohol and drugs. It would
thus encompass those persons suffering from mental illness, for example,
schizophrenia; it would also cover persons with a primary diagnosis of
personality disorder, brain injury, or learning disability.

The Richardson review proposed that there would be formal assessment before compulsory care/treatment could be imposed (here the discussion focuses upon the recommendations made regarding civil powers).
This assessment on the recommendation of three professionals could last
for up to seven days with provision for application for a further twenty-
one days to an independent reviewer. It also recommended that there
should be an application to an independent tribunal for the imposition of
care and of treatment of greater than 28 days. It would go further than the
existing powers to consider whether detention criteria are met on that day
to looking at the basis for continued use of compulsory powers. It would
consider evidence such as information from the formal assessment
process, and involve scrutiny of the proposed plan for continuing care and
treatment. The government in its response, concerned about the practical
and resource implications, invited consultation as to whether independent
review was needed after seven days.

One feature of the new reforms is that of the enhanced role of the
Mental Health Review Tribunal. The new Mental Disorder Tribunal
would play a part both in the admission of patients and also in relation to
appeal and discharge. The structure of this proposed tribunal was the
subject of consultation by the government.

While the 1983 and 1995 Acts provided some powers in relation to care
in the community context, these are, as noted above, limited in scope,
with no effective powers for compulsion. The Richardson review recommended that there should be power to make a compulsory order in the
community replacing the existing system under sections 2, 3 and 4 of the
1983 Act. The same criteria would apply whether the order was to take
effect in hospital or in the community. The proposal has the merit of being
very flexible; it allows for compulsory care to be provided, as now, on an
in-patient basis, and it also allows for continuing compulsory care following a period in hospital and for the initiation of compulsory care
outside the hospital setting. At the same time some have reservations
regarding the civil liberties implications.

The Richardson Committee emphasized a capacity-based test in relation to care and treatment decisions. It recommended that in authorizing
compulsory care and treatment, the tribunal should apply differential criteria in cases in which patients did or did not possess capacity. They proposed a higher threshold, which would have to be established in a situation
in which the patient did possess capacity with a treatability criteria. The
government was unhappy regarding the emphasis the committee had
placed on capacity, and saw the crucial issue in many cases as being that
of 'risk'. The government stated that issues relating to the safety of the

individual patient and the public are of key importance in determining the question of whether compulsory powers should be imposed (see Chapter 3). Although assessment of capacity would still be integral to assessment of needs it would not be a primary factor in determining whether a compulsory order should be made. The government proposed an alternative which, in contrast to the Richardson proposals, did not take into account different thresholds of risk in relation to different tests of capacity. The government propose that compulsory treatment may be imposed if there is:

- the presence of a mental disorder which is of such seriousness that the patient requires care and treatment under the supervision of specialist mental health services; and
- that the care and treatment proposed for the mental disorder and the conditions resulting from it is the least restrictive alternative available consistent with safe and effective care; and
- that the proposed care and treatment cannot be implemented without the use of compulsory power; and is necessary for the health or safety of the patient and/or is necessary for the protection of others from serious harm and/or is necessary for the protection of the patient from serious harm.

As far as compulsory treatments are concerned both Richardson and the government have proposed that treatment for mental disorder should be left undefined in contrast to the present situation. Certain treatments though would be subject to specific safeguards – largely those already covered by section 57 of the 1983 Act. Again, as with the present situation certain treatments such as psychosis and hormone implants would require the introduction of specific safeguards. However, the government controversially rejected the inclusion of ECT in this category (Laing, 2000).

The chair of the expert committee, Professor Genevra Richardson, has expressed her concerns regarding the government's response in terms of the limited time-scale for consultation and the fact that it ignores many of the main principles behind the structure of the proposals. Richardson commented that:

> The government sees the whole thing turning on the question of risk, with the safety of the public as the dominant issue, rather than the safety and interests of the patient, other patients or the care staff. They see our capacity/incapacity test as less able to control that risk than their test, and see no need to justify further the discrimination against people with mental illness. The question of patient autonomy is nowhere (Jackson, 2000).

It remains to be seen whether the proposals for reform of care and treatment of those with mental incapacity, mental illness and within the group classified as having a dangerous personality disorder will be given parliamentary time. Reform is to be welcomed, but the present proposals have considerable limitations. The balance too is very much on the axis of risk and of public safety rather than of patient autonomy. It is likely that these are issues that will almost certainly need to be revisited in the light of the Human Rights Act 1998.

References

Bartlett, P. and Sandland, R. (2000). *Mental Health Law Policy and Practice*. Blackstone Press.

Bate, P. (1995). Children on secure psychiatric units: out of sight out of mind. *J. Child Law*, 131.

Bingley, W. (1995). The Mental Health Act Commission. *Health Director*, 14.

Department of Health (1993a). *Legal Powers of the Care of Mentally Ill People in the Community*. DOH.

Department of Health (1993b). *Guidance for Staff on Relations with the Public and the Media*. DOH.

Department of Health (1999a). *Report of the Expert Committee: Review of the Mental Health Act 1983*. DOH.

Department of Health (1999b). *Reform of the Mental Health Act 1983: Proposals for Consultation*. DOH.

Department of Health/Home Office (1999). *Managing Dangerous Persons with Severe Personality Disorder*. Home Office.

Dimond, B. and Barker, F. (1996). *Mental Health Law for Nurses*. Blackwell Scientific.

Fennell, P. (1994). Statutory authority to treat. *Med. Law Rev.*, **2**, 30.

Gostin, L. O. (1985). *Mental Health Services Law and Practice*. Shaw and Sons.

Grubb, A. (2000). Incompetent patient (child): HIV testing and best interests. *Med. Law Rev.*, **8**, 120.

Gunn, M. J. (1986). Mental Health Act guardianship: where now? *J. Social Welfare Law*, 144.

Gunn, M. J. (1995). Mental health nursing law. In: *Nursing Law and Ethics* (J. Tingle and A. Cribb, eds). Blackwells, pp. 158–191.

Gunn, J. (1999). *Br. Med. J.*, **319**, 1146–7.

Gunn, M. J. and Rodgers, L. (2001). Mental health nursing law. In: *Nursing Law and Ethics*, 2nd edn (J. Tingle and A. Cribb, eds). Blackwell Scientific (in print).

Hoggett, B. (1996). *Mental Health Law*, 4th edn. Sweet and Maxwell.

Home Affairs Select Committee (2000). *Managing People with Severe Personality Disorder*, third special report. Home Office. Also at http://www.publications.parliament.uk.

Jackson, C. (2000). Playing fast and loose; Genevra Richardson has serious reservations about the government's proposed mental health legislation. *Mental Health Learning Disabil. Care*, **3(5)**.

Laing, J. (2000). Rights versus risk; reforms of the Mental Health Act 1983. *Med.Law Rev.*, **8**, 210.

Law Commission (1995). *Mental Incapacity*. Law Com. Report No. 231, HMSO.

UKCC (1996). *Guidelines for Professional Practice*. UKCC.

Unsworth, C. (1987). *The Politics of Mental Health Legislation*. Clarendon Press, p. 332.

Further reading

Brazier, M. and Bridge, C. (1996). Coercion or caring: analysing adolescent autonomy. *Legal Studies*, **16**, 84.

Grubb, A. (ed.) (1993). Treatment decision: keeping it in the family. In: *Choices and Decisions in Health Care*. Wiley.

McHale, J., Fox, M. and Murphy, J. (1997). *Health Care Law Text and Materials*. Sweet and Maxwell, Chapters 7 and 9.

Chapter 7

Confidentiality and access to health care records

Jean McHale

Introduction

Confidentiality has long been emphasized in nursing practice. The Nightingale oath provided that (Nightingale, 1859):

> ... every nurse should be one who is to be depended upon, in other words, capable of being a 'confidential' nurse ... she must be no gossip; no vain talker; she should never answer questions about her sick except to those who have a right to ask them; she must, I need not say be strictly sober and honest; but more than this, she must be a religious and devoted woman; she must have a respect for her calling.

Confidentiality is still a fundamental part of nursing today. However, as health care has grown in sophistication and complexity, so the boundaries of confidentiality have become increasingly difficult to define. Instead of receiving treatment all their life from one family doctor, today patients are usually cared for in a group practice. During their time with that practice they may be seen by many different doctors and nurses. If they are given care in hospital, the number of persons treating them will be considerably larger. The difficulty in maintaining confidentiality was graphically illustrated by Marc Siegler, an American physician and academic (Siegler, 1987). One of Siegler's patients threatened to leave hospital if he was not told just how many people did have access to his medical records. Siegler went away and came back with a figure of some 75 people – doctors, nurses, etc., who had legitimate access to his medical records; that did not include, of course, those who might have obtained unauthorized access. This patient was receiving relatively straightforward treatment. It is perhaps no wonder that, after being told this, the patient retorted, 'Perhaps you could explain just what you mean by confidentiality?'. The maintenance of confidentiality may also be particularly problematic as health care professionals may work caring for patients alongside other professionals drawn from, for example, social work, housing and education.

This chapter examines the nurse's obligation to maintain her or his patient's confidence (difficulties relating to disclosure of the health care professional's own medical information to patients are examined in a later chapter). The first part examines the general obligation of patient confidentiality, and the second considers those situations in which health care information may be disclosed. Next, the problems facing nurses when there are conflicts between maintaining patient confidentiality and upholding standards of care are discussed. Finally, safeguards for the confidentiality of health care records are discussed, including on what basis a patient may obtain access to such records.

General obligations

Nurses have an obligation to keep patient information confidential. This obligation covers both information disclosed to them directly and information which they obtain from other health care professionals when treating the patient. The obligation of confidentiality is contained in the nurses' professional ethical code. The United Kingdom Central Council for Nursing, Midwifery and Health Visiting code provides that the nurse must:

> ... protect all confidential information concerning patients and clients obtained in the course of professional practice and make disclosures only with consent, where required by the order of the court or where you can justify disclosure in the wider public interest.

The extent of this obligation is explored further in guidance issued by the UKCC (UKCC, 1996). Secondly, the nurses' contract of employment requires them to keep patient information confidential. Unauthorized disclosure may lead nurses to be disciplined by their professional body or to be dismissed by their employer. Thirdly, where information has been disclosed in breach of an obligation of confidence legal proceedings may follow, such as an injunction being obtained to stop further publication of the confidential information. For example, in *X* v. *Y* ([1988] 2 All ER 648) the medical records of two general practitioners who had developed AIDS were disclosed in a national newspaper. The court issued an injunction to stop further publication of the records. To bring legal proceedings for breach of confidence, the patient must show that a duty of confidence, either express or implied, has arisen, that the information was given in confidence and that disclosure was made in breach of that duty (*Att. Gen* v. *Guardian Newspaper (No 2)* [1988] 3 All ER 545). A duty of confidence would be implied in a situation in which a patient discloses information to a nurse because of her or his status as a nurse.

Nurses are thus obliged in both law and professional practice to keep the patient's confidence. However, this obligation is not regarded as absolute; in some situations nurses may legitimately break confidence. In addition, nurses may be required to break confidentiality by court order or by specific statutory provision. These issues will be examined further below.

Children and confidentiality

What right does a child patient have to confidentiality? It is ludicrous to suggest that a nurse shouldn't discuss a toddler's illness with the child's mother. However, children grow and begin to express the wish to control aspects of their own lives. If a 14-year-old girl approaches a school nurse and asks for advice regarding contraceptive treatment, what should the nurse do?

In *Gillick* v. *West Norfolk and Wisbech AHA* ([1986] AC 150), Mrs Victoria Gillick sought an assurance from her local health authority that her daughter would not be given advice concerning contraception/abortion or receive treatment without her consent. The authority refused to give the assurance, and Mrs Gillick went to court and asked for a declaration that the authority's decision and the guidance of the DHSS on which the authority's refusal was based were unlawful. She was unsuccessful in her application. In the House of Lords, it was said that the child is able to consent to medical treatment where he or she has sufficient maturity to do so.

While the *Gillick* case was primarily concerned with consent to treatment, nevertheless it appears to be the case that this approach would be followed in relation to confidentiality (Grubb and Pearl, 1986; Montgomery, 1987). A health professional should not usually disclose information in the case of a *Gillick* competent child to a third party without that child's consent. This does give rise to some difficult issues as to whether a child has sufficient competence to consent (see Chapter 6). Where the child patient is very young, disclosure of information to the parents may be an integral part of the child's care. Nevertheless, the nurse should think long and hard before deciding to disclose a child's medical information without the child's consent.

The incompetent patient

The extent to which an obligation of confidence is owed to a patient who is permanently incompetent, such as a mentally handicapped patient, is unclear. In the absence of decided authority, it is submitted that it is likely that the general position taken by the House of Lords in the context of consent to treatment in the case of *Re F* ([1990] 1 AC 1) should be followed, and that information may be disclosed only where it is in that patient's best interests to do so.

After the patient's death

The obligation of confidentiality continues after the patient's death. When Lord Moran, Winston Churchill's physician, published a book that discussed the decline of the great war leader (*Churchill – The Struggle for Survival*), he was roundly condemned by his contemporaries. As Mason and McCall Smith (1999i) note, confidentiality after death is something that may be of particular importance in the age of AIDS. However, while maintenance of confidentiality after death may be part of the professional's ethical obligation, it is less certain whether legal proceedings could be brought in such circumstances. An action for libel and slander cannot be brought after the death of the person who has been defamed. It has been suggested that a court might reject a claim of breach of confidence brought after the patient's death on the basis that the obligation only existed during that patient's lifetime (Kennedy and Grubb, 1994).

Grounds for disclosure

Patient care would be impossible unless some disclosure of information were made. Certain recognized exceptions do exist. Nevertheless, the nurse should be aware that all disclosures should be carefully justified.

Disclosing with consent

Disclosure is both lawful and complies with professional ethical codes if the patient has given consent to the information being passed on. Such consent must be freely and fully given. However, in practice this may not always be the case. As Mason and McCall Smith (1999ii) comment:

> What patient at a teaching hospital out-patients department is likely to refuse when the consultant asks 'You don't mind these young doctors being present, do you?' – the pressures are virtually irresistible and truly autonomous consent is impossible.

It can be argued that when patients enter hospital they imply consent to such information as is necessary for their treatment being passed to other health care practitioners. However, consent to disclosure should not always be presumed. The UKCC (1996i) state in their document *Guidelines for Professional Practice* that:

> It is impractical to obtain the consent of patient or client every time you need to share information with other health professionals or other staff involved in the health care of that patient or client. What is important is that the patient or client understands that some information may be made available to others involved in the delivery of their care. However, the patient or client must know who the information would be shared with.

The Department of Health (1996) has provided, in guidance:

> All NHS bodies must have an active policy for informing patients of the kind of purposes for which information about them is collected and the categories of people or organizations to which information may need to be passed.

The nurse must ensure that from the onset of care patients are aware that some information may be disclosed to third parties who are involved in their care. Where disclosure is necessary, then information should be disclosed on a 'need to know' basis. The Department of Health (1996) suggests that this includes NHS purposes where:

> … the recipient needs the information because he or she is or may be concerned with the patient's care or treatment (or that of another patient whose health may be affected by the condition of the original patient, such as a blood or organ donor).

Public interest exception

The courts have held that in some situations disclosure of confidential information is justifiable in the public interest. The UKCC Code also recognizes a public interest exception. What amounts to disclosure in the public interest by a health care professional was examined by the courts in *W* v. *Egdell* ([1990] ChD 359). A breach of confidence action was brought against a psychiatrist. He had been commissioned by W's solicitors to make a medical report on W's fitness for discharge from the secure hospital where he had been detained after he was convicted of manslaughter 8 years previously. The report was highly unfavourable to W, and W's solicitors withdrew their application to a Mental Health Review Tribunal. Dr Egdell told the solicitors that he believed that a copy of the report should be put on W's hospital file. The solicitors disagreed. Dr Egdell himself sent a copy to the hospital. This fact emerged at a subsequent Mental Health Review Tribunal hearing, and W brought an action for breach of confidence against Dr Egdell.

The case was first heard in the High Court. Scott J. rejected the claim that Dr Egdell was wrong to have disclosed the information. In his opinion the doctor owed a duty not only to W but also to the public. This required him to place before the proper authorities the result of his examination of W. He placed weight upon the fact that while in detention W had been seen by a number of psychiatrists. Each of these owed him a duty of confidence such that they could not, for example, sell the information to a newspaper, but at the same time the reports compiled about W were on file and were available to the Home Office. In the view of Scott J., the fact that these reports were on file had not inhibited W in his dealings with these psychiatrists. He did not believe that the report of Dr Egdell should be treated any differently.

W appealed to the Court of Appeal, where his appeal was rejected. Sir

Stephen Brown was broadly in agreement with the first instance decision. Disclosure of the information was in the public interest in ensuring the safety of the public as a whole. The effect of suppressing the material contained in the report would have been to deprive both the hospital and the Secretary of State of vital information. The other judge to deliver a full judgment in this case, Bingham J., was more cautious. He stressed that a patient such as W, who was held under a restriction order, had a very great need for recourse to an independent and discreet professional adviser. The confidentiality of such patients should only be broken if needed on the basis of the doctor's duty to society. On the facts of this particular case, Bingham J. held that disclosure had been justified. The decisive facts were that:

> Where a man has committed multiple killings under the disability of serious mental illness, decisions which may lead directly or indirectly to his release from hospital should not be made unless a responsible authority is able to make an informed judgment that the risk of repetition is so small as to be acceptable.

W v. *Egdell* clearly illustrates that confidentiality in law is far from an absolute obligation. In each case, the court will balance the public interest in ensuring confidentiality against the public interest in disclosure. In determining public interest, the courts will make reference to the guidelines set out by the health care professionals. Nurses are given some guidance as to circumstances that may justify disclosure in the public interest by the UKCC (1996ii) in its document *Guidelines for Professional Practice*. This states that:

> The public interest means the interests of an individual, or groups of individuals or of society as a whole, and would, for example, cover matters such as serious crime, child abuse, drug trafficking or other activities which place others at serious risk.

It is fairly certain that disclosure to the appropriate authorities of the fact that a patient has a mental illness which makes him a potential danger to the community will be held to be in the public interest. Similarly, if a nurse was told of child abuse and disclosed this information to an agency such as the NSPCC it is likely that a court would hold that the disclosure was in the public interest. Nevertheless, there are other situations in which it is not clear whether the public interest justifies disclosure. A nurse who discovers that a patient has committed shoplifting offences should hesitate long before disclosing that fact. Again, the nurse may face a dilemma if a patient divulges that he knows the identity of the person who stabbed him but does not want the nurse to give this information to the police because of fear of retaliation from a gang of thugs. In such a situation the nurse should attempt to persuade the patient to approach the police himself.

What if a patient who is diagnosed as HIV positive refuses to tell his wife? Should the nurse or any other health care professional inform the man's wife? The man may be frightened that his marriage will break up if his wife is told. The General Medical Council has advised doctors that disclosure may be justifiable if there is a serious and identifiable risk to a specific individual (GMC, 1995). The legal position here is unclear, but it is suggested that if disclosure did take place a court would be prepared to hold that the breach of confidence was in the public interest.

Police enquiries

A police constable comes into hospital reception. He wants to ask questions of the ward sister and to search through a particular patient's medical records. Can he do this?

First, if the ward sister is asked questions she is under no obligation to answer them. In English law there is no general obligation placed upon any citizen to answer questions put to them by the police (*Rice* v. *Connolly* [1966] 2 QB 416), although if a defendant keeps silent there is a possibility that an adverse inference may be drawn regarding the decision to keep silent (Criminal Justice Act 1994). There are also some exceptional situations in which disclosure is required by statute. For example, under the Prevention of Terrorism (Temporary Provisions) Act 1989, a person can be prosecuted if he or she withholds information relating to acts of terrorism (s18). Secondly, the police have no automatic right to demand access to a patient's records. Access to medical records by police conducting enquiries is regulated by statute. Usually, before the police may examine a patient's medical records they must obtain a warrant under the Police and Criminal Evidence Act 1984 (PACE) (s9–s11 and schedule 1). Before a police constable can gain access to premises such as a doctor's surgery or a hospital in order to search for information such as medical records/samples of human tissue, or tissue fluid taken for the purpose of diagnosis/medical treatment or held in confidence, he or she must apply to a circuit judge for a warrant. The police must show that there is a reasonable belief that the information needed is contained on the premises and that prior to the 1984 Act a statute existed under which the police could have obtained the information. There is, however, no duty upon the police when applying for a warrant to inform the person whose confidential information is sought about the application. Only the person who is holding the information – in the case of hospital medical records, an administrator – must be told. It is submitted that this is undesirable and that the patient should, wherever possible, have a voice at the hearing. It appears that the courts have been prepared to scrutinize carefully applications for medical records. For example, in *R* v.

Cardiff Crown Court ex parte Kellam ((1993) 16 BMLR 76), the court refused to allow police who were investigating a murder of a mental patient to obtain access to records of admission, discharge and leave of patients at the hospital.

In practice if, for example, the police ask a nurse for access to medical records, the UKCC (1996iii) advises that 'it may be appropriate to involve senior staff if you do not feel that you are able to deal with the situation alone'.

Civil law proceedings

If a patient is injured due to what he or she claims is negligent treatment, the patient will need to obtain evidence in the form of, for example, medical reports to establish a case. The patient's lawyers will ask for access to the records. If this is refused, then an application must be made to the court under the Administration of Justice Act 1970 for disclosure of documents. Section 32 makes particular reference to records that are sought in a personal injury action. Here, the court can order that reports are made available to the applicant, to his or her legal adviser or, if the applicant does not have a legal adviser, to his or her medical advisers (s33 and s34 Supreme Court Act 1981). As has been commented (Mason and McCall Smith, 1999iii):

> ... the court can deal with problems of confidentiality relating to irrelevant conditions – such as a past history of a sexually transmitted disease – by limiting disclosure to the other side's medical advisors, who must respect confidentiality save where litigation is affected.

In addition, disclosure of expert reports should be made at the pre-hearing stage (*Naylor* v. *Preston AHA* [1987] 2 All ER 353). (See Chapter 1 regarding the encouragement given to broader disclosure and agreement between experts prior to trial following the Woolf Report.) There are, however, exceptions to the general requirements of disclosure. For example, communications between a claimant and his or her lawyer are usually not required to be disclosed. Such communications are covered by what is known as 'legal professional privilege'. In very limited situations information may be withheld because it is in the public interest not to disclose that information (*Re HIV Haemophiliac Litigation* [1990] NLJR 1349).

Evidence in court

If a nurse is summoned as a witness in a court case, he or she must give evidence. There is no special rule of evidence – no evidential 'privilege' that would entitle the nurse to refuse to testify (McHale, 1993; *Duchess of Kingston's case* (1776) 20 State Trials 355). The nurse is protected, in disclosing in the courtroom, from an action being brought by a patient on the basis of breach of confidence (*Watson* v *McEwan* [1905] AC 480). If the nurse refuses to disclose any information in response to any question put to him or her, then a judge may find the nurse in contempt of court and may ultimately send the nurse to prison.

Public health disclosure requirements

In some situations, disclosure of medical information is required by statute as a public health measure in order to limit the spread of certain diseases. Notifiable diseases include cholera, plague, smallpox, typhus, and rabies (s11 Public Health (Control of Disease) Act 1984). Where a registered medical practitioner becomes aware or suspects that a patient he or she is attending is suffering from such an illness, the practitioner must notify the local authority of the patient's name, age, sex, the disease from which the patient is suffering, and the date of onset of the disease.

Release of information without patient's permission

The UKCC (1996iv), in its document *Guidelines for Professional Practice*, suggests that before information is disclosed without a patient's consent the nurse should consult with colleagues, and it may also be appropriate to consult an organization such as the UKCC. If it is decided to disclose, the UKCC suggests that the nurse should record the reasons for disclosure, and thus the justification for any action taken, in the appropriate record or in a special note in a separate file.

Unauthorized disclosures

Unauthorized disclosures should be minimized. It is unethical to discuss a patient's case outside the clinical setting with friends, or to discuss a case with colleagues in public where there is the chance of being overheard. In hospital, records should never be left lying around where unauthorized persons may read them. It is important to ensure that safeguards exist against disclosure, particularly where a patient is, for example, suffering from AIDS. A minimal number of clinical staff necessary to facilitate that patient's care should be informed that the patient is HIV positive. Nurses have also been advised by the RCN to avoid giving information over the telephone because of the problem of verifying the identity of the caller, and also the risk of being overheard (RCN, 1991).

Occupational health context

Nurses employed by organizations other than the NHS may face some very difficult disclosure dilemmas. Take, for example, the occupational health nurse employed by a large industrial firm. The nurse owes a duty to the employer, but at the same time, as a caring professional, is bound by professional ethical code. If the nurse intends that the information given by the patient being treated should be disclosed to the employer, then the nurse must make this clear to the patient before undertaking the consultation.

Genetic information and maintaining confidentiality

One category of personal information that has led to particular concern regarding disclosure is that of genetic information. The sequencing of the human genome has been hailed as one of the great scientific achievements in recent years. Nonetheless, there is concern that the enhanced availability of genetic information may lead to individuals being subject to discriminatory treatment by, for example, insurers and employers, on the basis that they have some propensity to develop disease in the future. There has been discussion regarding the prospect of the introduction of specific legislation governing control of disclosure of genetic information (Nuffield Council on Bioethics, 1993; House of Commons Select Committee on Science and Technology, 1995). At present insurers do not require individuals to obtain a genetic test before obtaining insurance; however, this situation may change in the future (Human Genetics Advisory Commission, 1997). The discriminatory use of genetic information in a situation in which the condition has not yet manifested itself is presently not protected by the Disability Discrimination Act 1995. This may be subject to challenge under the Human Rights Act 1998 in relation to Article 8 of the European Convention on Human Rights – the right to privacy of home and family life.

In the context of the family, genetics again provides potential for considerable dilemmas. Take a situation in which a woman is screened during pregnancy and this reveals that she is the carrier of a genetic disorder. This information may be of assistance to her sister, who is contemplating pregnancy. The woman may of course be perfectly happy for the information to be disclosed to her sister, but what if she objects? In such a situation, could the midwife legitimately take the decision to breach the patient's confidentiality? One approach is to say that this is not simply an issue of individual confidentiality but that, as the Nuffield Council on Bioethics noted, in certain clearly defined contexts it might be appropriate to treat the family as a unit (Nuffield, 1993). The Nuffield Council suggested that where disease would cause grave danger to family members, an attempt should be made to ensure that the information is disclosed voluntarily, but that in exceptional situations information could be disclosed by health professionals to other family members despite an expressed wish for confidentiality. It remains to be seen how a court would regard such a disclosure. In the past, cases have focused on matters such as whether harm will be caused – but can harm here be easily detected? As has been commented by Boddington, this differs substantially from a situation in which the disclosure relates to an infectious disease:

... steps to prevent the incidence of genetic disorder in the population consist, not exclusively but in the main, not in ensuring that individuals do not acquire the disorder but in ensuring that individuals who would have that disorder are not born in the first place. Thus the population is not being protected from an outside danger; it could be said that it is being protected from the costs of bearing certain individuals amongst its number and also that, for certain types of individuals with certain genetic conditions, it is itself a bad thing to be born. It is also of course quite fallacious to think of genetic disease as 'spreading' in the population in the way that an infectious disease might spread.

The woman may be objecting to disclosure for a number of different reasons. It may be the case that the reason for refusal of disclosure is malicious, or it could be the case that disclosure would reveal compromising information about paternity. Disclosure could harm the woman, not only because of the breach of confidentiality but also because of the impact on the relationship with the man involved. It is also the case that by informing the woman's sister she may be provided with information that she herself does not want. She may be herself making a conscious choice not to discover certain genetic information. There has been much discussion of the 'right not to know' our genetic information (Chadwick *et al.*, 1997). It is worth noting that the Council of Europe in the Convention for the Protection of Human Rights and Dignity of the Human Being with regard to the Application of Biology and Medicine provides that:

> Everyone is entitled to know any information collected about his or her health. However the wishes of individuals not to be so informed shall be observed.

Ultimately, of course, these are specific decisions to be made in relation to individual cases. There is no single rule that can be laid down, and were the matter to arise in the courtroom the court would obviously take into account all the circumstances in determining whether the public interest militated in favour of disclosure. Genetics is in its infancy, and the approach to such dilemmas may well change as there is greater knowledge of the development of certain diseases and disabilities and if there is the greater prospect for obtaining a cure for such conditions.

Legal obligation to break confidence?

Can the nurse ever be required to disclose information and be held liable in negligence if he or she does not do so? What if a patient tells a nurse of his or her wish to harm another person; should that nurse warn the person who might be in danger? This issue arose in the USA in the case of *Tarasoff* v. *Regents of the University of California* ([1976] 551 P 2d 334). Poddar, a university student, sought out patient care in a psychiatric hospital. He was suffering from deep depression as a result of being rejected by one Miss Tarasoff, with whom he had fallen in love. He told a psychologist at the hospital of his intention to kill Miss Tarasoff. After discussions with psychiatrists, the psychologist decided that Podder should be detained in a mental hospital. He told the campus police, who detained Poddar but later released him when he appeared to be rational. Two months after the consultation with the psychologist, Poddar killed Miss Tarasoff. The majority in the Californian Supreme Court held that the therapist was under a duty to warn both the victim and her family, and was liable for his failure to do so.

The *Tarasoff* case led to an outcry from psychiatric associations in the USA. The court reconsidered its decision some 18 months later, and modified the duty from one to warn the victim to one of exercising reasonable care for the victim's protection and taking steps reasonably necessary in the circumstances. In a memorable phrase, it was said that the 'protective privilege ends when the public peril begins'.

There are echoes of *Tarasoff* in the judgment of Scott J. in the English case of *W* v. *Egdell*, a judgment which received the approval of Sir Stephen Brown in the Court of Appeal. Scott J. held that:

> In my view a doctor called upon as Dr Egdell was to examine a patient owes a duty not only to his patient, but also to the public. His duty to the public would require him, in my opinion, to place before the proper authorities the results of his examination if, in his opinion, the public interest so requires.

What did Scott J. mean here by the duty to disclose? Will a court in future be prepared to find that a health care professional owes a duty of care to the person the patient claims that he or she is going to kill or seriously injure? At present it seems unlikely that an English court would impose such an obligation. The courts have been unwilling in the past to extend the scope of liability imposed upon third parties (*Smith* v. *Littlewood* [1987] 1 All ER 710; *Palmer* v. *Tees HA* [1999] Lloyds Rep Med 351 CA). Any obligation to disclose may limit an individual's privacy if practitioners feel that they must go ahead and disclose to avoid being sued in negligence.

Negotiated confidentiality

Confidentiality is an important obligation but, as has been seen, determining the boundaries may prove problematic. One suggestion that has been advanced is that the practice of 'negotiated confidentiality' could be adopted (Thompson, 1979; Sieghart, 1982). In this, the practitioner and patient discuss the extent to which patient information should remain confidential. They negotiate as to what information may be disclosed and what information may not. One major advantage is that negotiation removes much uncertainty – both parties know the ground rules for disclosure. However, such an approach is not without difficulties. It involves effort and understanding, and there is also the danger that when the negotiations were undertaken some criteria relating to disclosure had not been envisaged. Negotiation is also time-consuming, and it may not be a practical prospect in many situations.

Confidentiality – specific obligations

In addition to the general obligations spelt out above, certain specific obligations of confidentiality have been imposed by statute.

Human Fertilization and Embryology Act 1990

Few statutes expressly require patient confidentiality to be maintained, but one exception is the Human Fertilization and Embryology Act 1990. This Act regulates the provision of new reproductive technology services. Information relating to infertility treatment is particularly sensitive. Section 33 of the 1990 Act places a statutory ban upon the disclosure of information concerning gamete donors and patients receiving treatment under the Act. Unauthorized disclosure of such information by health care professionals and others has been made a criminal offence (1990 Act s40(1)(5)).

There are certain exceptions to the general obligation. The clinician at the *in vitro* fertility (IVF) unit may disclose information where the patient has consented to that disclosure to a specific person (1990 Act s33 (6B)), or where it is necessary to disclose the information to a person who 'needs to know' for the purposes of treating the patient, or where a medical emergency has arisen, or in connection with clinical or accounts audits (1990 Act s33(6c)). This statutory exception is itself the source of some controversy, particularly in view of the fact that it is now routine practice in IVF clinics to require patients to take HIV tests. It is questionable whether a patient's GP is entitled to know that his or her patient has tested HIV positive. This is another instance in which 'need to know' should be tightly interpreted.

Venereal disease

Legislation restricting disclosure of patient information also exists in the area of venereal diseases. The National Health Service Venereal Disease Regulations (SI 1974 No. 29) provide that health authorities should take all necessary steps to ensure that identifiable information relating to persons being treated for sexually transmitted diseases should not be disclosed. Such information may be disclosed where this is for the purpose of communicating the information to a doctor caring for the patient, or to a person working under the direction of that doctor to treat that condition or to prevent its spread.

Conflicts between confidentiality and the need to uphold standards of care – whistleblowing in the NHS

> A nurse is concerned by the poor staffing levels in her ward and is concerned at the standard of care being provided. She raises some concerns with her colleagues, but feels that what she has said has fallen largely on deaf ears. What should she do?

The whole issue of health care professionals wanting to go public and 'blow the whistle' on what they regard as being unacceptable standards of care has caused a furore over recent years. From the well-known case of Graham Pink, a nurse in Stockport (see below), to Stephen Boisin, regarding the deaths of children during cardiac surgery at Bristol Royal Infirmary, incidents of whistleblowing have rarely been far from the headlines.

The UKCC Code requires the nurse to report circumstances in which the standard of care given has fallen below levels that are acceptable.

> According the UKCC Code:
>
> As a registered nurse, midwife and health visitor you are personally accountable for your practice and, in the exercise of your professional accountability, must:
>
> 11. report to an appropriate person or authority having regard to the physical, psychological and social effects on patients and clients any circumstances in the environment of care which could jeopardise safe standards of practice;
> 12. report to an appropriate person or authority any circumstances in which safe and appropriate care for patients and clients cannot be provided;
> 13. report to an appropriate person or authority where it appears that the health and safety of colleagues is at risk, as such circumstances may compromise standards of practice and care.

In their document *Guidelines for Professional Practice* (UKCC, 1996v), the UKCC comments that this is a statement of the minimum action to be taken, and that (UKCC, 1996vi):

> You must not be deterred from reporting your concerns, even if you believe that resources are not available or that no action will be taken. You should make your report, verbally and/or in writing, and where available, follow local procedures. The manager (who may also be reg-

istered with us) should assess the report and communicate it to senior managers where appropriate.

This record may be of importance if subsequent action is taken against the nurse and he or she claims that the actions he or she took were affected by the fact that there were inadequate resources.

There may be instances in which the obligation of confidentiality owed by nurse to patient may conflict with the nurse's belief that standards of patient care had fallen. This problem arose in the case of Graham Pink. Pink was a charge nurse who believed that standards of hospital services provided to his elderly patients were unsatisfactory. Although he complained within the management structure, he did not believe that his complaints had been addressed. He was concerned about:

> ... avoidable injuries to patients (including a death); important observations for people on blood transfusions not carried out; patients offered a wash once a day. ... (Letter to the Chairman of Stockport Health Authority; *The Guardian*, 9 July 1991)

Thus, as a result of obtaining no response to his complaints, Pink made the decision to go public about his concerns: he wrote letters to *The Guardian* newspaper, and he gave an interview to a local paper. The Health Authority brought disciplinary proceedings against him on the basis of breach of patient confidentiality. Although the article did not name patients, relatives claimed that a patient could be identified from details of his case given in the press report. Pink was also charged with not reporting an incident in which a patient fell out of bed. At the disciplinary hearing the allegations were upheld against Pink, and when he refused to transfer to a post of community nurse he was dismissed (*The Guardian*, 18 Sept. 1991).

As the Pink case shows, the threat of dismissal for breach of confidentiality is a very real one. Pink challenged his dismissal at an industrial tribunal. A claim can be brought before a tribunal for unlawful dismissal on the grounds that the dismissal was unfair (s98 Employment Rights Act 1996). The tribunal decides whether the action taken by the employer was reasonable, and assesses the dismissal on the balance of competing equities. Pink's case was ultimately settled before any final decision was made by the tribunal.

If a nurse does not take action about what he or she regards as undesirably low standards, then the nurse runs the risk of being disciplined by the UKCC. The UKCC Code was claimed in his defence by Graham Pink. However, as Pink discovered, simply acting in accordance with the UKCC Code is by itself no defence should the employee's action breach the duty of employment.

NHS 'whistleblowing' guidelines

The government issued a document providing guidance for staff considering making complaints about what they regard as being poor standards of care (DOH, 1993). First, the guidelines stress that procedures should be set up to deal with staff grievances. Informal procedures should be available, but where these do not lead to a satisfactory resolution there should be formal procedures in existence to enable concerns to be aired. The formal complaints should be made either up the line management chain or to a designated officer, who may be the person designated to receive patient complaints. This has been criticized in that staff may be frightened to make such a reference because of the consequences for their own careers if they are regarded as being troublemakers. As Public Concern at Work (an organization funded by the Rowntree Trust to support whistleblowers both inside and outside the NHS) commented in relation to the draft guidelines (McHale, 1994):

> To require a concerned member of staff to confront his or her line manager on their judgment or priorities in this way is unlikely to be productive or conducive to a good working environment. Only the most exceptional manager would not, in such a situation, want to pull rank over the staff member concerned.

The guidelines distinguish between those health care professionals who are in a direct line management relationship and others not in such a relationship, such as consultants. In relation to the latter, it is suggested that they discuss their concerns with relevant colleagues and then take the matter up directly with the general manager or chief executive. This difference in approach may be seen as undesirable and indeed as divisive.

The guidelines suggest that if complaints are made to a designated officer and the matter is not resolved, then the issue should be referred to the chairman of the authority or trust for action to be taken. There is no external right of appeal, the highest level of appeal being within the existing management framework. The guidelines state that in some situations health care professionals may wish to consult with outside agencies. For example, where a nurse is concerned about the welfare of a patient detained under the Mental Health Act 1983, he or she may decide to take the complaint to the Mental Health Act Commission (see Chapter 6, p. 131).

The guidelines make reference to the fact that health professionals may raise concerns with the Health Service Commissioner (the Ombudsman). While at present the Commissioner may not receive general complaints from hospital staff concerning standards, nevertheless he has indicated that he is willing to receive complaints from staff if they are made on behalf of an individual patient, the patient himself is unable to complain, and there is no other person who could claim on the patient's behalf. In his 1991–1992 report, the Commissioner commented that he had undertaken an investigation of a complaint brought by a member of staff indicating that the level of care a patient was receiving was inadequate (Health Service Commissioner, 1992). Access to the Commissioner may indeed be a helpful way of airing staff concerns. However, the

Commissioner's office has only limited resources, and it may take a certain amount of time for a claim to be processed.

One welcome provision of the guidelines is the right to consult a professional agency such as a trade union or other representative agency (DOH, 1993, clause 23). Health care professionals may of course also raise their concerns with their MP. It is only at the very end of the guidelines that the question of disclosure to the media itself is considered. Such disclosure is regarded as a matter of last resort, and should the nurse make the decision to 'go public', as did Graham Pink, then the guidelines remind the nurse that he or she is at risk of disciplinary proceedings. The guidelines refer to the duty of confidentiality to preserve patient information and the duty of confidentiality and loyalty to the employer (DOH, 1993, clauses 8 and 9). Should a nurse find the internal mechanisms inadequate for dealing with concerns, then there is the option of going public, with the risk of legal and disciplinary proceedings should he or she do so.

The guidelines met with considerable opposition when they were originally published. Reg Pyne, former Assistant Registrar at the UKCC, called them 'seriously flawed' and 'oppressive' (Turner, 1994). While their publication can in one respect be regarded as an important step in recognizing that an important issue should be addressed, nevertheless, as was suggested above, in many ways they may be regarded as unsatisfactory.

Safeguarding whistleblowers in employment law – Public Interest Disclosure Act 1998

In response to the campaigns following celebrated cases such as that of Graham Pink, and the establishment of the organization Public Concern at Work, specific statutory protection was introduced in the form of the Public Interest Disclosure Act 1998. This safeguards a worker who makes what is known as a 'protected disclosure' under the Act (s43(B) Employment Rights Act 1996). Workers for the purposes of the Public Interest Disclosure Act 1998 are employees and also independent contractors who provide services outside a professional–client relationship (s43K Employment Rights Act 1996). Those who provide general medical, dental, ophthalmic and pharmaceutical services under NHS provision are specifically covered.

Protected disclosures include concerns regarding actual/apprehended breaches of law and dangers to health, safety and environment. Protection was already available in relation to disclosures concerning health and safety matters (Employment Rights Act 1996 ss 46 and 100). The worker must have a 'reasonable belief' that this is a protected disclosure (s43(B)(1) Employment Rights Act 1996). Disclosures made are protected if made in good faith to the employer, or to a person other than the employer if it relates to the conduct of that person, or concerns something for which that person has legal responsibility. In addition, a disclosure may be made to one of those bodies listed on a list produced by regulations under the Act by the

Secretary of State (S43(F) Employment Rights Act 1996).

There is also a second broad category of protected disclosures, and disclosures made to the media are likely to fall into this category. Protection is given to disclosures in this category where the disclosure has been made in good faith, the worker reasonably believes that the information disclosed and any allegations contained in it are substantially true, the disclosure is not made for any personal gain, and that in all the circumstances of the case it is reasonable for him to make the disclosure. In addition, the criteria in subsection (2) must be complied with. These are that the worker reasonably believes that the employer will subject him to a detriment if he makes the disclosure to his employer in accordance with section 43F, that he reasonably believes the evidence will be lost or destroyed if he makes a disclosure to the employer, or where there is no person who is prescribed under s43F to whom the worker could disclose in relation to this particular failure.

In this section, guidance is given as to what amounts to reasonableness in disclosure. Relevant factors include the person's identity and the seriousness of the failure, whether the failure is continuing or is likely to occur in the future, and whether the disclosure has been made in breach of a duty of confidentiality owed to the employer or to any other person.

Section 43H applies to disclosures that concern failures of an exceptionally serious nature, where the disclosure is made in good faith, the worker reasonably believes that the information that has been disclosed and any allegations contained in it are substantially true, the disclosure is not made for personal gain, and it is reasonable for the worker to make this disclosure in all the circumstances of the case. In determining the reasonableness of the disclosure for the purposes of this section, regard shall be had to the identity of the person to whom the disclosure is made (s42H (2)).

If a worker is dismissed for making a protected disclosure, this is automatically an unfair dismissal (s103 Employment Rights Act 1996). Protection is also given against victimization where this is 'on the grounds that a protected disclosure was made' (s47B Employment Rights Act 1996). This applies where the employer subjects the employee to action which is to his or her detriment, including failing to act (as, for example, in refusing promotion). The employer has the task of establishing the ground on which he or she subjected the employee to a detriment (s48(2) Employment Rights Act 1996). There is no limit on the award of compensation under the 1998 Act.

While such legislation gives some protection to the nurse it can be regarded very much as a measure of last resort. The prospects for reinstatement after the employment relationship has broken down are limited. It is preferable if concerns can be expressed by a culture of openness within the organization.

Gagging clauses

One of the concerns in the debate in the 1990s regarding whistleblowing in the NHS was the proliferation in the number of so-called 'gagging clauses'. These were contractual clauses imposed on NHS employees with the aim of stopping them from 'going public'. Such clauses are now prohibited by the Public Interest Disclosure Act 1998 in that they cannot stop a worker from making a protected disclosure (s43 J Employment Rights Act 1996).

Health care records – allowing patient access

In this section, the extent to which patients may access their own records and the particular obligations placed upon the nurse to maintain the security of these records against unauthorized disclosure to third parties is discussed. The 1980s saw a dramatic shift in policy, allowing patients access to their medical records. In the past, there was considerable opposition to patient access. There were several reasons for this. First, it was argued that the patient would have difficulty in understanding the records because they may have been compiled using technical terms or medical shorthand. Secondly, if health care professionals knew that a patient could gain access, they would not be so candid in their comments when compiling the records. Thirdly, it was argued that to allow access may be against the patient's interests because records may contain information that had been deliberately kept from the patient – for example, showing a terminal prognosis. However, these arguments met with criticism. It was claimed that access to records is a fundamental part of patient autonomy, and that the denial of access in the patient's best interests is a paternalistic approach. It was said that a blanket ban was wrong because, while some patients might be unable to cope with the information, this did not mean that all patients were unable to cope. If health care records were incomprehensible to patients this was not a basis for denying access; rather, it should be ensured that the records are comprehensible.

Statutory rights of access to health care records

Access to Medical Reports Act 1988

The Access to Medical Reports Act 1988 grants a statutory right of access to reports compiled for the purposes of employment or insurance (s2). Employers/insurers must obtain an individual's consent before obtaining the report (s3). This right covers only those reports made by a person who has had clinical care of the patient, and excludes one-off examinations specifically undertaken for the purposes of insurance by a clinician previously unknown to the patient. The patient who has requested that such a report be drawn up has the right to see the report. If the patient does not request the report, it cannot be sent off for 3 weeks (s4). If he or she believes it to be inaccurate, the patient may ask the doctor to amend it (s5). If the doctor refuses, then the patient can either refuse to allow the report to be sent to the employer or insurer, or can have his or her own comments added to the report.

Data Protection Act 1998

Prior to 2000, access to health care records was regulated predominantly under the Access to Health Records Act 1990 and the Data Protection Act 1984; the former applied to manually stored records created after 1991, while the latter related to those records stored electronically. The position has now changed (Data Protection Act 1998 (Commencement) Order 2000 SI 2000/183). The Data Protection Act 1998 gave effect to the European Directive on Personal Data, and repealed the Data Protection Act 1984 and most of the Access to Health Records Act 1990 (HSC 2000/009). It applies to access to both electronic and manual health records. Manual records are those that are part of a relevant filing system. This refers to information that is structured by reference to individuals (s1(1)). Information is also covered where this is part of an 'accessible record', which includes health records, defined in section 68(2) as:

any record which –

(a) consists of information relating to the physical or mental health of the individual, and
(b) has been made by or on behalf of a health professional in connection with care of that individual.

Health professionals include doctors, nurses, dentists, opticians and pharmacists (s69). The legislation covers processing of 'personal data' regarding 'data subjects' by 'data controllers'. 'Personal data' must relate to a living individual, and must identify that individual. Data controllers are required to comply with what are known as 'data protection principles', for example, in relation to the purposes for which data are processed, the accuracy of the data, and the fact that personal data shall be processed in accordance with the rights of data subjects under the legislation.

Enforcement

The legislation is subject to enforcement by the Data Protection Commissioner. Data subjects such as patients who believe that there is some error in the register may ask for the register to be rectified (s14), claim compensation for damage and distress (s10), and prevent processing of data that are likely to occasion distress or damage. In the case of a disputed decision between a person on whom a notice has been served and the Data Protection Commissioner, there is the provision for an appeal to the Data Protection Tribunal within 28 days of the notice relating to the disputed decision being served on the applicant (Data

Protection Tribunal (Enforcement Appeals) Rules 2000 SI 2000 No 189). At such an appeal hearing, the burden is on the Commissioner to satisfy the tribunal that the decision should be upheld.

Access rights

The data subject may apply for access to information under section 7 of the Act. The data controller must supply the information requested 'promptly', and there is a time limit imposed of 40 days (s7(8) and (10)). In a situation in which this information is not supplied, the data controller may be required to supply it by the court (s7(2)(a)). A fee may be requested, subject to a statutory maximum. Transitional provisions are applicable in situations where records are not exclusively automated or so intended up until 24 October 2001. The maximum fee where a permanent copy of the information is supplied is £50. However, where the request applies simply to data that form part of a health record, and the data were created in the 40 days that preceded the request and no permanent copy is going to be made, then no fee should be charged (Data Protection (Subject Access) (Fees and Miscellaneous Provisions) Regulations 2000, SI 2000 No 191). The subject may request a copy of the information which may include an explanation of any terms used.

Limitations on access rights

As with the Data Protection Act 1984 and the Access to Health Records Act 1990, access rights are not absolute. Access to health care records may be withheld in situations where the information is likely to cause serious harm to the patient's physical or mental health or condition or that of another person. Where the data controller is not a health professional, he or she must either consult the health professional who has responsibility for the patient's care or, if this person is not available, another health professional with sufficient experience and qualifications to advise on these matters. Access to information regarding the provision of treatment services and those born as a result of such treatment services and the keeping and use of gametes and embryos under the Human Fertilization and Embryology Act 1990 is also restricted (Data Protection (Subject Access Modification) (Health) Order 2000 SI 2000 No 413).

This clinical privilege to withhold information needs to be exercised with considerable sensitivity if the rights of the patient are to be adequately protected. As Brazier (1992) notes:

> What should not be forgotten is that a patient who genuinely would rather not know what was wrong with him will never ask for access to his records.

Information concerning identifiable third parties
Information relating to an identifiable third party may be withheld (s7(4)).
However, disclosure may take place where that person has given his or her
consent, or where it is reasonable in the particular circumstances to disclose without consent (s7(5)).

General exemptions
Data processed for research, statistical or historical purposes are exempt
from the access rights where the data are not being processed for the
purpose of supporting measures or decisions in relation to specific
persons. In addition, the processing itself must not be undertaken in
such a way that it causes the patient 'substantial damage or distress'.
Finally, in the case of research, any results of that research should not
be made available in a form in which the patient is identifiable (s33).
Professional regulatory bodies, such as the UKCC, are given some protection from access provisions where this is likely to prejudice the
proper discharge of their functions (s31(2)(a)(iii), s31(4)(b),
s31(4)(a)(iii)).

Incompetent patients
In contrast to the Access to Health Records Act 1990, which contained
specific provisions concerning the child patient, under the 1998 Act the
situation regarding mentally incompetent adults and child patients is
problematic because neither group is dealt with specifically in the legislation. It is unclear whether persons other than the data subject may make
an application for access under the legislation.

Residual access rights under the Access to Health Records Act 1990
While the majority of the provisions in the Access to Health Records Act
1990 have been superseded by the 1998 Act, access to the health records
of a deceased person are not covered by the 1998 Act. Personal representatives (s3(1)(f)) or persons claiming in relation to the deceased's estate
(s5(4)) will have to make an application under the Access to Health
Records Act 1990.

Ensuring the security of records

The nurse must ensure that patient records are kept secure from unauthorized access. This is particularly important in view of the fact that so
much information today is held on computer. The UKCC document
Guidelines for Professional Practice emphasizes the need to keep confidence. It states that (UKCC, 1996vii):

> As far as computer-held records are concerned, you must be satisfied
> that, as far as is possible, the methods you use for recording informa-
> tion are secure. You must also find out which categories of staff have
> access to records to which they are expected to contribute important

personal and confidential information. Local procedures must include ways of checking whether a record is authentic where there is no written signature. All records must clearly indicate the identity of the person who made that record.

Unauthorized access to information held on computer may constitute a criminal offence under the Computer Misuse Act 1990, although there are certain exceptions in relation to the situation in which a person accidentally exceeds his or her permission. The need to maintain controls over disclosure of computerized records has now further been developed with the Caldicott Review and subsequent developments.

The electronic patient record and the Caldicott Review

At present there are major developments within the NHS in relation to the use and transfer of patient information. The electronic patient record is being formulated along with the 'NHS net', which is an intranet for exchanging business and clinical data. An initial pilot study defined the electronic patient record as 'a dynamic collection of messages, held electronically, created by healthcare professionals principally to inform themselves and others about the provision of health care to an individual patient'. It is envisaged that eventually patients will possess an electronic health record, which will operate throughout their entire life. While such developments have considerable potential, they may also raise dilemmas concerning access and security of health information. The Caldicott Committee was established to undertake a review of the uses of patient-identifiable information flowing from NHS organizations to NHS and other bodies for purposes other than direct care or medical research, or where there is a statutory requirement for information (Caldicott, 1997). It recommended that data flow within the health service should be tested against basic principles of good practice. Individuals should be designated 'guardians' of health care information, and protocols developed governing the sharing of information between NHS and non-NHS bodies. Guardians should document all routine uses of person-identified information. Access to records would be on a strictly 'need to know' basis with confidentiality 'health checks' undertaken each year.

The committee's recommendations were accepted by the government, and Caldicott guardians were established nationwide. The document *Protecting and Using Patient Information: A Manual for Caldicott Guardians* (NHSE, 1999) provides that the guardian should be a member of the existing management board, a senior health professional, or an individual responsible for promoting clinical governance. A series of principles are set out in the document:

1. The proposed use and transfer of patient information must be justified
2. Patient information should not be used save where this is absolutely necessary
3. The minimum amount of identifiable patient information should be used
4. Patient information should be available on a strictly 'need to know' basis
5. All persons who handle patient information should know their responsibilities
6. All persons who handle patient information should understand and comply with the law.

All health authories, special health authorities, NHS trusts and primary care groups were required to appoint a Caldicott Guardian no later than 30 March 1999 (HSC, 1999/012). The intention was that during the first year there should be an audit, by the management, of procedures for protection and use of patient information. The guidance emphasizes that all NHS bodies must have an active policy for informing patients regarding the purposes for which information about them is collected, and the persons to whom such information may be passed. Protocols should be drawn up governing the disclosure of patient/client-identifiable information to other organizations. Where an individual wants information to be withheld, the guidance states that this wish should be respected. Protocols should govern disclosure of the information and its security. The guidance also notes the need to maintain security within the individual organization. There is also a new NHS Information Authority with the task of implementing information strategy including electronic records (NHS Information Authority (Establishment and Constitution Order) Order 1999 SI 1999 No 695). These guidelines are to be commended as a step in the right direction, alongside the safeguards of the data protection principles contained in the 1998 Act. Nonetheless, the boundaries of disclosure do need to be carefully monitored.

Liability for unauthorized disclosure of health information

There have been suggestions that if a practitioner goes ahead and discloses confidential information without the consent of a patient, the practitioner may be held liable in negligence for that disclosure. Carson and Montgomery (1990) gave an example of a case in which a doctor was held to be liable in negligence for revealing to the husband of his patient the fact that he considered that she was paranoid. He had not told the patient directly, because he thought that this would cause harm to the patient's mental state and to the doctor–patient relationship. It was held that the harm that took place was reasonably foreseeable in nature, even though the circumstances in which the husband revealed the information were not.

Should patients be allowed to retain their own records?

Health care records are usually held in hospitals, health centres or surgeries, although certain trials have been conducted to ascertain the feasibility of patients being given their own records on 'smart cards' – small cards on which data are electronically stored and which may be accessed by a special machine. However, the fact that a patient is simply given a smart card will not in itself facilitate access to records, because access is dependent upon the patient having means to access the electronic information on that card.

If the general principle of patient access is accepted, then why not allow patients to keep hold of their own records? There is, of course, the risk that patients would lose them, but studies undertaken seem to suggest that this is not the case (Gilhooley and McGhee, 1991). There are considerable advantages in patient-held records. For example, nurses would have immediate access to records if visiting patients at home; there would be no delay in transferring records when the patient moved GPs; time spent storing records would be saved in GPs' surgeries; and it would assist patients in correcting inaccuracies in records. It may also increase trust between patients and health care professionals. There is now a movement towards patient-held records, for example in relation to maternity care. As the UKCC (1998) has stated:

> Patients and clients increasingly own their own health care records and this should be encouraged as far as this is appropriate and as long as they are happy to do so. It enables them to be more closely involved in their own care and enables you to share with them the information that you consider relevant to your assessment and care of them. Patients and clients should be informed of the purpose and importance of the record and their responsibility for keeping it safe. These same principles apply equally to parent-held records.

However, as the UKCC notes, there are limitations to client-held records because the health professional may want to include information to be withheld from a client. The UKCC (1998) suggests that in some situations, in view of the concerns of the health professional, a supplementary record should be created, but that this should be very much the exception rather than the norm.

Conclusions

Reforming the law

The present law concerning patient confidentiality can only be gleaned by reference to a number of disparate sources. The boundaries of disclosure for the nurse are unclear, and there have been a number of proposals for reform in the area. In 1981, the Law Commission suggested that the law concerning breach of confidence should be placed upon a statutory footing (Law Commission, 1981). In 1995, the British Medical Association produced a draft Bill on confidentiality. The Bill was the result of deliberations by a working party, which included nursing input from the UKCC. A version of this Bill was introduced into the House of Lords by Lord Walton in 1996, and was given a second reading. The Bill applied to information relating to an individual's physical or mental health, and which is in the control of a health service body or qualified health professional. It set out the basis on which information could be lawfully disclosed and made unauthorized disclosure a criminal offence. The Bill ultimately fell, and at present comprehensive legislation in the area appears unlikely.

Specific proposals have been made in the context of genetic information – for example, the House of Commons Select Committee on Science and Technology called for the enactment of specific legislation governing the privacy of genetic information. The House of Commons Select Committee (1995) went so far as to recommend that (para 225):

> ... misuse of genetic information should be both a criminal and civil offence.

The coming into force of the Human Rights Act 1998 may lead to an alteration in the manner in which issues in this area are dealt with now that Article 8, the right to privacy, has finally become enforceable in the English courts. Nonetheless, while clarification of the boundaries of disclosure by Parliament and the courts is surely to be welcomed, ultimately the best safeguard of patient confidentiality is that of good professional norms.

References

Brazier, M. (1992). *Medicine, Patients and the Law*, 2nd edn. Penguin.
Boddington, P. (1994). In *Genetic Counselling Practice and Principles* (A. Clarke, ed.) Routledge.
Caldicott (1997). *Report on the Review of Patient Identifiable Information (The Caldicott Report)* (December). http://www.doh.gov.uk/confiden/crep.htm
Carson, D. and Montgomery, J. (1990). *Nursing Law*. Macmillan.
Chadwick, R., Levitt, M. and Schickle, D. (1997). *The Right to Know and the Right Not to Know*. Ashgate.
Department of Health (1993). *Guidance for Staff on Relations with the Public and the Media*. DOH.

Department of Health (1996). *The Protection and Use of Personal Health Information.* DOH.

General Medical Council (1995). *HIV and AIDS: The Ethical Considerations.* GMC.

Gilhooley, M. and McGhee, S. M. (1991). Medical records; practicalities and principles of patient possession. *J. Med. Ethics*, **17**, 138.

Grubb, A. and Pearl, D. (1986). Medicine, health, family and the law. *Family Law*, **16**, 227–240.

Health Service Commissioner (1992). *Annual Report for 1991–92.* HMSO, HC 82.

House of Commons Select Committee on Science and Technology (1995). *Human Genetics: The Science and its Consequences.* Third Report.

Human Genetics Advisory Commission (1997). *The Implications of Testing for Insurance,* http://www.dti.gov.uk/hgac.

Kennedy, I. and Grubb, A. (1994). *Medical Law, Text with Materials.* Butterworths.

Law Commission (1981). *Breach of Confidence.* Cmnd 838.

Mason, J. K. and McCall Smith, R. A. (1999). *Law and Medical Ethics,* 5th edn. Butterworths, (i) p. 213; (ii) p. 194; (iii) p. 208.

McHale, J. V. (1993). *Medical Confidentiality and Legal Privilege.* Routledge.

McHale, J. (1994). Whistleblowing in the USA. In: *Whistleblowing in the Health Services* (G. Hunt, ed.). Edward Arnold, pp. 133–145.

Montgomery, J. (1987). Confidentiality and the immature minor. *Family Law*, **17**, 101.

NHS Executive (1999). *Protecting and Using Patient Information: A Manual for Caldicott Guardians.* HNSME.

Nightingale, F. (1859). *Notes on Nursing.* Blackie reprint 1974, p. 70.

Nuffield Council on Bioethics (1993). *Genetic Screening: Ethical Issues.* Nuffield Council.

Royal College of Nurses (1991). *Guidelines on Confidentiality in Nursing.* RCN.

Seighart, P. (1982). Professional ethics: for whose benefit? *J. Med. Ethics*, **8**.

Siegler, M. (1987). A decrepit concept. *N. Engl. J. Med.*, **307**, 1518.

Thompson, I. (1979). The nature of confidentiality. *J. Med. Ethics*, **5**.

Turner, T. (1994). Paradox in practice. *Nursing Times*, **90(21)**, 18.

UKCC (1998). *Guidelines for Records and Record Keeping.* UKCC.

UKCC (1996). *Guidelines for Professional Practice.* UKCC, (i) para 52; (ii) para 56; (iii) para 59; (iv) para 61; (v) para 40; (vi) para 41; (vii) para 64.

Chapter 8

Clinical research and the nurse

Jean McHale

Nurses increasingly participate in clinical trials (Parabor, 1997). They may run their own trials or may undertake research as part of a diploma qualification or for a higher degree. They may be involved in a trial being run by a medical practitioner or by another nurse. Nurses may be members of a research ethics committee, which has the task of scrutinizing proposals for clinical research in a particular area. This chapter provides an account of the legal regulation of research and the obligation of the researcher to the research subject. The basic principles on which research should be conducted are outlined in the document *Guidelines for Professional Practice* (UKCC, 1996(i)).

In the first section of this chapter, consideration is given to the manner in which clinical research is regulated. In the second section, the role of research ethics committees in scrutinizing clinical trials and legal principles regulating clinical trials are discussed. In the final section, the question of negligence actions brought against nurses and others where research subjects are injured in a clinical trial are considered, along with the role of the nurse in policing unethical researchers.

Framework of regulation

The abuses of clinical research in Nazi Germany and in Japan during the middle years of this century resulted in pressure for the regulation of clinical research. International guidelines were developed, most notably the Nuremberg Code in 1949 and the Declaration of Helsinki in 1964. In this country there is no one piece of legislation governing the conduct of all research activity, although certain legislation does govern specific areas such as animal research (Animals (Scientific Procedure) Act 1986) and research undertaken on embryos (Human Fertilization and Embryology Act 1990). A number of guidelines have been published, for example by the Department of Health (DOH, 1991), the Royal College of Physicians

(RCP, 1996) and by the Royal College of Nursing (RCN, 1993). While these guidelines are not legally binding, they suggest conduct that amounts to good research practice and may be referred to in subsequent legal proceedings. The law governing research derives from general principles of civil law and criminal law, along with certain specific statutory provisions such as the Medicines Act 1968. Clinical research is undertaken across a vast area of scientific activity.

Below is a brief overview of some of the areas of current regulatory activity. Certain research gives rise to particularly difficult ethical issues requiring careful consideration – for example, embryo research, the use of fetal tissue and the research into gene therapy. Embryo research was considered by the Warnock Committee, and is regulated by the Human Fertilization and Embryology Authority under the Human Fertilization and Embryology Act 1990 (Harris and Dyson, 1987). Embryo research was eventually sanctioned after a heated ethical debate regarding the status of the embryo. As with abortion, ethical objections were raised regarding the use and consequent destruction of embryos for research purposes. The Act represents in many respects a compromise of views, allowing controlled research for a limited period of time in the early stages of development of the embryo. The Authority issues licences to researchers to undertake such research as falls within the criteria set out in the legislation. Researchers may undertake embryo experimentation if this comes within the criteria set out in the Human Fertilization and Embryology Act 1990, which include promoting advances in the treatment of infertility, increasing the knowledge of congenital disease, increasing knowledge about the cause of miscarriages, developing more effective means of contraception, and developing methods for detecting the presence of gene or chromosome abnormalities in embryos before implantation. The Act bans certain forms of experimentation, such as keeping or using an embryo after the appearance of the primitive streak (after 14 days of development), placing an embryo in an animal, or replacing the nucleus of a cell of an embryo with a nucleus taken from a cell of any person, embryo or subsequent development of an embryo (cloning through nuclei substitution) (s3(3) Human Fertilization and Embryology Act 1990).

Xenotransplantation is regulated by the Xenotransplantation Interim Regulatory Advisory Authority (UKXIRA, 1998). Gene therapy is overseen by a specially created government body, the Gene Therapy Advisory Committee, which imposes stringent requirements on researchers. The use of fetal tissue is regulated through the use of guidance issued following a government commissioned report into the issue by the Revd John Polkinghorne (Polkinghorne, 1989). This chapter focuses upon those clinical trials in which nurses are at present most likely to be directly involved, and discusses general principles of research activity on human subjects. As will be seen, the conduct of most clinical trials is subject to the consideration of non-statutory bodies – local research ethics committees.

Drug trials and innovative therapies

Before medicines are made available to the public, they must be licensed by the Department of Health or the Department of Agriculture (Medicines Act 1968). Unlicensed medicines may be used if the government has issued a clinical trial certificate. Such a certificate does not have to be obtained under what is known as the DDX provision if the trial is being conducted by a doctor, other than under arrangements with a manufacturer or supplier. If these requirements are not complied with, then criminal penalties may follow (Dodds-Smith, 1992). Although safeguards in the form of licensing exist in relation to experimental drug therapy, there are at present no equivalent safeguards as regards innovative therapy such as keyhole surgery. Kennedy and Grubb (1994) have suggested that, in view of the fine line between innovative therapy and research, innovative therapy should be classed as medical research in situations in which the main purpose of therapy is to acquire knowledge, as opposed to caring for the patient. In the light of much public concern regarding the use of certain new therapeutic techniques, notably keyhole surgery, the government indicated that it was considering the introduction of legislation in this area (*The Times*, 21 February 1995). The previous Conservative Government suggested that the Royal Medical Colleges should establish a committee on the safety and efficacy of medical intervention. New techniques would be referred to the committee, and small groups of experts would be given the task of deciding which techniques should be used and how their effectiveness should be assessed. The National Institute for Clinical Excellence is likely to perform such a role in the future (see Chapter 1).

Animal research

The Animals (Scientific Procedures) Act 1986 states that before research can be undertaken on animals, researchers must obtain a licence from the Home Secretary. A Home Office committee examines whether the benefits to be gained from research being undertaken upon these animals justify the suffering that may be occasioned. The practice and ethics of these procedures go beyond the scope of this book, and the reader is referred to further sources (see, for example, Fox, 1995).

Regulation of research: general principles

This chapter considers the basis of regulation of clinical research involving human subjects and legal principles governing the operation of clinical trials, as well as the criteria that the nurse should satisfy before embarking on a clinical trial. The principles of consent to treatment applicable in the context of research are considered, and the particular problems that arise in the context of certain groups of research subjects such as children and the mentally incompetent. A nurse researcher will also be bound to respect patient confidentiality, and particular applications of this are considered. This chapter concludes by examining the role and obligations of the nurse researcher on the wards.

Before a trial is undertaken, the researcher should obtain approval for the conduct of the trial from a research ethics committee. The main guidelines governing the operation of such committees are those issued by the Department of Health (DOH, 1991). These recommend that a local research ethics committee should be composed of between eight and 12 members drawn from hospital medical staff, nursing staff and general practitioners, and two or more lay persons (DOH, 1991i). The guidelines suggest that the chair or the deputy chair should be a lay person. Lay members import a degree of independence into the decision-making process. The Royal College of Physicians (1996) has stated that two measures are required to ensure ethical research practice: first, there should be adherence to good practice in research, and second, there should be some form of mechanism for investigating allegations into fraud (Lock, 1993). In 1997, a Committee on Publication Ethics was formed to assist in this regulation (Smith, 1997). While it is not mandatory by law for trials to be referred to local research ethics committees, many journals now require evidence of ethics committee approval before publishing the research.

Where it is proposed to undertake a trial over a number of research centres in different health authority areas, the proposal should be referred to one of a number of committees governing the approval of multi-centred trials (DOH, 1997).

Assessing the risk

A researcher must satisfy the committee that the project is ethical and that any risk posed to research subjects is of an acceptable level. Factors the committee must consider include any discomfort or distress the project may cause the research subject, any hazards that may arise during the project and precautions introduced to deal with them, and the extent to which the research subject's health will be affected by involvement in a trial. The Royal College of Physicians' 1996 guidelines helpfully state the following (RCP, 1996, para 7.3):

Benefit may be weighed against risk in two different ways. First and most obviously, the patient may benefit. This is typified in a therapeutic trial where at least one of the treatments offered may be beneficial to the patient. Benefits may be considerable, for example in cancer treatment, and may counterbalance even high risk to the individual. Second, society rather than the individual may benefit. In such situations, however large the benefit, to expose a participant to anything more than a minimal risk needs very careful consideration and would rarely be ethical.

What if a volunteer is prepared to accept a more than minimal risk in participating in a clinical trial? Some people will take risks of a very high order for altruistic reasons. A person may volunteer to be involved in a trial to help researchers develop a cure for a condition suffered by a close relative. It is unclear whether it is lawful for a research subject to consent to involvement in a very high-risk trial. As was noted earlier in relation to consent to treatment, English law does not allow a person to consent to any harm. If a research subject included in a high-risk trial dies, then there is the possibility that a researcher would be prosecuted for manslaughter.

There has been controversy as to whether women of childbearing age should be included in a clinical trial, and, in particular, concern as to the inclusion of women who are pregnant. That does not mean that trials cannot be undertaken on pregnant women. Indeed, trials into birthing techniques and the use of devices such as birth cushions require pregnant women, of course! Those proposing to undertake such a trial should bear in mind the Department of Health (1991ii) guidelines, which state:

> Where women are used as research subjects, the possibility of their being or becoming pregnant should always be considered. The recruitment of females of childbearing age should always be justified by the researcher.

Whether the possibility of risk to female volunteers of childbearing age from involvement in a clinical trial justifies their exclusion from such trials is the subject of much debate. While involvement may potentially harm such volunteers, it could be seen as paternalistic to ban involvement. Perhaps a better approach is to examine rigorously any trial where women of childbearing age are involved, and to ensure that all women are provided with full information as to any possible risks to their health from involvement in the trial if they become pregnant.

Inducements to participate

Many trials are undertaken using volunteers, and while some may be willing to give up their time out of altruism, many trials would simply not go ahead unless inducements were given. A small financial inducement may be given to compensate for time spent and potential inconvenience caused. However, while payment of small sums may be acceptable, there is a danger that an unethical researcher may offer large sums to encourage participation in a trial imposing an undue risk. Similarly, some payments to researchers may be unethical. If the researcher receives payment on the basis that the more patients are recruited the larger the fee, there is danger that researchers may place undue pressure on patients and others to be included in the research (DOH, 1991iii). Nonetheless, the level of any inducement given to the NHS body, health professionals, researchers or subjects to participate in clinical research is a factor that will be considered by a local research ethics committee when considering whether to approve a clinical trial (DOH, 1991iv). Inducements to research subjects may, of course, be other than financial. For example, pressure may be put on nurses by nurse researchers to participate in clinical trials because it is something that is expected of them. Such pressure is unjustifiable. It is important to ensure that subjects give full and free consent to entry into any trial.

Consent

As with any clinical procedure, it is vital to obtain consent from a research subject before a trial commences. The nurse may have the task of obtaining a patient's consent to participation in a trial or, even if not involved in initially obtaining consent, the nurse may be drawn into the process if a patient later approaches him or her and asks questions about the trial. Ensuring that research subjects are given adequate information is an important part of the role of a research ethics committee. What information must be given to the research subject in a clinical trial? A distinction should be drawn between therapeutic and non-therapeutic trials. Therapeutic research is research intended to benefit an individual patient, whereas non-therapeutic research is research that is unlikely to or will not benefit the research subject (whether a patient or a healthy volunteer) personally.

The Department of Health guidelines provide simply that the research subject should give written consent, and that the consent should be 'real'. While the guidelines state that a research subject should be given an information sheet before giving consent, they do not specify the content of such an information sheet. The research ethics committee looks at the information sheet compiled by researchers for research subjects, to see if it is satisfactory. The Royal College of Physicians (1991) recommends that information sheets should always contain statements regarding the nature of the investigation, the procedures involved, the risks and possible benefits to the subject or others, and the fact that a subject can decline to participate without giving reasons or incurring a penalty. In addition, if the research ethics committee decides that the risks warrant it, the Royal College of Physicians recommends that the sheet should include statements as to the availability of compensation and also an invitation to research subjects to ask for further information. These are sensible recommendations. An information sheet should provide as full and clear an explanation as possible. However, the nurse will not have fulfilled his or her legal obligations by simply handing over an information sheet. This issue is developed further below.

Providing full information recognizes the autonomy of the research subject. Without informed consent, research subjects may not realize that they are being subjected to procedures aimed at benefiting future patients rather than themselves. However, there are certain situations in which researchers may wish to withhold information from patients. For example, some patients included in a trial recover not because of the effect of new medication, but simply because they think that they have been given a new drug. This is known as the 'placebo effect'. In an attempt to overcome this problem researchers undertake randomized controlled trials, where research subjects are divided into two groups; one group is given the treatment, the other is given a placebo or dummy treatment. The patient does not know whether he or she is receiving the real or the dummy treatment. A variant on this is the 'double-blind' trial; in this type of trial, both the clinician and the research subject do not know whether the patient has been given the treatment or an inert substance. It is particularly important for patients to appreciate that they are being entered into a randomized clinical trial and that there is a risk of missing out on a standard course of treatment. When providing information about the trial, researchers must ensure that all subjects are told that they are free to withdraw at any stage (DOH, 1991v).

There are no statutes or decided cases in English law stating how much information subjects in clinical trials should be given. A research subject may claim that provision of inadequate information constitutes the tort of battery. As discussed in Chapter 5, regarding consent to medical treatment, the courts have stated that as long as a patient gives general consent to an operation being undertaken, then health care professionals will not be liable in battery (*Chatterson* v. *Gerson* [1981] QB 432 at 443). However, would the same test be applied to clinical research? In the Canadian case of *Halushka* v. *University of Satkatchewan* ([1965] 53 DLR (2d) 436 at 438), it was held that the failure of researchers to provide the subject with full information constituted a battery. Hall J.A. said:

> The subjects of medical experimentation are entitled to a full and frank disclosure of all the facts, probabilities and opinions which a reasonable man might be expected to consider before giving consent.

It is suggested that the adoption of such an approach – requiring a broad duty of disclosure to those entering a non-therapeutic trial – is desirable. What of patients included in therapeutic trials? The difficulty here is that if patients included in trials had to be given a full explanation, this would give such patients the right to receive more information than a patient receiving any other therapy. At present it seems likely that the courts would hold that a patient is entitled to the same level of disclosure whether therapy is given as part of treatment or as therapeutic research.

It may be necessary to undertake research using patients brought into casualty unconscious and in a critical condition. The Department of Health (1991vi) guidelines provide that research projects involving such patients should be examined with particular care. If it is possible to anticipate that a patient may be subject to an unexpected event, such as complications during childbirth, then the researchers should obtain the patient's consent before labour begins.

Duty to inform – negligence

While a research subject may have been given some information as to the trial such that an action in battery may be difficult to establish, a research subject may claim that a researcher acted negligently because inadequate information was provided as to the risks posed by involvement in the trial. In the context of medical treatment, as discussed earlier a nurse is not negligent as long as he or she gives the patient such information as would have been provided by a responsible body of professional nursing opinion (*Sidaway* v. *Bethlem Royal Hospital Governors* [1985] AC 871). Does the duty differ in relation to clinical research?

Two alternative approaches could be taken. Given the uncertain nature of clinical research and the risks involved, different standards of disclosure could be adopted for treatment and for therapeutic research, with the research subject entitled to receive more information than the patient. However, the dividing line between therapeutic treatment and therapeutic research is a very fine one, and this may be regarded as an unjustifiably narrow distinction to draw. Alternatively, a complete reassessment could be made of the legal obligation to disclose information to patients. It appears unlikely that the courts or Parliament will attempt such a reform in the near future. Such judicial or legislative reform may not prove necessary if clinical practice moves towards providing patients routinely with information regarding the risks of treatment (see Chapter 5).

A strong argument can be made in favour of full disclosure of all risks in the case of non-therapeutic trials. If a research subject is subjected to scientific tests for the benefit of the community as a whole, and not for his or her own personal benefit, then he or she should be told of the risks run by involvement in the project. What must be emphasized is that simply to provide a large amount of information about potential risks of entry into a clinical trial may be of little value. A nurse will not comply with his or her legal obligation by simply providing a patient with an information sheet. The RCN (1993) suggests that the researcher should:

> … explain as fully as possible, and in terms meaningful to the subjects, the nature and the purpose of the study, how and why they were selected and invited to take part, what is required of them and who is undertaking and financing the investigation.

The nurse can independently observe what information the patient has been given. He or she may be of the view that the information that has been given is inadequate. In such a situation, the nurse should raise the concerns with the researcher. It is certainly arguable that in a research situation the nurse may be justified in personally providing the research subject with more information. However, the nurse should only contemplate providing the patient with more information directly after having ascertained the position regarding disclosure. The question of unethical researchers is explored further in the section on policing trials later in this chapter. (See also the discussion of conflicts between nurses and other health care professionals over information disclosure on p. 107.)

Where a research subject asks questions about the research project, it is again unclear whether the researcher has to answer such queries fully. It is submitted that, as with medical treatment, any refusal to provide information would require careful justification in the case of a therapeutic trial, and that such a refusal would be unjustifiable in the case of a non-therapeutic trial.

Can patients be compelled to participate?

Consider a patient asked to participate in a clinical trial. The trial offers the prospect of a cure for what is otherwise an incurable condition. The patient refuses to be involved. Could the patient be compelled to participate? The law states that a competent adult patient has the right to refuse treatment, even if as a consequence the patient dies. In a number of controversial cases, treatment has been authorized despite patient refusal (see Chapter 6). Nonetheless, it is doubtful whether any court would authorize the inclusion of a competent but protesting adult in a research trial, even if the trial was clearly therapeutic. Indeed, to sanction such involvement would, it is submitted, represent an unjustifiable limitation on individual autonomy.

If a nurse or doctor in charge of a project appears to be putting pressure on a patient to participate, the nurse acting as patient advocate should make the patient aware of his or her right to refuse to be included in the trial. The nurse should also protest to the researcher about what he or she regards as bad practice. If a researcher continues to act in flagrant disregard of legal obligations, then the nurse should bring the matter to the attention of the appropriate bodies, including the research ethics committee.

Children and clinical trials

Wherever possible, clinical trials should be conducted using competent adults (DOH, 1991vii). However, in some situations it is necessary to include children in a clinical trial – for instance, if the trial involves a study into childhood diseases or concerns the suitability for administration to children of a drug that is currently used to treat adult patients. A research ethics committee assesses the risk level of trials, and the risk to a child of participation in a trial is something that they will be particularly concerned to assess.

Particular difficulties surround non-therapeutic trials. The Department of Health (1991viii) guidelines emphasize that to expose a child in a non-therapeutic trial to a risk other than merely negligible may be to act unlawfully. But is this right? We noted earlier that some are of the view that it is legitimate to include children in non-therapeutic procedures as long as this is 'not against' their best interests. It has been argued that just as parents are lawfully entitled to expose their children to certain quite risky activities, they should be entitled to expose them to the risks surrounding entry into a clinical trial (Nicholson, 1985). One approach is to limit the entry of child patients to those trials where there is minimal risk, an approach for example favoured by the British Paediatric Association (BPA, 1992). However, there is scope for disagreement regarding what constitutes 'minimal risk'. A scientist may rate a procedure as having a lower risk than would a patient assessing the same procedure (Nicholson, 1991). Research ethics committees need to be extremely sensitive to the different weightings that may be placed on risk levels by scientists and research subjects in scrutinizing research protocols.

If it is proposed to include a child in a clinical trial, from whom should patient consent be obtained – parent or child? As already discussed, in law, a child over 16 years can give consent to medical treatment and a child under that age may be competent to give consent (s8 Family Law Reform Act 1969). In *Gillick* v. *West Norfolk and Wisbech AHA* ([1985] 3 All ER 402), the House of Lords held that whether a child under 16 years was capable of consenting to medical treatment was dependent upon an assessment of the child's maturity. It seems likely that the *Gillick* approach would be adopted by a court if it was asked to consider whether a child could consent to involvement in a therapeutic research project. Application of this test is not straightforward. Researchers must carefully assess each child individually to determine his or her capacity to consent to be involved in a particular trial. It would be good practice for researchers to ensure that they have the written consent of those with parental responsibility, even if the child is competent to consent to involvement in the trial.

It is uncertain whether a child can consent to being included in a non-therapeutic trial. The courts may be prepared to adopt the *Gillick* test of competency and hold that a competent child may give a valid consent to involvement in a non-therapeutic research project. But would a child be competent to make that choice? It is important not to underestimate a child's powers of comprehension. Mason and McCall Smith (1999) comment that it would be very unusual for a child in his or her teens not to understand the implications of entry into a clinical trial.

Compelling a child to be involved

What can a nurse do if a child tearfully refuses to be involved in the project? Can the child be compelled on the grounds that it is in his or her best interests to be involved? The courts have indicated that if a competent child refuses treatment, the parents may authorize treatment on the child's behalf. Compelling a child's involvement in any clinical procedure is a very serious step. If such a conflict were to arise and the issue go to court, then it is submitted that a court would be unlikely to authorize a child forcibly to be involved in a therapeutic trial, save perhaps in an exceptional situation where the child is suffering from a condition with a terminal prognosis and the treatment represents the child's only chance of life. Even here, it would be exceedingly controversial to compel involvement. Can a very young child be forced to take part in a clinical trial? The Department of Health guidelines do not deal with this question, and the legal position is uncertain. Certainly, as far as possible the wishes of even a very young child should be given serious consideration in making this decision.

The incompetent adult

The nurse may be involved in a research project including mentally ill or mentally handicapped adults. Wherever possible, competent adult subjects should be used. However, as with the child subject, there may be situations in which research is inevitably on the mentally ill and incompetent because it relates to a condition specific to this subject group – such as research into a particular mental illness or the effects of a particular treatment. For example, a study into the side effects of antipsychotic drugs must be undertaken using clients who are receiving such medication. However, researchers must not forget that while persons may have some mental impairment, this does not mean that they are totally unable to give consent. The majority of psychiatric patients are as capable of giving consent as other patients (Royal College of Psychiatrists, 1990). Admittedly, some patients will never reach that level of competence. Nevertheless, including such patients in a research project may be of very real benefit to them or to groups of other patients in the future.

As stated in Chapter 6, relatives and other persons have no power to give consent in law on behalf of a mentally incompetent person. The House of Lords in *Re F* ([1990] 2 AC 1) stated that treatment may be given where the health professionals believe that it is in the best interests of an incompetent patient. While the question of therapeutic research was not discussed in *Re F*, it appears likely that such research may be justified if it can be shown that it is treatment for 'life, health, well-being'. The difficulty lies in determining what amounts to treatment in the 'best interests' of the patient. In *Re F*, Lord Brandon said:

> The operation or other treatment will be in the best interests of such patients if, but only if, it is carried out either in order to save their lives or in order to ensure improvement/prevent deterioration in their physical/mental health.

As far as non-therapeutic research is concerned, at present it appears that it is unlawful to undertake this on a mentally incompetent patient. It can be argued that such research is not in the best interests of a mentally incompetent adult within the definition of the House of Lords in *Re F.*

Concern as to the vulnerability of the mentally incompetent adult and the need to ensure that procedures are undertaken only when necessary is reflected in *Mental Incapacity*, the report of the Law Commission (1995). It accepted that in certain limited situations non-therapeutic research could be undertaken, but only if subject to safeguards. First, all non-therapeutic trials on mentally incompetent adults should be referred to a specially created committee, a mental incapacity research committee. Such a committee would examine whether intended research projects satisfied a number of criteria (draft Bill clause 11(3)):

1. that it is desirable to provide knowledge of the causes or treatment of, or of the care of people affected by, the incapacitating condition with which any participant is affected;
2. that the object of the research cannot be effectively achieved without the participation of persons who are or who may be without capacity to consent, and
3. that the research will not expose a participant to more than a negligible risk, will not be unduly invasive or restrictive of a participant and will not unduly interfere with a participant's freedom of action or privacy.

The committee was to approve trial proposals in principle; involvement of a particular individual in a trial was a matter to be assessed separately. First, some of the participants may give consent themselves. The Law Commission gave the example of proposed research upon members of a residential home who have Alzheimer's disease. If individuals are unable themselves to give consent, the Law Commission recommended that research may be undertaken where there has been court approval, the consent of an attorney or manager, a certificate from a doctor not involved in the research that the person's participation is appropriate, or in cases where the research is designated as one that does not involve direct contact (draft Bill clause 11(1)(c) and (4)). This final consideration refers to covert observation, photography or the inspection of written records. Allowing automatic approval for such observational studies is exceedingly controversial. Much may depend upon the condition of the individual patient, and any decision to include a person in such a project should be made on the basis of what constitutes that person's best interests.

In 1997 the government, in their document *Who Decides?* (1997), announced their intention to enact some of the provisions of the Law Commission, but were not convinced of the fact that there was the need for an additional committee, although they did consult on this issue (para 5.41). These proposals were not included by the government in their document *Making Decisions* (Lord Chancellor's Department, 1999.

The Council of Europe Convention on Human Rights and Biomedicine (1997) now provides that non-therapeutic research on incompetent patients may be undertaken if:

i) the research has the aim of contributing through significant improvement to the understanding of the individual's condition, disease or disorder, to the ultimate attainment of results capable of conferring benefit to the person concerned or to other persons in the same age category or afflicted with the same disease or disorder or having the same condition

ii) the research entails only minimal risk and minimal burden for the individuals involved, and that in addition research of comparable effectiveness cannot be undertaken on a competent adult and that the appropriate consent has been obtained.

At present the UK has not become a party to this Convention, but it is likely to have some influence, at the very least in the context of directing ethical guidelines in this area in the future.

Reforming the consent process in clinical trials

In May 2000, the UK government announced that it would be conducting a review into the consent process for clinical research in the NHS. This was in response to the study undertaken at the North Staffordshire Hospital NHS Trust by Professor David Southall. A trial was conducted upon neonates who suffered respiratory failure, considering the effect of treatment using continuous negative extrathoracic pressure (CNEP) rather than standard ventilation. Parents whose two children received the procedure complained. The first child died whilst on a ventilator, and 10 months later a second child was discovered to have brain damage. In neither case, it was claimed, had it been explained to the parents that this was an experimental procedure. The review of the trial conducted by Professor Rod Griffiths, a director of public health in the West Midlands regional office of the NHSE, was highly critical (Griffiths, 2000). It stated that 'the apparent lack of adequate explanation, of choice and consequent properly elicited and recorded consent and involvement in later decision making' was unacceptable. The professor heading the trial had not 'ensured that each member of staff who might be involved in the project was trained or supervised to ensure that they were doing what the research project said they should'. The ethics committee that approved the trial was also the subject of criticism. It was claimed that the committee had not examined the proposal sufficiently – while in fact, failures of management and supervision were, in the view of the report, 'virtually built into the design'. The report commented that:

> In effect the combination of a slightly complacent local research ethics committee, an enthusiastic and assertive researcher, and a vacuum in research governance in the trust led this trial to run in a less than adequate way.

Both consultants were subject to disciplinary action, while it appears that nurses who were involved in the trial were also subject to investigation by the UKCC. The report recommended that formal guidance on research governance within the NHS should be developed. Until this is developed at NHS level, the report recommended that the Trust should develop its own guidance. It also recommended that there should be co-operation between the Department of Health and professional and regulatory bodies to consult and produce agreed guidelines that clarify issues of consent for participation in clinical trials. It proposed that the Department of Health should consider the establishment of a surveillance system to look at unexpected outcomes from non-drug treatments, and also recommended that an audit of the efficacy of the CNEP procedure should be undertaken.

The panel's report went beyond the CNEP procedure to look at broader issues, such as the use of video surveillance in relation to the detection of Munchausen's syndrome by proxy. This concerned the use of covert video surveillance of children and their parents in hospitals in cases where the parents were suspected of abuse (Evans, 1995; Gillon, 1995; Southall and Samuels, 1995). The report proposed that there should be an expert multi-disciplinary panel to look at this issue and provide guidelines on the use of covert video surveillance.

Research involving human tissue samples

Much valuable clinical research would be impossible without the use of data from human tissue samples. The retention and use of tissue and organs has attracted much controversy, as it has been discovered over the last couple of years that hospitals up and down the country have maintained large stores of bodily parts, allegedly without patient consent. The question of retention of such materials after a coroner's post-mortem has been undertaken was considered by Professor Ian Kennedy and the team involved in the inquiry at Bristol Royal Infirmary (Kennedy, 2000). They recommended that this area be subject to a major review, which should take the form either of a new code of practice or of legislation. It empha-sized the importance of gaining consent from relatives for the retention of body tissue after the post-mortem had been completed. The legal issues surrounding this whole area are uncertain. There is no property in a dead body (*R* v. *Kelly* [1998] 3 All ER 741), and yet it is the case that property interests have been recognized in bodily parts and products (*R* v. *Welsh* [1974] RTR 478 ; *R* v. *Rothery* [1976] RTR 478). Particular difficulties are likely to arise in the future in the form of the retention and use of materials extracted from body tissues in DNA banks (Martin and Kaye, 1999). Such materials can reveal considerable information about the research subject. The need for confidentiality of such information goes without saying, but other important issues of consent arise. It is suggested that it is not sufficient today to assume that, for example, spare body tissue has been 'abandoned by the patient and that there is thus no legal or ethical issue arising regarding its subsequent use' (McHale, 2000). It is desirable to obtain specific consent from the patient for the use of such material now and also in the future. It may be questionable as to what extent general blanket consents given by patients regarding the use of their bodily materials or of indeed to genetic information derived from that bodily material will necessarily be valid. The legal status of spare bodily parts and products, and the boundaries of research in the area of genetics, need urgent legal clarification. Without such clarification we are likely to be faced, as has happened in the USA, with patients challenging the use of their bodily materials without their consent, particularly in situations where there has been commercial exploitation of such bodily materials (*Moore* v. *University of California* [1990] 793 P 2d 479).

Confidentiality and research information

Nurses must always bear in mind that patient information is to be treated as confidential. Research projects may involve highly sensitive clinical information – for example, a study examining counselling provision for persons who are HIV positive. The nurse, as we saw earlier, is obliged by his or her contract of employment and by the UKCC professional ethical code to maintain patient confidentiality. The RCN (1993) has stated that:

> ... usually this means that data are analysed and reported in such a way that particular individuals, small groups or even organizations cannot be identified unless they have given prior agreement, the full information being only known to the research team.

Research may be undertaken using existing medical records. In principle, the patient's consent to disclosure should be obtained; however, if the sample is very large, tracing all patients may be totally impracticable. Nevertheless, the Department of Health guidelines stress that if a patient has previously indicated that he or she did not want medical information released for the purposes of medical research, this request should be respected (DOH, 1991).

It is important that information generated during a clinical trial is kept just as confidential as any other clinical information; the researcher must respect the confidentiality of information given to him or her by staff and patients. Unauthorized disclosure is not only ethically unjustifiable, but it may also prejudice further research. If a study is undertaken into working practices on the wards, it is important to ensure that nurses can speak frankly. They may not be willing to be so frank without a guarantee of anonymity being provided and adhered to. No individual should be identifiable from the published results without consent. Use of anonymized information is presently unlikely to require subsequent consent from the subject (*R* v. *Department of Health ex parte Source Informatics* (1999) 52 BMLR 65 CA). The Department of Health guidelines emphasize that identifiable data should be destroyed at the end of the project if no longer needed by the researcher (DOH, 1991). If the researcher wants to keep the data, he or she must be prepared to justify this to the research ethics committee/relevant NHS body and to the research subject.

The Department of Health recommends that persons should not be included in the trial unless they agree that information can be disclosed to their GP. On the face of it, this may seem a perfectly reasonable suggestion. Without that information, a GP subsequently treating the patient may not realize that certain symptoms are related to involvement in a clinical trial. However, this does not mean that it is desirable for all information to be automatically transferred. What if, for example, tests are undertaken and it is found that the research subject has tested HIV positive? The subject may be unwilling for this information to be passed on to the GP. The author suggests that any rule requiring disclosure to a GP should not be absolute in nature.

Intervention with care of the patient on the ward

While observing practice on the ward, the nurse researcher may come across situations in which patient care falls below what is regarded as being an acceptable standard (Dines, 1995):

A nurse researcher is interested in the feeding problems of stroke patients. She is using non-participant observation as her research method. She is seated inconspicuously wearing a white coat in the ward; it is a mealtime. A stroke patient nearby is propped up against his pillows and reaches for his milky tea. He takes the spouted beaker to his lips but spills the drink down his pyjama jacket. No nurse is in sight, what should the nurse researcher do?

Some time later the sister appears; she is updating the fluid balance charts. Observing the empty beaker she congratulates the patient on drinking his tea and charts the fluid intake. What should the nurse researcher do?

Should the nurse intervene? As Dines notes, the nurse faces a dilemma. By intervening she would be unable to observe what action the ward sister would take in that situation – a matter which is part of her research. However, if the nurse failed to act and the patient became dehydrated, would she be negligent? In this situation a court would have to consider whether she owed a duty to the patient on that ward. The nurse is not responsible directly for the clinical care of that patient, and there is no general duty to act as a 'Good Samaritan'. If the nurse researcher were held to be under a duty in such a situation, the court would assess whether the conduct was negligent by reference to a responsible body of professional practice. Some guidance to the approach of one body of professional opinion in such a situation can be gleaned from a publication of the RCN (1993), which suggests that:

The nurse who is undertaking a research project in an exclusively research role has no responsibility for the service, care, treatment or advice given to patients or clients unless stipulated within the design of the research. Otherwise, any intervention in a professional capacity should be confined to situations in which a patient or client requires to be protected or rescued from danger.

However, it is uncertain what is meant here by 'protection from danger'. Does this mean immediate danger, or something that becomes dangerous because it is repeated – for example, the patient regularly spilling a drink and losing fluid?

The RCN (1993) has said:

A nurse in a research situation still holds expert knowledge and may at times feel impelled to action for a patient's benefit.

Whether the nurse is held to be negligent may depend on factors such as the risk to the patient by her non-intervention. Take the example given at the start of this section. If the nurse continued to observe the patient losing fluids and saw that no check was made by the sister and the patient was placed at grave risk of dehydration, then it is arguable that by not acting to warn the nurse on the ward the nurse researcher would be negligent.

Compensating research subjects and policing trials

This section considers the liability of nurses, whether as researchers or as ethics committee members, when trials go wrong (Guest, 1997). The role of the nurse in policing unethical behaviour in a trial is also discussed. As noted above, the general principles of law apply to clinical trials. If a research subject is not told of a particular risk of involvement in a trial and that risk materializes and the subject is injured, he or she may bring an action in negligence or battery against the researcher. If a research subject is injured during a trial due to the researcher's lack of care, then again an action for negligence may be brought.

No national scheme of compensation exists for those injured in clinical trials, and researchers must be adequately insured. However, some special compensation provision exists for certain trials. The Association of British Pharmaceutical Industries (ABPI) guidelines provide that researchers should make contractually binding undertakings with research subjects in non-therapeutic trials to pay compensation in the event of injury (Hodges, 1991). The Association does not require contractually binding undertakings to be made with research subjects in therapeutic trials, although it suggests that assurances should be given that compensation would be paid in the event of harm resulting. While there are no contractual sanctions for breaking an undertaking, to break it would lead to criticism and make it very difficult for the researcher to arrange insurance cover from the Association in the future. This scheme has not, however, met with universal approval.

There has been some criticism of the operation of indemnity schemes by the ABPI in that it has installed threshold limits before claims can be brought (Burris, 1995). If the research is commissioned by the Medical Research Council, there is no automatic entitlement to compensation, although the Council has indicated that compensation payments may be made on an *ex gratia* basis.

Liability of ethics committee members

If a research subject is injured in a clinical trial, then it is possible that an action could be brought against individual members of the research ethics committee on the grounds that they were negligent in approving the conduct of the trial. It has been suggested that, at least in theory, each individual ethics committee member owes a duty of care to each research subject (Brazier, 1990). Any costs of legal proceedings brought against a nurse employed by the NHS who sits on a research ethics committee will be covered by NHS indemnity insurance. The Department of Health has stated that it will cover the costs of a research ethics committee member as long as he or she has not been guilty of misconduct or gross lack of care. It should be noted that although an action in negligence is a theoretical possibility, in practice bringing such a claim might be difficult. A research subject would have to show that it was the negligence of a particular committee member in approving the trial that caused the injury he or she had suffered.

What can be done if it is thought that the trial is being conducted unethically?

If the nurse believes that a trial in which he or she is involved is being conducted unethically, the nurse may raise this with the person in charge of the trial. But what if no notice is taken of what the nurse has said? He or she can draw the matter to the attention of the research ethics committee who approved the trial. The committee may decide to take action, but in practice it has few powers. It may ask the researchers to report to them and then withdraw authorization from the trial. If the unethical researcher is a nurse, it may be thought appropriate to refer the researcher's conduct to the UKCC, who may decide to take disciplinary proceedings. In the case of a doctor, misconduct may be referred to the General Medical Council. As in the report regarding the research undertaken by Professor David Southall, conduct of a particular trial may also be the subject of an inquiry.

If a nurse conducting a trial departs from an agreed trial protocol and has acted unethically, it may limit the nurse's chances of obtaining approval for another clinical trial. However, there is no national code stating how research ethics committees should scrutinize projects once these are up and running. While some committees have follow-up procedures and write to the researcher to find out how the project has progressed, others do not. It is therefore arguable that the rights of the subject in the trial are being neglected. Neuberger (1992) has suggested that new powers be given to committees to carry out spot checks. In addition, questionnaires could perhaps be given to research subjects to discover how a trial has been conducted. However, to expect the research ethics committee to undertake detailed policing of the many trials they scrutinize is clearly unrealistic. Committee members are unpaid, and systematic scrutiny with spot checks, etc., would really require full time officers to be appointed. The administrative workload would increase, as would the cost. In a National Health Service subject to considerable budgetary restraints, such innovations are unlikely – at least in the immediate future.

References

Brazier, M. (1990). The liability of ethics committee members. *Professional Negligence*, **6**, 186.

British Paediatric Association (1992). *Guidelines for the Ethical Conduct of Research Involving Children.* BPA.

Burris, J. M. (1995). The compensation of patients injured in clinical trials. *J. Med. Ethics*, **21**, 166.

Department of Health (1991). *Guidelines for Local Research Ethics Committees.* DOH, (i) para 2.5; (ii) para 4.5; (iii) para 7.86; (iv) para 3.15; (v) para 3.7; (vi) para 3.9; (vii) para 4.1; (viii) para 4.4.

Department of Health (1997). Ethics Committee Review of Multi-Centre Research: Establishment of Multi-Centre Research Ethics Committee (HSG(97)27).

Dines, A. (1995). An ethical perspective – nursing research. In: *Nursing Law and Ethics* (J. Tingle and A. Cribb, eds). Blackwell Scientific, p. 257.

Dodds-Smith, I. (1992). Clinical research. In: *Doctors, Patients and the Law* (C. Dyer, ed.). Blackwell Scientific.

Evans, D. (1995). The investigation of life-threatening child abuse and Munchausen's syndrome by proxy. *J. Med. Ethics*, **21**, 9.

Fox, M. (1995). Animal rights and wrongs: medical ethics and the killing of non-human animals. In: *Death Rites: Law and Ethics at the End of Life* (R. Lee and D. Morgan, eds). Routledge.

Gillon, R. (1995). Editorial: Covert surveillance by doctor for life-threatening Munchausen's syndrome by proxy. *J. Med. Ethics*, **21**, 131.

Griffiths, R. (2000). *Report of the Review into the Research Framework in North Staffordshire.* http://www.doh.gov.uk/wmro/northstaffs.htm.

Guest, S. (1997). Compensation for subjects of medical research; the moral rights of patients and the power of research ethics committees. *J. Med. Ethics*, **23**, 181.

Harris, J and Dyson, A. (1987). *Experiments on Embryos.* Routledge.

Hodges, C. (1991). Harmonisation of European Controls over Research Ethics Committees – Consent, Compensation and Indemnity. In *Pharmaceutical Medicine and the Law* (A. Goldberg and I. Dodds Smith, eds). Royal College of Physicians.

Kennedy, I. (2000). The Inquiry into the Management and Care of Children Receiving Complex Heart Surgery at Bristol Royal Infirmary; Interim Report – Removal and Retention of Human Material.

Kennedy, I. and Grubb, A. (1994). *Medical Law Text with Materials*, 2nd edn. Butterworths.

Kirk, E. (1995). Research and patients. In: *Nursing Law and Ethics* (J. Tingle and A. Cribb, eds). Blackwell Scientific.

Law Commission (1995). *Mental Incapacity*. Report No. 231, HMSO.

Lock, S. (ed.) (1993). *Fraud and Misconduct in Medical Research*. British Medical Journal Press.

Lord Chancellor's Department (1997). *Who Decides?* LCD Cm 3803.

Lord Chancellor's Department (1999). *Making Decisions*. LCD Cm 4465.

Martin, P. and Kaye, J. (1999). *The Use of Biological Sample Collection and Personal Medical Information in Human Genetics Research*. Wellcome Trust.

Mason, J. K. and McCall Smith, R. A. (1999). *Law and Medical Ethics*, 5th edn. Butterworths, p. 372.

McHale, J. (2000). Waste, ownership and bodily products. *Health Care Analysis*, **8**, 123–135.

Neuberger, J. (1992). *Ethics and Health Care; The Role of the Research Ethics Committee*. Kings Institute.

Nicholson R. (1985). *Medical Research and Children*. MRC.

Nicholson, R. (1991). The ethics of research with children. In: *Protecting the Vulnerable* (M. Brazier and M. Lobjoit, eds). Routledge.

Parabor, K. (1997). *Nursing Research, Principles, Process and Issues*. Macmillan.

Polkinghorne, J. (1989). *Review of the Guidance on the Research Use of Fetuses and Fetal Material*. Cmnd 762.

Royal College of Nursing (1993). *Ethics Relating to Research in Nursing*. Scutari Press, para 3.14.

Royal College of Physicians (1986). *Research on Healthy Volunteers*. RCP.

Royal College of Physicians (1991). *Report of Working Party on Research on Patients*. RCP, para 7.12.

Royal College of Physicians (1996). *Guidelines on the Practice of Ethics Committees in Medical Research Involving Human Subjects*, 3rd edn. RCP.

Royal College of Psychiatrists (1990). Guidelines for psychiatric research involving human subjects. *Psychiatric Bull.*, **48**.

Silverman, W. A. (1989). The myth of informed consent. *J. Med. Ethics*, **15**, 251.

Smith, R. (1997). Misconduct in research: editors respond. *Br. Med. J.*, **315**, 201.

Southall, D. P. and Samuels, M. P. (1995). Some ethical issues surrounding covert video surveillance – a response. *J. Med. Ethics*, 104.

UKCC (1996). *Guidelines for Professional Practice*. UKCC.

UKXIRA (1998). *Guidance on Making Proposals to Conduct Xenotransplantation on Human Subjects*. United Kingdom Xenotransplantation Interim Regulatory Authority.

Chapter 9

Reproductive choice

Jean McHale

Today, patients have an increasing range of reproductive choices. Nurses may play a direct part in guiding some of these choices – for instance, in the case of the teenager who approaches the nurse for advice regarding contraception, or the mother wondering whether her mentally handicapped daughter should be sterilized. In others, nurses may not be direct participants in the process unless a patient specifically approaches them for advice. Nevertheless, it is important for nurses to be aware of the legal framework within which these choices are made and clinical procedures are undertaken. This chapter begins with an examination of the legality of the provision of contraceptive services and the question of sterilization of the mentally incompetent adult. Secondly, the regulation of the new reproductive technologies such as IVF and the prospects for cloning are considered. Thirdly, the role of the law in regulating conduct during pregnancy is explored. Finally, the legality of abortion and the involvement of nurses in the abortion process are discussed.

Provision of contraceptive services

Nurses may be involved in providing contraceptive advice and treatment, whether in a family planning clinic or in the hospital setting. Statute states that the Secretary of State for Health has a duty to meet reasonable requirements relating to the provision of contraceptive advice/treatment of persons in England and Wales (s5 (1) b National Health Service Act 1977).

While in the past the legality of undertaking sterilization operations for contraceptive purposes was questioned, today such operations are generally accepted to be lawful (*Bravery* v. *Bravery* [1954] 3 All ER 59, pp. 67–8). As with any surgical procedure, before sterilization is undertaken the patient's own consent must be obtained; the spouse or partner has no right to participate in the consent process and may not veto the operation. The implications of the operation and the fact that there is a possibility of failure are indicated on the NHS consent form, but these should also be drawn explicitly to the patient's attention, otherwise there is the possibility that a negligence action will result (*Thake* v. *Maurice* [1986] 1 All ER 497 and see also *McFarlane* v. *Tayside Health Board* [1999] 4 All ER 961 HC).

One major point of controversy has concerned provision of contraceptive advice and treatment to teenagers. As seen in Chapter 7, this issue came before the courts in the case of *Gillick* v. *West Norfolk and Wisbech AHA* ([1986] AC 150). If a young girl approaches a nurse seeking contraceptive advice/treatment, the nurse must assess whether the girl has sufficient maturity to appreciate the nature of the advice/treatment sought and whether she is capable of making an informed choice.

Sterilizing the mentally incompetent

A mother is worried that her mentally handicapped daughter, who is in her early teens, is vulnerable to seduction. She believes that her daughter should be sterilized for her protection. She discusses her concerns with the district nurse who is helping her to care for her daughter. What should the nurse do?

In the case described, the mother genuinely believes that sterilization is in her daughter's best interests. However, while the girl may have the mental age of a young child, she may develop maternal feelings and in the future be capable of being a loving mother. There is also a danger in assuming that sterilization will be a panacea, when in fact by removing the risk of pregnancy the girl may be placed at risk of undetectable abuse. If parents and health care professionals disagree as to whether sterilization should be undertaken, then this issue should be referred to the court. The court will determine whether the proposed sterilization operation is lawful by assessing whether the procedure is in the girl's best interests.

Use of a 'best interests' test leaves much discretion in the hands of the courts. In *Re D*, D, an 11-year-old child from a poor background, suffered from Sottas syndrome ([1976] 1 All ER 326). This condition results in accelerated growth during infancy, epilepsy, generalized clumsy appearance, behavioural problems and certain aggressive tendencies. D had reached puberty, and while she had not shown any marked interest in the opposite sex, her protective mother was concerned about the consequences if she became pregnant. She wanted her daughter sterilized, and her doctor supported her opinion.

Heilbron J. refused to authorize the sterilization. She said that the evidence showed that there had been improvement in D's mental and physical condition, and her future prospects were unpredictable. Nevertheless, it was likely that in the future she would be able to make her own choice. Should she then realize the impact of what had happened to her, she might feel frustration and resentment. The judge emphasized that the decision to undertake sterilization for non-therapeutic purposes on a minor was not a matter for clinical judgment alone.

In cases following *Re D*, the courts have, however, shown far less hesitation before authorizing sterilization. In *Re B* ([1987] 2 WLR 1212), B was a 17-year-old woman who had a mental age of 5–6 years and was also epileptic. Evidence was given to the effect that she did not understand and was unable to learn the causal connection between intercourse, pregnancy and the birth of children. However, she had the sexual inclinations of a normal 17-year-old. It was claimed that there was only a 40 per cent chance of establishing an acceptable regime with oral contraceptives, and there would be side effects. Because she suffered swings of mood and had considerable physical strength, administration of a daily dose of medication may have been impossible. B was also obese and this, coupled with the irregularity of her periods, may have made early detection of pregnancy difficult. B's mother and the local authority sought an order from the court authorizing sterilization. The court granted the order. Lord Hailsham said that the case was clearly distinguishable from *Re D*. He said (p. 216):

> To talk of a basic right to reproduce of an individual who is not capable of knowing the causal connection between intercourse and childbirth, the nature of pregnancy and what is involved in delivery and is unable to form maternal instincts or to care for a child is to wholly part company with reality

Lord Templeman stated that in his opinion sterilization of a woman under 18 years should only be undertaken with the leave of the High Court. In this case, it would, he said, be cruel to expose her to an unacceptable risk of pregnancy. Lord Oliver also distinguished from *Re D*. He said:

> ... the right to reproduce is only valuable if accompanied by the ability to make a choice and in the instant case there is no question of the minor being able to make a choice or indeed to appreciate the desire to make one. All the evidence indicates that she will never desire a child and that reproduction will be positively harmful to her.

The decision of the House of Lords in *Re B* has been the subject of much critical comment. For example, Lee and Morgan (1987) have asked why B was able to manage the hygienic mechanics of menstruation but not contraception, and why she was able to understand the link between pregnancy and babies but not that between sex and pregnancy. Emphasis was placed in the case upon B's mental age. However, it has been suggested that this hides the complexity of the issue. For instance, a woman may have a mental age of 5 years in relation to some functions, while at the same time having far higher comprehension levels in relation to other tasks. Reference was made in *Re B* to a Canadian case, *Re Eve* ([1986] DLR (4t) 1), in which the court held that non-therapeutic sterilization of a mentally incompetent adult was never justifiable. The House of Lords, however, disagreed, and said that it was wrong to draw a distinction between therapeutic and non-therapeutic sterilization. It is perhaps ironic in view of this that, as will be seen below, later courts appear to have drawn just such a distinction when considering whether all sterilization operations should require judicial approval.

There are perceptible advantages in the postponement of the sterilization decision until a mentally incompetent woman is older. Assessment of her physical and mental development may then be made on the basis of conclusive evidence, as opposed to guesswork. In B's case there was some urgency in performing the operation before she reached her eighteenth birthday, because at that time the legality of treatment of the mentally incompetent adult was unclear. This issue was finally resolved in 1989 by the House of Lords in *Re F* ([1990] AC 1). The House of Lords held that a mentally incompetent adult woman could be sterilized if it was in her best interests, but it stated that it would be desirable for the medical team to obtain a declaration from the court before such an operation was undertaken.

The majority of the cases concern females; however, in *Re A (medical treatment: male sterilization)*([2000] FCR 193) the Court of Appeal was asked to rule upon the sterilization of a 28-year-old man with Down's syndrome. He was assessed as borderline between having significant and severe intelligence impairment. While incapable of making a decision regarding sterilization himself, he was sexually aware and active. His mother supported his sterilization. The Court of Appeal held that the sterilization should not at present go ahead. Dame Elisabeth Butler Sloss P. indicated that at a time when there was soon to be direct application of the European Convention of Human Rights in English law, the court should be slow to take a step that may infringe the rights of those unable to act for themselves. The Court of Appeal emphasized that the patient's best interests were something different from the interests of carers or others, but left open the extent to which the interests of third parties should be weighed in the balance when determining what was in the patient's best interests. It was noted that such a decision should not be authorized on eugenic grounds. Moreover, a decision to sterilize a female patient involved different considerations, and in the context of a man there were no direct consequences other than the fact that he may contract a sexually transmitted disease. It is likely that the court will be presented with human rights based arguments in future cases concerning the decision to sterilize. The argument advanced that male patients may be treated differently is one which should be used with caution. It is important that the decision to sterilize female patients should be taken with caution.

A Practice Note has been issued providing guidance as to how cases should be handled (Practice Note: Official Solicitor: Sterilization [1996] 2 All ER 111). Guidance states that the application will be made to the High Court, patients will be represented and the Official Solicitor will attempt to ascertain the patient's views in an interview. Evidence will be required as to the patient's capacity, the risks of pregnancy, the consequences of pregnancy for the woman's health and alternatives to sterilization. The courts have indicated that sterilization of a mentally incompetent woman undertaken for therapeutic purposes, such as the performance of a hysterectomy upon a woman suffering from extensive menstruation, does not require judicial approval (*Re E (a minor)* [1992] 2 FLR 585). Cases involving non-therapeutic sterilization will, however, continue to be referred to the courts. It is important to ensure that such decisions are made on the basis of the woman's best interests rather than what is convenient for the carers.

In a number of cases, the judges, when authorizing sterilization, have emphasized the possibility of surgical reversal of the sterilization operation (*Re P (minor) (wardship: sterilization)* [1989] 1 FLR 182, [1989] Fam Law 102 and *Re M (a minor) (wardship: sterilization)* [1988] 2 FLR 497). However, as Brazier (1990) has argued, while leading experts may achieve a high level of reversals, this does not mean that all clinicians can achieve this. Also, it is highly questionable whether an operation to reverse the sterilization of a mentally handicapped person would be a priority in a financially constrained NHS.

The nurse acting as patient advocate may play an important role, particularly in ensuring that in those situations in which sterilization has not been referred to the courts, it is being undertaken for therapeutic purposes and is in the patient's best interests. An alternative approach to that presently adopted with regard to therapeutic sterilization operations is that of at least requiring some form of second opinion to be obtained. This type of approach was favoured by the Law Commission (1995) in their report, *Mental Incapacity*.

Modern reproductive technology

Developments in medical technology have, in the last half century, given much hope to the infertile. For example, a woman who is unable to conceive may receive *in vitro* fertilization treatment (IVF), which involves the egg being fertilized outside the womb and then implanted into the uterus. However, use of such techniques has not been free of controversy. In response to debate generated, the government established a committee, the Warnock Committee, to examine the use of new reproductive technologies. This committee reported in 1984 (Warnock Committee, 1984). It recommended that use of these technologies be subject to regulation. Today, modern reproductive technologies are regulated by statute in the form of the Human Fertilization and Embryology Act 1990. This Act established the Human Fertilization and Embryology Authority (HEFA), whose functions include the licensing of clinics providing fertility treatment (Lee and Morgan, 1991). It also grants licences for the conduct of embryo research. Not all forms of assisted conception must be licensed by the Authority; for example, artificial insemination of a woman with her partner's sperm does not need licensing. The licensing of certain technologies, is prohibited; for example, human embryos may not be placed in an animal, and nor can 'cloning' – where this amounts to replacing the nucleus of an embryo – be undertaken (s3(3)).

A right of access to assisted reproductive services?

A 39-year-old woman and her partner are presently unable to conceive. The woman has up until now postponed having a family due to her busy career. They seek access to infertility treatment.

There is no automatic right of access to infertility services. A woman seeking access to IVF, for example, would have to satisfy the clinic that she was a suitable case for receiving such treatment. Her eligibility is determined by reference to criteria set out in the Code of Practice produced by the HEFA (1998), and criteria considered would include a child's need for a father, the applicants' medical histories, and their commitment to bringing up children (HEFA, 1998). That does not mean that single women would be precluded from access to infertility treatment, but the clinic would scrutinize the application and consider, for example, whether there would be any male influences in the child's upbringing (HEFA, 1998, para 3.18). Individual clinics also produce their own criteria for the approval of treatment, and these include restrictions by reference to the age of the woman seeking treatment. Many clinics do not allow women over 35 years of age access to infertility treatment on the grounds that the success rates of treatment on older women are limited.

While there is the potential for persons denied access to IVF services to challenge this refusal in the courtroom, in practice such challenges are unlikely to be successful. For example, in *R* v. *Ethical Committee of St. Mary's Hospital, Manchester* ([1988] 1 FLR 512), R was unable to conceive. Her application to adopt a child had been rejected because of her criminal record relating to prostitution and brothel keeping. She sought IVF treatment, however a consultant at the IVF clinic rejected her application. This decision was supported by the hospital's infertility ethical committee. (Bodies undertaking infertility treatment must establish ethical committees to which problematic decisions relating to access to such treatments may be referred.) Schiemann J. said that the committee was in essence an informal body. If the committee in a particular case refused to give advice to a consultant or did not come to a majority view on a decision, he did not see that the court could compel it either to give advice or to enter into a particular investigation. Schiemann J. did not rule out the possibility of judicial review:

If the committee had advised, for instance, that the IVF unit should in principal refuse treatment to anyone who was a … Jew or coloured, then I think that the court might well grant a declaration that that was illegal.

However, he stressed that the committee was a talking shop for professionals, and a court should be cautious before intervening. It appears that such challenges are unlikely to be successful in the future unless they are manifestly unreasonable/indefensible. This was illustrated in the later case of *R* v. *Sheffield HA ex parte Seale* ([1994] 25 BMLR 1). S, a 36-year-old woman, was denied IVF treatment. It was said that there was a need to ration resources, and treatment was generally less effective in those women who were over 35 years of age. The court was not prepared to overrule the clinic's decision to refuse her treatment on the basis that it was irrational. The 39-year-old career woman in the example given at the start of this section would be likely to be able to afford the cost of private medical care. Nonetheless, clinics do have a discretion, and there is no automatic right to access treatment services. The Human Rights Act 1998 provides the prospect of persons denied access to treatment seeking redress from the courts. They are likely to argue for a right to reproduce in relation to Article 8 of the European Convention of Human Rights – the right to privacy – and Article 12 – the right to marry and found a family. Nonetheless, the scope for success in such litigation may be questioned. The right to reproduce is an uncertain concept, and judicial enforcement of expenditure of NHS resources in this manner is unlikely.

Posthumous conception and the use of stored gametes

The Act expressly regulates the donation, storage and use of gametes and embryos for the purposes of treatment and research (see Chapter 8, p. 165), and makes these subject to consent procedures (s14 HFE Act 1990; HEFA Code of Practice 1998 paras 5.9–5.11; 8.10). Storage means of course that gametes/stored embryos may be sought for use after one partner has died. The Act does not ban such conception, although it does provide that a child born through the use of such techniques is legally fatherless (s28). The question of the use of posthumous conception arose in the well-known case of Diane Blood. Mr and Mrs Blood had been planning to start a family when Mr Blood contracted meningitis. Sperm was removed from him while he was in a coma. Subsequently his widow sought to have use of the sperm in order that she could be artificially inseminated (*R* v. *Human Fertilization and Embryology Authority ex parte Blood* [1997] 2 All ER 687). In the *Blood* case itself the HFEA refused to allow the treatment to go ahead because the treatment was not sanctioned under the statute, as there had been no prior consent given for the use of the sperm from her deceased husband after his death. The Court of Appeal upheld this decision. However, the HFEA also refused to allow the sperm to be exported to enable Mrs Blood to be treated in Europe. The Court of Appeal ruled that the HEFA had not taken into sufficient account, when exercising their discretion to allow the sperm to be exported, the fact that restrictions placed upon the export could be regarded as being contrary to principles of free movement in European law (Articles 59 and 60 EC Treaty). The HFEA was asked to reconsider the issue. They did, and allowed the export to go ahead. One of the interesting issues flowing from this case is how it illustrates the way in which the principles of European law are beginning to have an impact in the area of health care law (see Chapter 1). The question of consent to use of gametes was explored in a review chaired by Professor Sheila McLean (McLean, 1997). She recommended that the consent requirement should remain. Reasons for this included the need to provide good practice and because of the question of genetic identity. However if a person was unconscious and the necessary treatment would render them sterile removal of gametes may be legitimate to provide them with the opportunity to become a parent.

Parentage and the 1990 Act

The Human Fertilization and Embrology Act itself provides guidance as to parentage consequent upon the use of new technologies beyond the situation of posthumous conception. This is of course necessary, since the genetic composition of the fetus may well be different to that of the couple seeking treatment because donor gametes have been used. Donor anonymity is guaranteed, so that sperm donors, for example, cannot subsequently be traced, although some genetic information is available to the child on reaching maturity (section 31). The Act provides that the gestational mother is in law the mother, even if donor eggs have been used. In the case of the father, this depends on whether the couple are married, in which case the husband is deemed to be the father, although this is a rebuttable presumption (s28(2)). In the case of an unmarried couple, then the man will be treated as the father if they both go together for treatment (s28(3)). (For parenting issues consequent upon surrogacy, see p. 192.)

As far as the use of sex selection is concerned, this is not banned by the Human Fertilization and Embryology Act 1990. Use of such techniques are, however, controversial. The Council of Europe, in their Convention on Human Rights and Biomedicine (to which the UK has yet to become a signatory) provides in Article 14 (non-selection of sex):

> The use of techniques of medically assisted procreation shall not be allowed for the purpose of choosing a future child's sex, except where serious hereditary sex-related disease is to be avoided.

The Code of Practice issued by the Human Fertilization and Embryology Authority provides that couples contemplating use of modern reproductive technologies should be given counselling as to the implications of undertaking such therapy (HEFA, 1998, Chapter 6). Nurses may be involved in such counselling.

Conscientious objection

Nurses may object to their participation in the use of certain techniques such as IVF, which involve gamete or embryo manipulation, on religious or cultural grounds. Section 38 of the 1990 Act gives nurses and other health professionals the right to refuse to participate in such treatments by expressing a conscientious objection.

Surrogacy

A surrogate is the term used to describe a woman who carries the child of another. This practice has been undertaken for centuries. Recently, however, surrogacy has been linked with modern reproductive technologies. It is argued that surrogacy can be both a necessary and a helpful method of alleviating infertility. It may assist women who have suffered repeated miscarriages, and might be appropriate in a situation in which a woman was medically unable to cope with the trauma of pregnancy although she was capable of caring for a child once born. In practice, it appears that surrogacy is regarded as appropriate only in exceptional cases. The British Medical Association (BMA, 1990) has recommended that surrogacy:

> ... should only be considered as a last resort where the commissioning couple suffers from infertility due to a medically recognized disorder and where all appropriate means for enabling them to have a child have been tried and failed.

There are several reasons why surrogacy is seen as problematic. First, there may be conflicts between the natural mother and the commissioning parents, with the surrogate seeking to keep the child. Allowing surrogacy subject to a legally enforceable agreement would have the effect that a newborn could be forcibly removed from the surrogate to the commissioning parents. Secondly, much discussion about surrogacy has concerned the commercialization of the practice. It has been argued that making money out of the surrogate process is ethically unacceptable. The Warnock Committee was opposed to the commercialization of surrogacy (Warnock Committee, 1984). The Surrogacy Arrangements Act 1985 provides that it is an offence to arrange a commercial surrogacy agreement (s2 (1)) or to advertise surrogacy services (s3). No prosecutions have as yet been brought under the Act. The legislation is targeted at surrogacy agencies; the commissioning mother and the surrogate do not commit an offence under this statute (s2(2)). While the law does not ban surrogacy agreements, they are however unenforceable. For instance, if a surrogate decided to keep the child, the commissioning parents could not demand that the child was handed over by her (s36(i) Human Fertilization and Embryology Act 1990).

A number of non-profit-making surrogacy agencies were established following the legislation, notably the agency COTS. It was claimed that some surrogates were being paid considerable sums of money in the form of 'expenses'. The legitimacy of such payments was the subject of consideration in a review commissioned by the Department of Health and chaired by Professor Margaret Brazier (DOH, 1997). The review was opposed to the commercialization of surrogacy, and argued that while expenses could be recoverable they should be reclaimable only where these were documented as relating to costs consequent to pregnancy and birth.

Where children are born as a consequence of consensual surrogacy arrangements, the surrogate is legally the child's mother, as she is the gestational mother (s27 HFE Act 1990). However, in such a situation the commissioning couple can apply either to adopt the child or for a special order under section 30 of the Human Fertilization and Embryology Act 1990, which has the effect that the commissioning couple can become parents if it is a consensual non-commercial arrangement, the child has had a home with the commissioning couple, and the application has been made within 6 months of the birth. The Brazier Review has recommended that there should be consideration given to a new Surrogacy Act replacing both s30 and the 1985 Act which would also include a Surrogacy Code. These recommendations have not yet been taken forward by the Government

Cloning

One of the most heated recent debates in relation to the use of new human reproductive technologies has arisen in the context of cloning. In 1997, Ian Wilmut cloned Dolly the sheep at the Roslin Institute in Edinburgh. Cloning involves various techniques. One such technique is 'embryo splitting', which is the replication of the process that occurs naturally, leading to the production of twins. Embryonic cells are separated at a very early stage before they have had a chance to differentiate. Another method is that of 'nuclear replacement' – replacing the nucleus of an embryo/unfertilized egg with a nucleus taken from another.

Cloning may be undertaken for therapeutic purposes, such as tissue and organ replacement (see Chapter 10) and for reproductive purposes – the creation of a new human being e.g. enabling an infertile man to have genetically related children. Although the Human Fertilization and Embryology Act 1990 prohibits cloning where this is the replacement of the nucleus of an embryo, it appears that other cloning methods are possible under English law (Mason and McCall Smith, 1999; p. 187). Following Dolly, the House of Commons Science and Technology Committee Enquiry examined the issue. Their report was published in March 1997 (House of Commons Select Committee on Science and Technology, 1997), and proposed that Parliament should confirm a ban on reproductive cloning. It also proposed that 'experimental human beings' should not be created. The Minister of State for Health supported this in June 1997.

There are a number of reasons why there has been opposition to cloning. First, it is a costly technology and one that is likely to lead to considerable wastage of eggs and a high degree of risk. Dolly was the only normal lamb born from 276 similar attempts. Only 29 of these cases led to implantable embryos, and all of these except Dolly resulted in defective pregnancies and grossly deformed births. Other concerns relate to the life expectancy of the clone, which may be reduced due to the fact that a clone could be born prematurely aged because its genetic material would already be as old as the being from whom the genetic material had been removed. Some concerns have also been expressed regarding whether cloning might produce resultant health defects. In 1999, a 2-month-old cloned calf died after it developed blood and heart problems (*BMJ*, 1999). Numerous ethical and social issues have also been identified. It has been suggested that cloning may amount to using individuals as a means to an end, and as such is wrong. Could cloned children be in effect regarded as commodities? There may be the prospect that human rights or dignity may be infringed by the prospect of two or more persons being in existence with identical genetic composition. However, proponents of cloning have argued that nature already provides for monozygotic twins, who have identical composition. It has also been suggested that a clone would not be identical to the individual from which it was cloned, because this does not take into account social, cultural and environmental issues, which play a very important part in an individual's development (Harris, 1998).

There has been considerable opposition to reproductive cloning in particular. Warnock was of the view that this should not be permitted. In introducing the report of the Human Genetic Advisory Commission and the Human Fertilization and Embryology Authority, Sir Colin Campbell stated that:

> We want to stop the wild and irresponsible notion of cloning whole human beings but allow procedures that in 5 to 10 years time may lead to the curing of diseases.

Ruth Deech, the chair of the HEFA, suggested that:

> The Human Fertilization and Embryology Act 1990 empowers the HEFA to forbid human reproductive cloning in the UK and we have no intention of changing our minds on that decision. Nevertheless the government may wish to consider the possibility of legislation explicitly banning reproductive cloning.

At the same time as the UK debate was being undertaken, the international response to cloning was proving hostile. In January 1998, 19 members of Council of Europe signed an agreement in Paris to the effect that it prohibited:

... any intervention seeking to create a human being genetically identical to any other human being, whether living or dead, by whatever means.

In 1998, the European Union called upon member states to ban cloning. A protocol to the Council of Europe Convention on Human Rights and Biomedicine contains a prohibition on cloning of humans (Council of Europe, 1998). Cloning has been seen by some as constituting a serious violation of human rights, being contrary to the principle of equality, permitting eugenic and racist selection, and offending against human dignity. Debates have also raged in the USA. In 1997, President Clinton announced an enquiry into the ethical and legal implications of cloning, to be carried out by the National Bioethics Advisory Commission, and it was also stated that 'no federal funds shall be allocated for cloning of human beings'. It was also proposed that there should be a moratorium on non-federal-funded research.

The National Bioethics Advisory Commission's conclusion to their review of the legal and ethical implications of cloning was that, at the present time:

... it is morally and ethically unacceptable for anyone in the public and private sector, whether in a research or clinical setting, to attempt to create a child using nuclear cell transfer cloning.

This is on the basis that use of such techniques at the present time is not safe. However, the Commission stated that appropriate legislation should include a 'sunset clause', which will enable Congress to review the legislation after a specified period of 3–5 years, and at this point a decision can be reached as to whether the prohibition is still needed. In February 1998, a bill to ban human cloning was shelved in Senate following much controversy as to what constitutes a human life, which is entitled to legal protection.

In July 1999, the UK government confirmed that in its view human reproductive cloning is ethically unacceptable. A new expert advisory group has been established with the task of assessing the potential benefits of cloning for therapeutic purposes. The government also said that a 6-month study would be undertaken on therapeutic applications of cloning, leading to further consideration of the issue (see also Chapter 10, p. 239). Development of therapeutic cloning in the UK seems likely, although the prospects for reproductive cloning are unlikely in the near future.

Regulating the conduct of the mother during pregnancy

Nurses and midwives have long played an important role during pregnancy and in childbirth. Today midwives are involved not only in the delivery itself but also, through antenatal classes, in the process of health education regarding birth. While over time the guidance and advice given to pregnant women has increased, few active constraints are imposed during pregnancy. While there is an active debate in the USA as to the extent to which women should be constrained by law during pregnancy, attempts to use the law to regulate behaviour in the period prior to birth in this country have been unsuccessful (Robertson, 1995). This is illustrated by the case of *Re F (in utero)* ([1988] 2 All ER 193). The court was faced with the issue of whether a fetus could be made a ward of court. F's mother had led a nomadic existence around Europe. She had disappeared, and those caring for her were concerned that the fetus in her womb would suffer harm if the woman did not seek medical attention. The court, however, refused to make the child a ward of court, stating that the court's jurisdiction under wardship did not extend to an unborn child.

It is unlikely that at present English law will be used to compel behaviour during pregnancy (contrast this with the attitude of the law regarding childbirth itself; see p. 197). Were such compulsion to be sanctioned, this would require radical re-evaluation of the role of the nurse and midwife in caring for the mother.

Freedom to choose where to give birth

During the last century, the birth process has become increasingly medically dominated. Much use is made of technological interventions in pregnancy, and today only around 1 per cent of women give birth in their own homes. There are a number of reasons why this is the case. It may be regarded as 'safer' for the mother, and hospital births may be more convenient for the hospital team. Some suggest that the increase in surgical interventions during pregnancy is motivated by fear of a 'malpractice crisis', with doctors increasingly prepared to advise patients to undertake Caesarean sections to avoid the risk of litigation should the pregnancy prove problematic. Indeed, the need for the number of Caesarean sections presently undertaken has been questioned. In some instances a Caesarean section may be the only alternative, otherwise the mother, child, or both may be at risk of death. A child may be in the breech position, and if the child's head becomes stuck then brain damage may result. At the same time, there are risks attached to the performance of a Caesarean section. Evidence has been given to the effect that, for example, the operation may put a woman at a 6–11 times greater risk of death during childbirth or due to haemorrhage. In addition, if the woman becomes pregnant again, the risk of rupture to the scar on the uterus may mean that another Caesarean operation will be required (Anderson and Strong, 1988).

There is some evidence of a shift in policy regarding the conduct of childbirth. A report issued by a House of Commons Committee stated that 'the policy of encouraging all women to give birth in hospital cannot be justified on grounds of safety' (House of Commons Health Committee Session 1991–92 Maternity Services). A government committee chaired by Lady Cumberlege published a report in 1993 called *Changing Childbirth: Report of the Expert Maternity Group* (Cumberlege, 1993). The report identified three key principles: the woman should be the focus of maternity care provision; maternity services should be readily and easily accessible to all; and services must be effective and efficient.

Today, the law regulates childbirth in two specific ways: first by statute in the form of the Nurses, Midwives and Health Visitors Act 1997, and secondly through common law interventions regarding enforced Caesarean sections.

Care during birth

It is a criminal offence under s16 of the Nurses, Midwives and Health Visitors Act 1997 for a person other than a registered midwife or registered medical practitioner to attend a woman in childbirth. This provision is aimed at protecting the mother and ensuring that she has expert care to hand when she needs it. There is an exception for sudden and urgent necessities, as in the situation where a midwife is summoned but the mother gives birth, with the assistance of her partner, before the midwife arrives. Student midwifes are allowed to attend a mother in childbirth as part of their training, but they must be supervised by a qualified practitioner (s16(2)(b) Nurses, Midwives and Health Visitors Act 1997). The practitioner supervising the midwife remains accountable for the conduct of the birth.

Birth plans and compelling a Caesarean section

Today it is common for women to agree with their midwife a plan for the conduct of their birth, and this states such matters as whether a woman will receive pain relief, etc. However, what if in a particular situation a midwife believes that it is necessary for the health of the woman to depart from the birth plan? Treating in the face of a previously stated refusal may, as seen earlier, render the midwife or doctor liable in the tort of battery (see Chapter 5). In some situations it may not prove practical to adhere to the birth plan. A woman states her wishes as regards a natural 'low tech' birth, but then complications develop; should the birth plan be followed? It could be argued that it should not if all the possible eventualities have not been foreseen. Any birth plan drawn up should be undertaken only after the implications of refusal of certain types of treatment and the problems should an emergency arise have been pointed out to the woman. Where it is proposed to go ahead in the absence of express consent, then wherever possible a court order should be sought.

A pregnant woman is told that she needs a Caesarean section and that without it both her life and the survival of the fetus are in grave danger. The woman says that she is opposed to blood transfusions being given on religious grounds, and tells the midwife that she is totally opposed to a Caesarean section. What can be done?

Such a problem came before the English courts in the 1992 case of *Re S* ([1992] 4 All ER 671). S was 6 days overdue giving birth. The health care team wanted to undertake a Caesarean section because, as the fetus was in transverse lie, any attempt at a normal birth carried a very grave risk of rupture to the uterus. S, who was a born again Christian, refused the operation because it would have involved a blood transfusion, which was against her religious beliefs. The hospital sought a declaration from the court, which was granted by Sir Stephen Brown. The decision – notable for its brevity – has been criticized (Grubb, 1993), not least for the fact that Sir Stephen Brown made reference to a case in the USA, *Re AC* ([1990] 573 A.2d 1235 at 1240), in which a court had been prepared to authorize a Caesarean section on a pregnant woman. While some courts in the USA have been prepared to order enforced treatment upon pregnant women, *Re AC* is very far from a clear authority supporting the use of enforced Caesareans. On appeal in *Re AC*, after the death of the woman on whom the Caesarean had been ordered, the court stated that the operation should not have been authorized.

Following *Re S*, the Royal College of Obstetricians and Gynaecologists published a consultation paper (RCOG, 1994) stating that:

It is inappropriate and unlikely to be helpful or necessary to invoke judicial intervention to overrule an informed and competent woman's refusal of a proposed medical treatment even though her refusal may place her life and that of her fetus at risk.

Despite this, in a number of subsequent cases judicial intervention was sought and the courts authorized the performance of Caesarean sections upon women who had refused such procedures (*Tameside* v. *Glossop* ([1996] 1 FCR 753; *Rochdale NHS Trust* v. *C.* [1997] 1 FCR 274; *Norfolk & Norwich NHS Trust* v. *W* [1996] 2 FLR 613). These cases attracted a storm of controversy, and thus it was hardly surprising when attempts were made to challenge these decisions in the courts. The Court of Appeal was given an opportunity to rule upon this issue in *Re MB* ([1997] 2 FLR 426). MB attended an antenatal clinic when she was 33 weeks pregnant, and refused to have blood taken from her because she had a fear of needles. She subsequently agreed to a Caesarean section when she found that the fetus was in the breech position and was at risk of harm due to oxygen starvation. However, she then refused consent, subsequently agreed to the anaesthetic, and then refused it again. The hospital sought a court order, which was given by Hollis J. He found that MB was incompetent because of the effects of the needle phobia on her decision-making powers. An appeal to the Court of Appeal that night was rejected. The Caesarean operation was carried out the following day when she agreed to the anaesthetic.

Subsequently, MB challenged the legality of the procedure. In the Court of Appeal (Butler Sloss, Saville and Ward L.J.J.), the right of the competent patient to refuse treatment was confirmed. The Court of Appeal upheld earlier cases such as *Re F (in utero)*, *Paton* v. *British Pregnancy Advisory Authority* ([1978] 2 All ER 987) in confirming that the fetus has no independent status in English law. They were of the view that Sir Stephen Brown in *Re S* had reached an incorrect conclusion. Thus even at the point of birth itself the court could not intervene in the face of refusal of medical intervention by a competent woman with the aim of safeguarding the position of the fetus.

Nonetheless, it was also recognized that, in an emergency, treatment could be given where a patient lacks capacity, as long as this was on the basis of necessity, the procedure not extending beyond what was reasonably required by the patient. It was noted that difficult issues arose regarding the determination of capacity. Butler Sloss L.J. quoted from Lord Donaldson in *Re T* that the doctor must assess carefully whether in that case the patient had the capacity relative to this particular decision. In *Re MB*, the Court of Appeal upheld the decision of the judge at first instance to the effect that MB lacked capacity. While MB was competent to consent to the Caesarean section itself, she was not competent to refuse because she was 'at that moment suffering an impairment of her mental functioning which disabled her. She was temporarily incompetent'. In this case it was her phobia of needles that impaired her ability to decide.

Having found MB to be temporarily incompetent, the Court of Appeal then considered whether the procedure itself could be authorized by reference to the test of best interests set out by the House of Lords in *Re F C* [1990] AC1. Here, 'best interests' equates to what a responsible body of medical practice would regard as being in the best interests of the patient in accord with the *Bolam* test *(Bolam* v. *Friern Hospital Management Company* [1957] 2 All ER 118). In *Re MB* (p. 439), Butler Sloss L.J. stated that:

> In considering the scope of best interests, it seems to us that they have to be treated on similar principles to the welfare of a child since the court and the doctors are concerned with a person unable to make the necessary decision for himself.

The Court of Appeal held that the treatment was in MB's best interests in this emergency situation. It took into consideration the fact that agreement had initially been given by MB for the Caesarean section. Furthermore, evidence from the consultant psychiatrist was to the effect that if the child had been born handicapped or had died, MB herself would have suffered long-term harm. In contrast, little harm would be caused by the administration of the anaesthetic against her wishes.

While the decision of the Court of Appeal in *Re MB* does confirm the pregnant woman's autonomy in principle, it does leave open a number of important issues. How will temporary issues of capacity be addressed? What is the scope of the best interests test today, and what are the differences in practice between children and incompetent adults? Nonetheless, one of the most important aspects of the decision in *Re MB* is that it provides guidance for future cases in this area in that it sets out the procedure that should be undertaken. This includes the requirement that the woman should be represented in all cases save where, in exceptional circumstances, she does not wish to be so (p. 445). This recommendation goes some way to meeting concerns as to the manner in which such proceedings have been brought. This guidance has been subsequently incorporated into a NHS circular (*Consent to Treatment*, NHS EL (97) 32).

Caesarean sections and the Mental Health Act

In parallel to the cases discussed above regarding Caesarean sections, there have been a number of cases involving the use of the Mental Health Act 1983. Section 63 of the Act provides that:

> The consent of a patient shall not be required for any medical treatment given to him for the mental disorder from which he is suffering.

But how far does this provision extend? Would it sanction the Act being used to authorize the performance of Caesarean sections? This issue came before the courts in *Tameside and Glossop Acute Hospital Trust* v. *CH* ([1996] 1 FLR 762; see also Grubb, 1996). CH was detained under section 3 of the Mental Health Act 1983. She was suffering from paranoid schizophrenia. She was then discovered to be pregnant. It was held that she lacked capacity to consent or refuse treatment, and the Caesarean section could be authorized as the performance of a Caesarean section was treatment for 'mental disorder' and thus fell within the scope of section 63 of the Mental Health Act 1983. If a stillbirth had occurred, her health would have deteriorated. In addition, she needed strong antipsychotic medication, which could not be given to her when she was pregnant. The court followed the approach in *B* v. *Croyden HA* ([1995] 1 All ER 683); namely that section 63 of the 1983 Act encompassed matters that related to the 'core treatment'. In *B* v. *Croyden*, the court authorized the force-feeding, through a nasogastric tube, of a patient with a personality disorder and intended self-harm.

However, a more restrictive approach was taken by the Court of Appeal in the case of *St Georges NHS Trust* v. *S* ([1998] 3 WLR 936). S was diagnosed as suffering from severe pre-eclampsia on registering as a patient at a new NHS practice when 8 months pregnant. She was advised that she should have an early delivery. S, who had intended a home delivery, refused treatment. She asserted that nature should take its course, although she was informed as to the risk of death and disability to herself and the fetus. Her GP then called a psychiatrist and approved social worker. S was detained in hospital under section 2 of the Mental Health Act 1983, and was subsequently transferred to another hospital. She repeated her refusal, both orally and in writing, and sought legal advice. Without the knowledge of S, or of her legal advisers, the hospital authority made an *ex parte* application to the High Court for a declaration to the effect that it would be lawful to undertake treatment, including a Caesarean section. Meanwhile S had been in touch with solicitors with the intention of bringing an appeal before a Mental Health Tribunal.

The declaration was granted, and S gave birth to a daughter. The detention under the Mental Health Act was terminated, and S discharged herself. While detained in hospital, S was not offered treatment for her mental disorder. An action was subsequently brought for judicial review to challenge the legality of the action taken.

As in *Re MB*, the Court of Appeal (Butler Sloss, Judge and Robert Walker L.J.) again emphasized the fact that the competent adult is entitled to refuse treatment. They addressed the question of the status of the fetus. Judge L.J. stated (p. 957) that:

> In our judgment while pregnancy increases the personal responsibilities of a woman it does not diminish her entitlement to decide whether or not to undergo medical treatment. Although human and protected by the law in a number of different ways as set out in the judgment in *re MB* ... an unborn child is not a separate person from its mother. Its need for medical assistance does not prevail over her rights.

The Court held that a battery had been committed on S. Judge L.J. stated (p. 953) that:

> ... how can an enforced invasion of a competent adult's body against her will even for the most laudable of motives (the preservation of life) be ordered without irredeemably damaging the principle of self-determination?

The Court examined the provisions of section 2(2) of the Mental Health Act 1983, which had been used to authorize the admission of S. The Court of Appeal emphasized that the criteria for detention under the section were cumulative. In this case, the doctors had been justified in their assessment that the woman was suffering from depression which constituted 'mental disorder'. However, S was not being detained in order for treatment to be given for her mental disorder. It was noted that detention under the Mental Health Act had to be linked to the mental disorder, and the fact that, as here, the treatment was for the purposes of pregnancy was not sufficient justification for the detention.

Thus the courts have affirmed that for treatment to be lawful under section 63 it must be crucial to the mental disorder. In this case, the treatment was not treatment for mental disorder within the provisions of the statute. However, as Bailey Harris has commented, it is the case that questions regarding the connection between the disorder and the treatment proposed are likely to arise in the future (Bailey Harris, 1998). One further point here is that there had also been an irregularity in the documentation used by the hospital. Forms had not been completed when the woman was transferred between hospitals, as was required by regulations made under section 19 of the Mental Health Act. This would in any event have entitled S to discharge herself from hospital. S was thus competent; she had been unlawfully detained, and the procedure was a battery. Finally, the Court of Appeal criticized the procedure adopted in the case of the application to the court, which was made without the knowledge of S and her legal advisers. As in *Re MB*, they set out guidelines regarding the conduct of proceedings for a declaration.

Both *Re MB* and *St Georges NHS Trust* v. *S* provide a welcome clarification of the legal position in the area. The autonomy of the patient is confirmed. The operation of the Mental Health Act 1983 in such cases is made clear. The refusal of treatment by the competent pregnant woman is upheld. Guidance has been provided by the courts in these cases as to the correct procedures that should be adopted when making an application for a declaration. The decisions highlight the need for information to be given to the pregnant woman and her advisers. Too often in the past the woman has been without legal advice or, as in *St Georges NHS Trust* v. *S*, is simply not informed of the steps being taken. Admittedly there is a danger that the involvement of the legal process may be regarded as detracting from patient care, leading to polarization of the views of the parties, women, midwives and doctors. Nonetheless, it is suggested that certain decisions, because of their inherently problematic nature, cannot be left for resolution by the parties. The decision-making process may in fact be benefited by the involvement of an independent arbiter. In addition, the acute dilemma facing health care professionals in such a highly emotionally charged situation, in which they realize that medical intervention would almost certainly enable the fetus to be born healthy, should not be underestimated. It also provides safeguards for the patient in ensuring accountability. Difficulties are, however, likely to arise in the future regarding the definition of incapacity itself and those situations in which a pregnant woman is declared to be incompetent, enabling treatment to be given without her consent.

Patient refusing care with dependant family

No English court has yet been faced with the question of whether to authorize treatment on the basis that the patient who is refusing care has a dependant family. The issue has arisen in the USA, where the courts have been prepared to uphold the right of the patient to refuse treatment regardless of the impact upon the patient's family (*Norwood Hospital* v. *Munoz* [1991] 564 NE 2d 1017). It is submitted that this is the correct approach to take and that, whatever the consequences, if a competent patient makes a clear refusal of treatment, then that refusal should be respected.

Postnatal care

The nurse or health visitor may be involved in providing postnatal care to mother and baby. What if the nurse believes that a mother who is being attended is abusing drugs and that the home is unsuitable? In this situation, the nurse should bring the matter to the attention of her line manager initially. It may then be decided to refer the issue to Social Services. They may decide to take action and, if necessary, use one of the orders available to them under the Children's Act 1989 (for fuller discussion see Chapter 6).

Liability for injuries in relation to conception and childbirth

Negligence of health professionals, whether in providing advice regarding sterilization or during the conduct of childbirth, may lead to litigation. The process of childbirth is fraught with difficulties, and mistakes are easily made. In the debates on the existence of a malpractice crisis in health care, obstetrics and gynaecology are frequently cited as examples. The general principles of negligence are discussed in Chapter 2. Here, a few specific points are briefly considered.

Where a child is born handicapped as a result of conduct which it is claimed is negligent, then a claim may be brought against a nurse or doctor. The Congenital Disabilities (Civil Liability) Act 1976 allows an action to be brought by a child who has suffered a disability (s1(3)). This Act was passed following the debate and legal action that arose from the use of the drug Thalidomide. This drug was given to pregnant women to counteract morning sickness, and it was alleged that as a consequence children had been born handicapped. An action can only be brought under the 1976 Act if the child is born alive and has lived for at least 48 hours (s4(2)). It must be shown that the disability that the child has suffered was the result of an occurrence that affected the mother's or father's ability to have a child, or affected the mother during pregnancy, or affected the mother or child during birth. Situations in which an action may be taken include a child being born handicapped due to negligence during the birth. To bring a claim under the Act, it must be shown that the nurse or midwife owed the mother a duty of care (s4(2)). Any damages awarded under the Act may be reduced if the parents were contributorily negligent in the harm caused.

In practice it seems that liability is difficult to establish, with few claims having been brought. Many of these claims will fail on the grounds that the negligence itself did not cause the harm suffered. It is perhaps of interest, in view of the earlier discussion as to the obligation of the pregnant woman towards her fetus, that an action may not be brought by a child against his or her mother for negligent conduct under the 1976 Act. The one exception to this is in a situation in which the fetus is injured by the negligence of the mother when driving a car and the mother knew or ought reasonably to have known that she was pregnant (s2 Congenital Disabilities (Civil Liability) Act 1976).

An action at common law cannot be brought on behalf of the child on the basis that the injuries the child suffered were such that he or she would be better off never having been born. The Court of Appeal rejected such a 'wrongful life' claim in the case of *McKay* v. *Essex Area Health Authority* ([1982] 2 All ER 771), on the basis that the court could not assess the award of damages satisfactorily to assess the difference between never having been born and a life of disability. In addition, it was argued that to allow such damages here could encourage health care professionals to advise on an abortion, rather than risk subsequent litigation where a child was born handicapped. Parents can, however, bring claims for the cost of bringing up a severely disabled infant born due to medical negligence during pregnancy or childbirth. The possibility of such litigation illustrates the importance of risk management and following protocols where available (see Chapter 10).

Abortion

Background to the existing law

Abortion is one of the most controversial of all clinical procedures (Keown, 1988; Dworkin, 1993). It was made a criminal offence in England by the Offences Against the Person Act 1861 (s58 and s59). In addition, the Infant Life Preservation Act 1933 made it an offence to destroy the life of a child capable of being born alive. This remained the position until 1967, subject to a limited exception being recognized for abortions undertaken to preserve the life of the mother or to ensure that she was not rendered a 'physical and mental wreck' (*R* v. *Bourne* [1939] 1 KB 687). In 1967, after much heated debate, the Abortion Act was passed, largely through the efforts of the Liberal MP David Steel. This legislation was amended in 1990 by clauses inserted into the 1967 Act by the Human Fertilization and Embryology Act 1990. The introduction of abortion legislation was accompanied by a heated ethical debate. On the one hand, the use of abortion was strongly advocated by those who supported a 'pro-choice' approach. Abortion was, however, opposed by those who can be loosely grouped under the heading 'pro-life', and who regarded the abortion process as that of the killing of a human person or potential person (Dworkin, 1993). The legislation, as can be seen below, has provided no absolute rights to any of the parties to the abortion process. There is no right to abortion on demand, the father has no rights, and nor has the fetus. In many respects the abortion decision can be viewed as one characterized by medical determination and domination.

Nurses should be broadly aware of the law as it relates to abortion, and particularly the Abortion Act 1967, for a number of reasons. Acting in their role as patient advocate, nurses may be involved in counselling and advising women who are contemplating an abortion. Also, nurses may have fundamental religious objections to abortion. When can they legitimately refuse to participate?

When is an abortion lawful?

An abortion is lawful if authorized by two registered medical practitioners who are of the opinion, held in good faith, that one of the four grounds laid down in the Abortion Act 1967 has been met.

Social abortions

First, an abortion is allowed if the woman is less than 24 weeks pregnant and if continuation of the pregnancy would involve a risk, greater than if the pregnancy were terminated, of injury to her physical or mental health or that of any child in her family (s1(1)a). This category – the so-called 'social ground' – is the provision under which most abortions are authorized. It leaves considerable room for the exercise of medical discretion. For example, there is controversy as to whether the psychological pressure placed upon women in certain cultural groups to have a male child provides sufficient justification for the abortion of a female fetus. 'Social' abortions can only be undertaken in the first 24 weeks of pregnancy, but the Act does not state from when this time runs. There are a number of possibilities (Murphy, 1991), such as the date of the woman's last period, the date of implantation, or the date of fertilization.

Other grounds for abortion

The other grounds for abortion under the 1967 Act are not subject to an express time limit. An abortion may be undertaken if termination of pregnancy is necessary to prevent grave permanent injury to the physical or mental health of the pregnant woman (s1(1)b). An abortion is also lawful if continuation of the pregnancy involves a risk to the life of the pregnant woman greater than if the pregnancy were terminated (s1(1)c). Finally, an abortion may be undertaken if there is a substantial risk that if pregnancy were to continue the child would be born seriously handicapped (s1(1)d). The statute does not define 'seriously handicapped'. It is unclear whether this refers to a handicap that the child would be born with if the pregnancy continued, or if it extends to conditions such as Huntington's Chorea, which will not develop until a person is around 40 or 50 years old (Morgan, 1990).

Emergency abortions

The Act states that an abortion must be authorized by two medical practitioners (s1(1)). However, one doctor may authorize an abortion if it is the only way of averting an immediate risk to the woman's life or grave permanent injury to her (s1(4)).

No right to an abortion

It must be stressed that there is no right in English law to abortion on demand. The ultimate decision regarding the performance of an abortion is a matter of clinical judgment after discussion between the doctor and the patient. Just as a woman has no right to demand an abortion, neither does her husband or partner have any legal right to be consulted or to veto the abortion decision (*Paton* v. *Trustees of the British Pregnancy Advisory Service* [1978] 2 All ER 987; *C* v. *S* [1988] QB 135). Also, English law does not recognize the fetus as possessing legal rights (*Paton* v. *British Pregnancy Advisory Service*). It can only be speculated as to what the impact of the Human Rights Act 1998 will be in this area. It is likely that at some point the abortion legislation may come under scrutiny in the courts in relation to a woman's claim of the application of the right to privacy under Article 8, and claims in relation to the interests of the fetus in the context of the right to life in Article 2 of the European Convention of Human Rights.

Selective reduction

The development of IVF treatment led to a difficulty relating to abortion. In the course of IVF treatment, in order to increase the chance of a successful implantation, more than one embryo is usually transferred into the womb. In some situations, this may result in a number of embryos becoming implanted. Such a multiple pregnancy may constitute a serious risk to the mother's health. The amendments made to the Abortion Act 1967 in 1990 include a provision to the effect that it is lawful to remove one or more embryos as long as one of the grounds for abortion under the 1967 Act is met (s5(2)). These provisions do not only apply to multiple pregnancies arising as a result of infertility treatment. There was considerable controversy regarding a press report that a consultant had performed selective reduction on a woman with twins who sought an abortion under the 'social' grounds of the legislation (*The Guardian*, 1996).

Abortion on teenagers and incompetent adults

While a competent adult patient can clearly consent to an abortion, difficulties may arise if it is proposed to undertake an abortion upon a teenager or a mentally incompetent woman. A teenager may be competent to consent herself if she is regarded as of sufficient maturity under the *Gillick* test (see Chapter 6). However, what if she refuses an abortion? While in theory the parental power of consent may override the refusal of a competent child, if a teenager wants to keep her baby then any dispute between her and her parents should be immediately referred to the court. It would, it is suggested, be unlikely that the court would force a girl to undergo an abortion.

While it may be seen as good practice to seek court approval before an abortion is performed on a mentally incompetent woman, there is, strictly speaking, no need for such an order to be made before the abortion goes ahead (*Re SG* [1991] 6 BMLR 95 (Fam Div)). The decision to undertake an abortion upon a mentally incompetent adult must be reached on the basis of what are her best interests. The nurse as patient advocate may play an important role in ensuring that the patient's interests are properly taken into account in making this decision.

The Law Commission (1995), in its report *Mental Incapacity*, expressed concern that abortions were being undertaken on young women with learning disabilities without proper investigation into their ability to consent, and their best interests. It suggested that, before an abortion is performed upon a mentally incompetent woman, there should be a requirement for a certificate to be obtained from an independent medical practitioner stating that the abortion is in the woman's best interests. The government, in the document *Who Decides* (Lord Chancellor's Department, 1997), was not convinced by this solution and was of the view that the existing legislative safeguards were adequate.

Where should the abortion be carried out?

Section 1(3) of the Act provides that abortions must be undertaken in an NHS hospital or in a place that has been approved by the Secretary of State for the purposes of undertaking abortions. This provision created difficulties in relation to the abortion pill, the drug RU486, as it was intended that this would be administered to patients at GPs' surgeries. To cover this, section 1(3)(a) was enacted, which provides that:

> The power under subsection (3) of this section to approve a place includes a power in relation to treatment consisting primarily in the use of such medicines as may be specified in the approval and carried out in such manner as may be so specified, to approve a class of places.

This power has not yet been exercised; thus at present RU486 may be lawfully administered to patients only in hospital. Even if a GP's surgery is approved as a relevant place, this only covers the initial administration of the drug. The patient is then usually discharged. At this time the drug is still acting. Surely each patient's home cannot be included in any designation! These problems require urgent consideration by Parliament.

The role of the nurse in prostaglandin abortions

While the 1967 Act provides that the pregnancy must be terminated by a registered medical practitioner, the nurse plays a major role in certain abortion procedures. In prostaglandin abortions, the doctor inserts a catheter into the womb via the cervix in order to create a space between the womb and the amniotic sac containing the fetus. This may cause abortion. If not, various other steps are undertaken, such as attaching a catheter to a pump propelling prostaglandin into the womb. These procedures are mostly carried out by a nurse or midwife. However, the legislation makes no reference to the nurse, simply referring to the doctor's role in the process. The Royal College of Nursing went to court to obtain an order to clarify the legality of the nurse's involvement in the abortion process (*RCN* v. *DHSS* [1981] AC 800). The House of Lords held that the doctor need not do everything with his own hands. Lord Diplock stated that Parliament had contemplated that, as with other hospital treatment, abortion would take place as a team effort; junior doctors, paramedics, nurses and other members of the health care team would each undertake those tasks that would be, in accordance with a responsible body of medical practice, entrusted to a member of staff possessed of their respective skills. The involvement of the nurse in the process was lawful.

Conscientious objection

Abortion is an exceedingly sensitive ethical issue on which many people hold very strong beliefs. The 1967 Act itself takes account of this. Section 4 of the 1967 Act provides that:

1.   Subject to subsection (2) of this section no person shall be under any duty, whether by contract or by any statutory or other legal requirement, to participate in any treatment authorized by this Act to which he has a conscientious objection.

Provided that in any legal proceedings the burden of proof of conscientious objection shall rest on the person claiming to rely on it. ...

The section does, however, go on to provide that:

2.   Nothing in subsection (1) of this section shall affect any duty to participate in treatment which is necessary to save the life or to prevent grave permanent injury to the physical or mental health of a pregnant woman.

Thus, a nurse who is a devout Roman Catholic may refuse to participate in an abortion procedure save in an exceptional situation, such as where a woman is brought in bleeding profusely from the uterus and it is clear that without an abortion she will die.

While the Act gives the nurse the right to refuse to be involved in clinical procedures, the statutory right of conscientious objection does not extend to those persons more remotely connected to the abortion process. In *Jannaway* v. *Salford AHA* ([1988] 3 All ER 1079), a secretary who was a Roman Catholic refused to type a letter referring a pregnant woman to a consultant with a view to securing an abortion. Ultimately she was dismissed. She claimed that the dismissal was unfair and that the conscientious objection provision under section 4 protected her. Her claim was rejected in the House of Lords. Lord Keith said that 'participation' for the purposes of section 4 meant actual participation in the treatment administered in a hospital or other approved place.

Liability if the 1967 Act is not complied with

There has been some discussion as to whether the procedure set out in the 1967 Act has to be complied with before, for example, an intrauterine device is inserted after intercourse, or before the 'morning after' pill is given. In some situations, failure to comply with the Abortion Act 1967 may result in a criminal prosecution. Section 58 of the Offences Against the Person Act 1861 states that it is an offence to use an instrument with the intention of procuring a miscarriage. What constitutes 'carriage' for these purposes is somewhat unclear (Montgomery, 1997), but advice has been given by the Department of Health that postcoital contraception should only be administered in a period of 72 hours after conception.

Today, abortion may also be undertaken through administration of the drug RU486. This drug is clearly abortifacient, since it operates after the ovum has become implanted. It is almost certain that it must be given in accordance with the 1967 Act.

Failure to comply with the 1967 Act may also place those performing the abortion at risk of prosecution under the Infant Life Preservation Act 1929 for the offence of child destruction. Section 1(1) of this Act provides that:

Any person who with intent to destroy the life of a child capable of being born alive by any wilful act causes the child to die before it has a life independent of its mother shall be guilty of the offence of child destruction and shall be liable on conviction to life imprisonment.

but that:

... no person shall be found guilty under this section unless it is proved that the act which caused the death of the child was not done in good faith for the purpose only of preserving the life of the mother.

No offence will be committed under this Act as long as the provisions of the Abortion Act 1967 have been complied with. Were a prosecution to be brought under this section, a court would have to consider whether the fetus was 'capable of being born alive'. Some guidance as to what this term means was given in the case of *C* v. *S* ([1988] QB 135). Here, the court rejected the claim that a fetus of 18–21 weeks was 'capable of being born alive'. Lord Donaldson said that while at 18–21 weeks the cardiac muscle is contracting and primitive circulation is developing – and therefore the fetus could be said to be developing real and discernible signs of life – nevertheless it was unable to breathe either naturally or with the aid of a ventilator.

The mature fetus

If a hysterectomy is undertaken in the later stages of pregnancy, the fetus may be born alive. An infant who has taken breath and shown signs of life after being expelled from the womb is entitled to a full birth certificate and to be fed and cared for. If a nurse leaves the infant to die, then a prosecution for murder or manslaughter may result. For example, in R v. *Hamilton* (*The Times*, 16 September 1983), an infant was discovered after abortion to be 33 weeks rather than 23 weeks old. The infant, clearly alive after delivery, was left in the sluice room for some 15 minutes before being transferred to the intensive care unit. The infant survived. Dr Hamilton was charged with attempted murder although, ultimately, the magistrates decided that there was no case to answer. The nurse, as patient advocate, should be concerned to safeguard the rights of the infant patient. If the nurse finds that a baby has been born and is at risk of death, he or she must immediately take steps to secure the infant's survival. The nurse should also report the condition in which the infant was found, and any perceived deficiencies in care.

One reason why abortion may be undertaken late in pregnancy is because of delay in the initial referral. Clarke quotes a Royal College of Gynaecologists' study which found that 20.5 per cent of women who had abortions between 20 and 23 weeks had been referred at 12 weeks but had then experienced delay in obtaining a consultation and appointment for treatment (Clarke, 1987). As far as possible, any delay in the time from the initial point at which a woman sees her doctor to any abortion should be minimized.

Registration of births and stillbirths

When a woman gives birth, whether to a living infant or to a stillbirth, then the doctor or the midwife who has attended the woman is under a statutory duty to inform the responsible medical officer of that fact (s124 NHS Act 1977; Notification of Births and Deaths Regulations 1982; SI 1982 No 286). A stillbirth is the term used to describe a child born dead after 24 weeks of pregnancy and which did not breathe or show any sign of life (s41 Births and Deaths Registration Act 1953, as amended by the Still Birth Definition Act 1992).

The Births and Deaths Registration Act 1953 requires the mother or father to inform the Registrar of a birth within 42 days (s2). If either of them is unable to do so, then there is a duty upon the occupier of the house, any person present at the birth or any person who has charge of that child to give the Registrar that information (s2(1)(2)). A midwife may be such a person. If the birth has not been registered within 42 days, then the Registrar can compel any qualified informant to come before him or her to provide information and to sign the Register, having first given the informant 7 days' notice in writing. Where a stillbirth is being registered, the informant must provide the Registrar with a certificate stating that the child was not born alive. This certificate should have been signed by a registered medical practitioner or by a certified midwife who was present during the birth or who subsequently examined the dead body. A birth is classified as a stillbirth where the fetus is more than 24 weeks old (Still Birth (Definition) Act 1992).

References

Anderson, G. and Strong, C. (1988). The premature breech; Caesarean section or trial of labour. *J. Med. Ethics*, **18**, 18.

Bailey Harris, R. (1998). Pregnancy, autonomy and refusal of medical treatment. *Law Q. Rev.*, **550**, 554.

Brazier, M. (1990). Sterilization: down the slippery slope. *Professional Negligence*, **6**, 25.

British Medical Association (1990). *Surrogacy: Ethical Considerations. Report of a Working Party on Human Infertility Services.*

British Medical Journal (1999). Cloning may cause health defects. *Br. Med. J.*, **318**, 1230.

Clarke, L. (1987). Abortion – a rights issue. In: *Birthrights* (R. Lee and D. Morgan, eds). Routledge.

Council of Europe (1998). *Additional Protocol to the Convention for the Protection of Human Rights and Dignity of the Human Being with regard to the Application of Biology and Medicine, on the Prohibition of Cloning of Human Beings.* Paris. Council of Europe.

Cumberlege, Lady (1993). *Changing Childbirth: Report of the Expert Maternity Group.* DOH.

Department of Health (1997). *Surrogacy: Report for Health Visitors of Current Arrangements for Payments and Regulations* (1998) Cm 4068. (Brazier Review).

Dworkin, R. (1993). *Life's Dominion: An Argument About Euthanasia and Abortion.* Harper Collins.

Grubb, A. (1993). Treatment without consent: adult. *Med. Law Rev.*, **1**, 931.

Grubb, A. (1996). Treatment without consent: pregnancy (adult). *Med. Law Rev.*, **3**, 191.

The Guardian (1996) 'No new issue' in abortion of twin. 5 August.

Harris, J. (1998). *Clones, Genes and Immortality.* Oxford University Press.

HEFA (1998). UK authorities recommend human cloning for therapeutic research. *Br. Med. J.*, **317**, 1613.

Hewson, B. (1996). Women's rights and legal wrongs. *NLJ*, **146**, 1385.

HEFA (1998) *Code of Practice.* Human Fertilization and Embryology Authority.

House of Commons Science and Technology Committee (1997). *The Cloning of Animals from Adult Cells.* The Science and Technology Committee Fifth Report of Session 1996–97, HC 373-1.

Keown, J. (1988). *Abortion, Doctors and the Law.* Cambridge University Press.

Law Commission (1995). *Mental Incapacity.* Report No. 231, HMSO, para 6.10.

Lee, R. and Morgan, D. (eds) (1987). A lesser sacrifice: sterilization and the mentally handicapped woman. In: *Birthrights.* Routledge.

Lee, R. and Morgan, D. (1991). *The Human Fertilization and Embryology Act 1990.* Blackstone Press.

Lord Chancellor's Department (1997). *Who Decides?* LCD.

Lord Chancellor's Department (1999). *Making Decisions.* LCD.

Mason, J. and McCall Smith, R. A. (1999). *Law and Medical Ethics* (5th edn). Sweet and Maxwell.

Montgomery, J. (1997). *Health Care Law.* Oxford University Press, p. 362.

Morgan, D. (1990). Abortion – the unexamined ground. *Crim LR* 687.

Murphy, J. (1991). Cosmetics, eugenics and ambivalence; the revision of the Abortion Act 1967. *J. Social Welfare Fam. Law*, **1**, 375.

Robertson, J. (1995). *Children of Choice.* Princeton University Press.

Royal College of Obstetricians and Gynaecologists (1994). *A Consideration of the Law and Ethics in Relation to Court-authorised Obstetric Intervention.* RCOG.

Warnock Committee (1984). *Report of the Committee of Inquiry into Human Fertilization and Embryology.* HMSO, Cmnd 9314.

Chapter 10

The end of life

Jean McHale

The nurse frequently plays an important role in caring for patients at the end of life whether, for instance, in the area of palliative care and the hospice movement, or in the intensive care unit. Many difficult issues arise at the end of life. A patient who is terminally ill and who is in considerable pain may tell the nurse that he wants to die. What should the nurse do? The midwife presents a mother with a child who is grossly handicapped and the mother screams for the child to be taken away from her. How far is the medical team required to keep that child alive? A young man is killed in a road accident, and the man's father approaches the nurse for advice as to whether his son's organs could be used for transplantation. While the nurse may be the primary carer and required to take primary responsibility at the end of life, in many situations he or she will be acting as part of a treatment team. This area also gives rise to a number of difficult issues for the nurse as patient advocate.

This chapter considers a number of important legal questions regarding the end of life. It begins by examining the approach taken in English law to issues of active and passive termination of life. There has been much discussion as to whether there is a 'right to die'. As will be seen, in English law there is presently only a right in the sense that a patient can choose to end his or her own life – English law does not sanction active euthanasia, although in certain situations withdrawal of treatment is lawful. This is an area of law that is likely to come under scrutiny now that the Human Rights Act 1998 has come into force. Arguments are likely to rage about the boundaries of the right to privacy and autonomy of the individual and the principle of the right to life.

The second section of the chapter considers the definition of death. In the final section, the legal regulation of organ transplantation is examined and some proposals for law reform are considered.

Ending life – criminal liability

> A seriously ill patient may plead with a nurse that he has suffered
> enough and that he wants someone to 'put him out of his misery'.
> What action should the nurse take?

However grave the patient's agony, if the nurse complies with his request
to 'put him out of his misery', he or she may be prosecuted for murder.
English law does not recognize active euthanasia. In *R* v. *Carr* (*Sunday
Times*, 30 November 1986), Dr Carr had injected a massive doses of phe-
nobarbitones into a patient with inoperable lung cancer. The judge, Mars
J., emphasized that every patient was entitled to every hour that God had
given him, however seriously ill that patient might be. The jury eventually
acquitted Dr Carr.

However, in 1992 Dr Cox was prosecuted for and convicted of
attempted murder (*The Times,* 22 September 1992). (He was not charged
with murder because, at the time of the investigation, the body of the
alleged victim had been cremated and thus the exact cause of death could
not be established.) Dr Cox had been treating a 70-year-old woman who
was terminally ill, with rheumatoid arthritis, and also suffering from
gastric ulcers, gangrene and pressure sores. She expressed a wish to die.
When repeated doses of heroin did not ease her agony, Dr Cox gave her a
dose of potassium chloride – a poison. Dr Cox was convicted and sen-
tenced to 1 year's imprisonment suspended for 12 months.

In July 1997, Dr David Moor was charged with the murder of an 85-
year-old retired ambulanceman, George Liddell (*BMJ*, 1999a, 1999b). It
was alleged that he had caused the death through the administration of a
large dose of morphine. In a TV interview, Dr Moor had said that he had
been involved in helping patients to die. He had stated that he 'would be
very surprised if I had to defend myself in court'. At the trial, Mr Liddell's
relatives spoke up in support of the doctor. His 66-year-old son said at the
trial:

> When I eased him forward he started to cry. It was a long and pro-
> tracted cry. This was more than I could stand. I have never heard any-
> thing like it before.

Dr Moor was acquitted. The judge told the jury that:

> You may consider it a great irony that a doctor who goes out of his way
> to care for George Liddell ends up facing the charge he does.

In *R* v. *Arthur* (*The Times*, 5 November 1981), the non-treatment of an
infant resulted in a criminal prosecution. A baby, John Pearson, was born
with Down's syndrome but apparently suffering no other complications.

Dr Arthur, a paediatrician caring for the child, wrote in the notes, 'Parents do not wish it to survive, nursing care only', and he prescribed a strong painkilling drug, DF118 – a drug not normally given to infants. The baby died a few hours later. Dr Arthur was charged with murder, but this was later reduced to a charge of attempted murder. While he was eventually acquitted, the case left open many difficult issues as to what care a child must be given and whether the health care professional can cease treatment if it is believed that further care is hopeless. The judge in *R* v. *Arthur* described the doctor's conduct as being a 'holding operation'. However, it has been suggested that the administration of the drug DF118 – an appetite suppressant – amounted to a positive act. This case must now be considered in the light of the *Bland* decision, where the court indicated that a decision to cease life-sustaining treatment will not necessarily give rise to criminal liability (see below).

Generally, there will only be liability in criminal law where a nurse or doctor has undertaken a positive action. The law does not usually impose liability for omissions. Nonetheless, as will be seen below, there may on occasions be only a narrow line between these two categories.

The nurse as whistleblower where a doctor has deliberately ended a patient's life

A nurse strongly suspects that a doctor has deliberately ended the life of an elderly patient on her ward; what should the nurse do?

In two cases in which doctors were prosecuted for allegedly ending the life of a patient, the prosecutions followed action taken by the nursing staff. Dr Arthur was prosecuted after a nurse who was a member of a pro-life organization made a report. Dr Cox's prosecution followed a report made by a nurse, Sister Hart, regarding his conduct. She stated that she was required by the UKCC code to speak out – relying on clauses 2 and 11. Nurses may be subject to disciplinary proceedings if they fail to report such an incident (Fletcher *et al.*, 1995). Nurses are also given some statutory protection under the Public Interest Disclosure Act 1998 (see p. 153).

What should a nurse do if, as in the case of Sister Hart, he or she knows that the patient's life has been ended but that the patient has expressed a wish to die? Does the duty that the nurse owes to the patient mean that the fact that this patient had expressed a wish to die should be taken into account? While obliged to act in the patient's interests, it must be the case that the nurse should be prepared to report what is a serious breach of criminal law.

Parental obligations to their children

The law places parents under particular obligations in relation to the care of their children, and holds them accountable not only for their actions but also for their omissions. If parents, perhaps motivated by some personal ethical belief, fail to seek medical care for a gravely ill child and as a result the child dies, they may be prosecuted under section 1 of the Children and Young Persons Act 1933, which makes it an offence to neglect the care of the child. A prosecution may also be brought for murder or manslaughter. In *R* v. *Senior* ([1899] 1 QB 283), the parents were members of a religious sect that objected to the use of medical assistance and medicines. Their child fell ill, but they did not seek medical help and the child died of diarrhoea and pneumonia. Evidence was given to the effect that had the child received medical treatment, then she would probably have lived. Although no medical care had been given, the child had been generally well treated. It was held that the parents' actions amounted to neglect under section 1 of the Prevention of Cruelty to Children Act 1896 – the statutory predecessor to the 1933 Act – which provided that:

> If any person ... who has the custody, charge or care of a child ... wilfully neglects ... such child in a manner likely to cause such child injury to its health that person shall be guilty of a misdemeanour.

In this case the parents were found guilty of manslaughter, because their actions had caused or accelerated the child's death. More recently the courts have held that neglect by itself will not necessarily mean that a prosecution for manslaughter will succeed (*R* v. *Lowe* [1973] QB 70). However, in 1993 parents who believed in homeopathic remedies and who failed to seek conventional medical help for their child, who subsequently died, were convicted of manslaughter (*The Independent*, 29 October 1993).

Administration of painkilling drugs

The nurse charged with ending the life of a suffering patient cannot plead that this was a 'mercy killing'. No such defence is recognized in English law. However, in some situations administration of strong painkilling drugs is justifiable even though repeated doses will, over time, have the effect of cutting short the patient's life. In *R* v. *Bodkin Adams* ([1957] *Crim Law Review* 365), Dr Bodkin Adams was prosecuted for murder. Dr Adams had cared for many elderly patients, and had been a beneficiary in the wills of a number of those patients. One 81-year-old widow who had suffered a stroke was prescribed heroin and morphia by Dr Adams and later died. Dr Adams was named as a beneficiary under her will. At the trial the judge, Devlin J., said that there was no special defence of mercy killing, but that a doctor was entitled to do all that was proper and necessary to relieve his patient's suffering, even if the measures used had the effect of incidentally shortening that patient's life. Brazier (1992) has stated that:

This analysis introduces into the law the double-effect principle much debated in philosophical circles, whereby if an act has one of two inevitable consequences, one good and one evil, the act may be morally acceptable in certain circumstances.

The doctrine of double effect has been used in the context of abortion. The approach taken in *R* v. *Bodkin Adams* has been questioned. The UKCC (House of Lords, 1994a) has commented that:

> ... to prohibit euthanasia ... yet permit the use of narcotics to alleviate pain even at doses which will dramatically shorten life or even bring it to a close within a very short period, is no longer a sustainable position.

Reg Pyne, former assistant registrar of the UKCC, suggested that nurses generally saw the doctrine of double effect as hypocritical (House of Lords, 1994b). The first duty of the nurse and other health care professionals is to care for the patient. A decision to administer strong painkilling drugs is not to be taken lightly. However, if that decision is made and the incidental effect is that a patient's lifespan is reduced, then at present that will not amount to murder in English law.

Suicide

While euthanasia is unlawful, a patient may take his or her own life. Suicide has not been a crime in this country since the Suicide Act 1961 came into force. As noted in Chapter 5, a patient may refuse life-saving treatment – and indeed, to treat a patient who has refused such treatment without his or her consent may lead to an action in the tort of battery and possibly to a criminal prosecution. However, if the patient asks a nurse to bring some lethal drug and to sit with him or her while dying, the nurse must not do so. Section 2(1) of the Suicide Act 1961 provides that assisting suicide is an offence. To establish a prosecution it must be shown that the defendant knew that the person was intending to commit suicide, assented to this, and encouraged the person in the attempt (*AG* v. *Able* [1984] 1 All ER 277).

Should euthanasia be legalized?

As with abortion, euthanasia is an exceedingly emotive subject (Dworkin, 1993). It has been argued that recognition of active voluntary euthanasia is simply a logical extension of the right to commit suicide, and that it is part of giving respect to the autonomy of the individual. Furthermore, it has been suggested that the present position, which sanctions the withdrawal of treatment while at the same time rejecting active euthanasia, is inconsistent and illogical. A number of unsuccessful attempts have been made over the years to legalize euthanasia in this country. In other jurisdictions legislation has been introduced which has sanctioned some medical assistance in dying, although not without much controversy and debate. In Australia, Northern Territory passed the Rights of the Terminally Ill Act 1995. This provided that a person could request assistance to terminate life. The request had to be voluntary, the patient of sound mind and over 18 years of age, and suffering from an illness that the medical practitioner believed would result in the death of the patient. The assessment of the need for assistance was to be confirmed by a second medical practitioner, and the request would not be effective if medically acceptable palliative care options were available. The legislation required notification of the criteria under the statute. During the period in which the Act was in force, seven patients used the Act and four died under its provisions (*BMJ*, 1998). This statute proved controversial, and was the subject of challenge in the Australian Federation; it was struck down by Parliament in 1997. In the USA, there was extensive media debate over the actions of Dr Jack Kevorkian, a doctor who made no secret of his role in assisting patients to die and who was ultimately prosecuted and convicted (Brody, 1999). In the state of Oregon, the Death with Dignity Act 1997 allowed doctors to prescribe patients lethal drugs for self-medication. This statute was the subject of much heated debate. Finally the Pain Relief Promotion Act was passed in 1999, and this had the effect that federally controlled substances – including morphine – could not be used for assistance in suicide, thus rendering the Death with Dignity Act largely ineffective (*BMJ*, 1999c). The introduction of euthanasia legislation is presently under consideration in Belgium (Nys, 1999).

While it has been argued that recognition of voluntary euthanasia is something that accords respect to the autonomy of the individual patient, nevertheless some strong voices have been raised in dissent. One fear is that of the 'slippery slope'. It is argued that it is easy to 'slip' from recognition of voluntary active euthanasia to involuntary euthanasia undertaken without an individual's consent, for convenience or other purposes. Critics of euthanasia point to the experience in the Netherlands. In that country, while euthanasia itself is unlawful, legislation provides that prosecutions will not be brought against doctors who terminate the lives of their patients as long as they comply with certain procedures. Claims have been made that procedures have not been complied with and that abuses have occurred (Keown, 1991). The 'slippery slope' argument was one factor that influenced the Select Committee of the House of Lords to reject the introduction of euthanasia legislation in this country (House of Lords, 1994a). A further difficulty relates to who would administer euthanasia. Should it be the same persons who normally care for patients? Were this to be introduced, it would have considerable implications for the role of the nurse. Recognition of active termination of life is opposed by those who see the function of health care as one of 'curing', not killing. In 2000, a special conference of the British Medical Association into the question of the introduction of physician-assisted suicide stated that (BMA, 2000a):

It would alter the relationships between: doctors and patients; doctors and significant others; and doctors and society.

During the previous year there was considerable press coverage of the prosecution for murder of Harold Shipman, a general practitioner who had prematurely ended the lives of a large number of predominantly elderly patients. There was no suggestion that these were 'mercy killings', but the ease with which the incidents had occurred and the length of time over which they took place without Shipman being detected, as well as the impact this had upon public confidence in the medical profession, would suggest that while the euthanasia debate is likely to continue in this country, any alteration of the law to sanction active euthanasia appears unlikely in the near future. Nonetheless, the present legal position is likely to come under some challenge now that the Human Rights Act 1998 has come into force, as it may very well be argued that the present legal position infringes the right of the patient under Article 8 of the European Convention on Human Rights – the right to the privacy of home and of family life.

Withdrawing treatment

While a health professional may not end a patient's life with a positive action, in some situations it is lawful to withdraw treatment in a hopeless case. This section considers the well-known case of Tony Bland, and the situations in which treatment may legitimately be withdrawn. It should be noted here that 'withdrawal' includes not only the decision to, for instance, remove a feeding tube, but also the decision not to administer a particular treatment should a relapse take place.

The Bland case

The case of *Airedale NHS Trust* v. *Bland* ([1993] AC 879) concerned Tony Bland, who was injured at the disaster at the Hillsborough football ground in 1989. His chest was severely crushed, and as a result he suffered hypoxic brain damage and entered a persistent vegetative state (PVS). He was fed through a nasogastric tube. After several years, during which he showed no noticeable sign of improvement, an application was made for a court order allowing the withdrawal of treatment. The order was granted. The judges in the House of Lords emphasized the fact that English law did not authorize euthanasia; however, there were situations in which there was no longer a duty to continue all treatment. The court recognized that there was a distinction in law between actions and omissions, and that usually failing to act was not culpable in criminal law. The House of Lords classed withdrawal of tube feeding where continued treatment was no longer in that patient's best interest as being an omission, not an act. In a case such as *Bland*, continued treatment was of no benefit to him as there was no prospect of his condition improving. What amounted to the patient's 'best interests' was to be assessed by reference to a responsible body of professional practice, the *Bolam* test (see Chapter 2). While obtaining a court order is a civil procedure, in practice a successful murder prosecution involving medical staff who remove an artificial feeding tube after a court order has been obtained is highly unlikely. Indeed, an attempt to bring a prosecution after the death of Tony Bland was unsuccessful (*R* v. *Bingley Magistrates Court ex parte Morrow* 13 April 1994, unreported).

The *Bland* case does not simply recognize that there may be a point at which it is legitimate to discontinue treatment and remove artificial feeding. It was suggested in the House of Lords that in some situations there may be a duty to do so. Lord Browne Wilkinson held that:

> If there comes a stage where the responsible doctor comes to the reasonable conclusion (which accords with the views of a responsible body of professional medical opinion) that further continuation of a life support system is not in the best interests of the patient, he can no longer lawfully continue that life support system; to do so would constitute the crime of battery and the tort of trespass to the person.

The exact scope of this duty is yet to be determined. It should be noted that it may be in the patient's best interests to discontinue treatment even though the relatives believe that treatment should be continued (*Re G* [1995] 2 FCR 46). One emotive question that remains to be answered after *Bland* is whether spoon feeding is classed, along with feeding through a nasogastric tube, as medical treatment.

Unauthorized termination of treatment

While a health care professional may be authorized to remove a patient from life support systems, that does not mean that any person switching off such a machine will be held to have simply omitted to act. If a mother comes into the ward and turns off the life support system because she believes that her son has suffered enough, and has not obtained a court order, she may be prosecuted for murder.

Applying Bland

In *Bland*, the diagnosis was clear. The relatives and health care professionals were in agreement. Nevertheless, the House of Lords noted that this was an exceptional case, and that subsequent cases should be referred to the courts. In a number of later cases withdrawal of treatment has been authorized, but difficulties remain. In *Frenchay* v. *S* ([1994] 2 All ER 403), S had taken an overdose and suffered consequent brain damage. The consultant caring for him said that S was in a persistent vegetative state and had no chance of recovery. S was being fed through a gastronomy tube in the stomach wall, and this tube became dislodged. The question was, should it be reinserted? The parents were divided as to whether treatment should be continued, while the health care professionals caring for S were opposed to the continuation of treatment. On appeal, the Court of Appeal upheld the decision of the judge at first instance, supporting withdrawal of further treatment. The case of *Frenchay* differs from that of *Bland* in certain respects. In *Frenchay*, there was no question of removing the feeding tube, as it had already become dislodged. In *Bland*, great emphasis was placed upon the fact that the patient was in an irreversible condition. One controversial aspect of *Frenchay* is that it was suggested that the diagnosis of PVS was by no means conclusive. In addition, the court in *Bland* had stated that there should be clear evidence as to the patient's medical condition, preferably from two doctors. Here, because the tube had become dislodged, the urgency of the case led to evidence being given by only one doctor. The *Frenchay* case may not be an isolated one, and it is likely that many of these decisions concerning treatment withdrawal may arise in similar emergencies. This may be particularly problematic, since recent research has questioned the efficacy of diagnosis of PVS in many cases (Andrews *et al.*, 1996). It appears that a considerable number of patients have, in the past, been the subject of misdiagnosis. A Practice Note which provides guidance as to the conduct of cases concerning withdrawal of treatment states that a patient should be in a PVS for a period of more than 12 months before diagnosis is made (Practice Note (Vegetative State) [1996] 2 FLR 375).

In *Bland*, it was suggested that whether a patient had fallen into a hopeless condition should be assessed by reference to the *Bolam* test – the view of a responsible body of professional practice (discussed further in Chapter 2 in the context of negligence). However, in *Frenchay*, Sir Thomas Bingham M.R. indicated that the courts would be prepared to review the doctor's assessment as to what was in the patient's best interests. This is a different approach, which may involve considering factors such as the quality of life the patient would enjoy were treatment to be continued. It appeared to be a shift away from *Bland* in that the court is undertaking the task of determining what amounts to 'best interests' rather than leaving this as a matter of judgment for health professionals (Kennedy and Grubb, 1994).

There are very difficult decisions concerning the withdrawal of treatment in a situation in which the patient is not in a PVS but is gravely handicapped and incompetent. Prior to *Bland*, a number of cases came before the courts regarding the decision to withhold treatment from handicapped children. If a child is born suffering from a serious handicap and, after counselling, the parents say they cannot cope and they do not want treatment to be continued, what can be done? This may be a situation in which it is sought to withdraw treatment. Such decisions are not to be taken lightly. Counselling should be given as to the nature of the handicap, prognosis and future survival rates. Handicaps can vary dramatically, from a Down's syndrome baby with a duodenal atresia where a simple operation to remove the complication can ensure that the child survives well into his or her thirties, to the anencephalic infant born without the upper hemispheres of the brain and for whom the prospects of survival are likely to be no more than a few weeks.

Where there is doubt as to whether treatment should be continued, it is advisable for an application to be made to the court to approve a course of non-active treatment. If such an order has been obtained, then any subsequent criminal prosecution, if death results, would be unlikely. The court makes an order as to future treatment on the basis of what is in the child's best interests. At first sight this may be regarded as similar to a *Bland*-type case. But there are differences. In *Bland*, the situation was hopeless with no prospect of recovery in the case of an adult unconscious patient. Ascertaining 'best interests' in the case of individuals who are incapacitated because of grave handicap may be more difficult. The court may in effect be assessing what is and what is not an adequate quality of life.

In *Re B* ([1981] 1 WLR 1421), a baby was born with Down's syndrome and a duodenal atresia. The parents did not want her to have an operation to correct the atresia, and believed that it would be better for her to die within the next few days. The hospital, however, informed the local authority and B was made a ward of court. The issue of whether to continue treatment was left to the court to determine. At first, the court authorized the operation. However, later B was removed to a different hospital where differences arose as to whether treatment should be given, and this led to the matter being referred back to the court. The Court of Appeal authorized the operation. Lord Justice Templeman said:

> There may be cases, I know not, of severe proved damage where the future is so certain and the prognosis so uncertain and where the life of the child is so bound to be full of pain and suffering that the court might be drawn to a different conclusion, but in the present case the choice which lies before the court is this: whether to allow an operation to take place which may result in the child living for 20 or 30 years as a mongoloid or whether (and I think that this must be brutally the result) to terminate the life of a mongoloid child because she also has an intestinal complaint.

The court decided that the operation should go ahead, as once B had the operation she was perfectly capable of living a full life to the normal Down's syndrome lifespan. In a number of subsequent cases, the courts have shown themselves willing to approve an order not to pursue active treatment. These cases extend beyond the very young infant to include children of some 3 or 4 months old. In *Re C* ([1989] 2 All ER 782), the Court of Appeal approved an order in respect of an infant born prematurely, suffering from severe hydrocephalus with severe mental and physical handicaps. She was not gaining weight, and the medical prognosis was that her condition was hopeless. On appeal, while the court approved the decision to cease active treatment, it said the following words (in the original order of the judge):

> The hospital authority be at liberty to treat the minor to allow her life
> to come to an end peacefully and with dignity ...

should be deleted because of the risk that misunderstanding would be
caused by the phrase 'allow her life to come to an end'.

The meaning of 'best interests' was explored further in the case of *Re
J* ([1990] 3 All ER 930) as discussed earlier. J was born nearly 13 weeks
prematurely, weighing only 1.1 kg. At birth, J was put on a ventilator and,
although later taken off the ventilator, he suffered relapses and had to be
reventilated. He was seriously brain damaged and appeared also to be
blind and deaf. In addition, it was likely that he would be totally paralysed. An application was made for an order to the effect that if J again suffered a collapse he should not be ventilated. The Court of Appeal made
the order. Lord Donaldson M.R., referring to a Canadian case, suggested
that in deciding whether to withdraw treatment, 'the court must decide
what the patient would choose if he was able to make a sound judgment'.
This child endured a very poor quality of life. He had already been ventilated for very long periods and had an exceedingly unfavourable prognosis. In reaching his decision, Lord Donaldson emphasized the fact that
mechanical ventilation was an invasive procedure that would cause the
child distress. Lord Donaldson's approach has been criticized. As Wells *et
al.* (1990) commented, it is artificial to use a subjective test in relation to
neonates and young children because there is no way of knowing what
they would have wanted. Much uncertainty, however, remains in this area.

The nurse may play an important role in ensuring that any decision to
withdraw treatment is carefully made. Any decision reached must be on
the basis of the best interests of the child, as opposed to what may be convenient for parents or for health care professionals. If the nurse believes
that a child is not being given suitable care, this must be reported to the
appropriate authorities.

Withdrawal of ventilator support

The question still arises regarding whether it would be possible to withdraw a patient from a ventilator if that patient has not been declared brainstem dead. Health care professionals would need to assess whether withdrawal from the ventilator can be said to be in the patient's best interests.
In 1996, the court authorized the withdrawal of ventilator support from an
infant brain-damaged by meningitis. The girl was blind, deaf and unable
to respond to her parents (*Re C (a baby)* [1996] FLR 43).

Conflicts between health care professionals and parents in rela-
tion to treatment decisions at the end of life

The courts have usually upheld medical opinion over parental opinion in
such situations. However an exception to this arose in the case of *Re T*
(1997). Here, the prognosis was that without the operation the child

would not live for more than 2½ years. A liver transplant operation had a good chance of success – a 90 per cent success rate was quoted. Nonetheless, in the Court of Appeal it was stated that here 'best interests' entailed respecting the mother's interests that the child should not undergo the pain/distress of this particular surgery. They emphasized that the child's welfare was dependent upon his mother. One doctor was of the view that there would be great problems undertaking treatment without parental support. However, this case may in many ways be regarded as exceptional. The parents were at the time living in another Commonwealth country, and had had to come to England for treatment to be undertaken. There was some suggestion that had a different approach been undertaken, the parents would have moved outside the jurisdiction.

What if the parents want treatment continued in the face of clinical opinion that the situation is hopeless? In *Re C (a minor)* [1998] Lloyd's Rep Med I (Fam. Div.) C was 16 months old and suffering from spinal muscular atrophy type 1– a progressive condition with no curative treatment. The child was regarded as being in what was known as a 'no chance' condition under the Royal College of Paediatricians and Child Health guidelines. However, the child was conscious – she was able to recognize her parents and smile. The child's parents, who were orthodox Jews, believed life should be preserved. It was proposed to remove the child from the ventilator, and if she suffered a further relapse she would be left to die. While the parents supported the decision to see if the child could survive without a ventilator, they wanted her to be attached to the ventilator if she relapsed. Sir Stephen Brown P indicated again that following the approach of the parents meant that the doctors would have been compelled to undertake a course of treatment, which they were unwilling to do. The court would not make an order requiring the doctors to treat. There has been some academic criticism of the case. Ian Kennedy commented that the guidelines from the Royal College of Paediatricians had been subject to a critical reception from the health care professions, and that 'particular exception was taken to some of the language used to categorize' and the 'no chance' category was regarded as insensitive (Kennedy, 1997).

A very heated conflict arose with family members in *R* v. *Portsmouth Hospitals NHS Trust ex parte Glass* ([1999] Lloyd's Rep Med 367). Here, D was 12 years old and had been born with severe mental and physical disabilities, which included cerebral palsy, hydrocephalus and epilepsy. He was suffering from various postoperative infections, and hospital staff were of the view that D was dying. They wanted to administer diamorphine with the aim of alleviating distress. The family was opposed to this, and a violent incident followed in the hospital. Criminal and civil proceedings were launched consequent upon this incident. D was discharged and was treated by his GP. The Trust wrote to the hospital and stated that should the child again fall ill, it would be better for D to be treated in another hospital. An application was made for judicial review. One aspect of the claim was that they asked for a declaration regarding treatment/withdrawal of life-sustaining treatment. Judicial review was refused because not only was this particular case not susceptible to judicial review, but also it would be difficult to frame the action in meaningful terms in a hypothetical situation.

Withdrawal of treatment from adult patients not in PVS

After *Bland*, there has been increasing judicial willingness to sanction withdrawal of treatment even though patients fall outside the PVS guidelines. In *Re D (Medical Treatment)* ([1998] 1 FLR 411), the patient had suffered severe head injuries following a road accident. She returned from hospital to live with her parents, who were caring for her. She was both physically and mentally disabled. She could communicate, but when she realized that her condition could not improve further then she became depressed and expressed serious dissatisfaction with her quality of life. She spoke about her death and funeral arrangements. In September 1995 she suffered an unexplained insult to the brain, and in March 1996 she was diagnosed as being in PVS. She was kept alive by a tube providing artificial nutrition and hydration, and on 18 March 1997 this became dislodged. A court order was sought, but the Official Solicitor opposed this, saying that she did not come within the criteria as set out by the Medical Royal Colleges. The court granted the declaration. She did not fulfil the 1996 guidelines (e.g. could track objects with her eyes and exhibit a menace response, and nystagmus occurred in response to ice water); however, the judge did accept the views of the experts – namely that she was indisputably in a PVS state. There was no evidence before the court that the defendant had any life whatsoever; she was suffering a living death – i.e. it was not in her best interests to be kept alive artificially. Subsequently, the case of *Re H (a Patient)* ([1998] 2 FLR 36) was heard. H was 43 years old and had suffered serious brain damage in a road traffic accident. She was kept alive via artificial feeding, and was unaware of her environment. In this case, it was thought best for feeding to be withheld. The consultant clinical psychologist found that there was a visual tracking movement and believed that H could focus on an object and be aroused by clapping – i.e. not all the Royal College of Physicians guidelines on the permanent vegetative state were fulfilled. However, experts were of the view that H was in PVS. Sir Stephen Brown made the order, and indicated that the sanctity of life was not paramount:

> I am satisfied that it is in the best interests of this patient that the life-sustaining treatment should be brought to a conclusion.

The trend away from PVS continues, with recent guidelines issued by the BMA on the *Withholding and Withdrawal of Life-Prolonging Medical Treatment* (BMA, 1999). These state that oral nutrition in the form of spoon feeding or moistening of the patient's mouth for comfort forms part of what they regard as 'basic care', and thus should not be withdrawn. As far as the basis for withholding/withdrawing treatment from patients was concerned, they stated that in a situation in which treatment was 'unable to achieve its intended clinical goal or the patient's imminent death is inevitable, active treatment may provide no benefit and may be withheld or withdrawn' (BMA, 1999, para 17.3). The BMA set out a series of factors to be taken into account when considering whether the provision of life-prolonging treatment should be withdrawn. Taking account of these and other relevant factors, decisions must be made in each case that can be justified in terms of the benefit to the individual patient.

Factors to be taken into account when considering whether the provision of life-prolonging treatment should be withdrawn include (BMA, 1999):

- the patient's own wishes and values (where these can be ascertained)
- the clinical judgment and effectiveness of the proposed treatment
- the likelihood of the patient experiencing severe unmanageable pain or suffering
- the level of awareness the individual has of his or her own existence and surroundings as demonstrated by, for example,
  - an ability to interact with others – however expressed;
  - the capacity for self-directed action or ability to take control of any aspect of his or her life
- the likelihood and extent of any degree of improvement in the patient's condition if treatment is provided
- whether the invasiveness of treatment is justified by the circumstances
- the views of the parents, if the patient is a child
- the views of people close to the patient, especially close relatives, partners and carers, about what the patient is likely to see as beneficial.

The BMA has indicated that where there is a question of withholding artificial nutrition/hydration and the wishes of the patient are unknown and death is not imminent, this should be subject to formal clinical review by a senior clinician with experience of the condition from which the patient is suffering, and who is not part of the clinical team (para 22.1(a)). Moreover, legal advice should be sought and indeed a judicial declaration may very well be needed (para 22.1(b)). The guidelines also emphasize that to the extent to which the patient is capable of understanding what is going on, every effort should be made to explain the particular decision to the patient (para 22.3).

Reforming the law

After the *Bland* and *Cox* cases, a Select Committee of the House of Lords was appointed to consider the issue of euthanasia and withdrawal of life-saving treatment (House of Lords, 1994a). As we saw above, the committee rejected an extension of the law allowing active euthanasia. They suggested that 'treatment limiting decisions' of incompetent patients should be taken by all those involved in the patient's care and the patient's close relatives. If there was no agreement as to what care to pursue, then the issue could be referred to a new forum. The basis for withdrawing treatment should be that 'treatment may be judged inappropriate if it will add nothing to the patient's well being as a person'. The Law Commission recommended that discontinuation of artificial sustenance to an unconscious patient who has no activity in the cerebral cortex and no prospect of recovery should require either court approval (consent of an attorney or manager) or, if allowed by an order of the Secretary of State, a certificate by an independent medical practitioner (draft Bill clause 10(2)). They were uneasy as to the use of 'best interests' as the test to apply in making the decision to withdraw treatment. This was because, while it could be said not to be in the patient's best interests to continue treatment, it could be argued not to be in the patient's best interests to end the treatment. Nevertheless, they went on to recommend that the factors in the 'best interests' checklist should be considered when making this decision (see Chapter 5).

With respect, this appears to be in effect performing mental gymnastics. Their proposal that approval may be given by one of three possible decision makers also creates difficulties. Surely there are different policy reasons for leaving this decision to a court than there are for leaving it to a medical practitioner? The government, in their document *Making Decisions*, took a different approach from that of the Law Commission on this issue. They recommended that this matter should remain one for the court to determine, and one not capable of being delegated to a court-appointed manager save in the situation in which there was a specific power given to a proxy decision maker appointed by the patient (Lord Chancellor's Department, 1999); Chapters 2 and 3).

Living wills

A patient is involved in a motorway crash and is brought into hospital unconscious. It appears that there are serious physical injuries and it is likely that, should the patient recover, he will be paralysed and severely brain damaged. The relatives say that the patient has made a living will, and that this states that in such a condition the patient would not have wanted to have treatment continued. What should be done?

A living will (or advance directive) is a statement made by a patient before he or she becomes incapable of making decisions, effectively stating the treatments the patient would not want pursued should he or she become incapacitated. Judicial acceptance has been given to advance refusals of treatment (*Re T* [1992] 4 All ER 649). One common form of such advance refusal is the card carried by Jehovah's Witnesses. A living will is in some respects an extension of such a card. However, although a living will may provide a useful guide as to what treatment should or should not be given, it is important to note that such a document may not authorize an action that is currently unlawful – for example, euthanasia. In addition, a patient cannot use a living will to require the health care team to continue all possible treatments regardless of expense and efficacy. The UKCC (1996) has noted, regarding living wills, that:

> Although not necessarily legally binding, they can provide very useful information about the wishes of a patient or client who is now unable to make a decision and should therefore be respected.

At present there is no legislation governing living wills, and many uncertainties remain regarding their application. The courts may accept them in principle, but it has been suggested that a number of safeguards are required to ensure that the living will properly reflects the patient's wishes. The Law Commission (1995i) recommends that there should be a rebuttable presumption that living wills are valid if in writing, signed by the maker and witnessed. However, the Law Commission does not believe that a patient should have the right to refuse all treatment. It suggests that a patient should not be able to refuse basic care, by which is meant care to ensure basic bodily cleanliness and direct oral hydration and nutrition (Law Commission, 1995ii). The BMA (BMA, 1999) has recommended that a valid advance directive should be upheld (para 10.1), stating that this will be valid where the patient was competent when they made the directive, where they were free from pressure, and where they were offered sufficient accurate information to make an informed decision. The BMA also states that (para 10.2):

> The patient must have envisaged the type of situation which has subsequently arisen and for which the advance directive is being invoked.

Death of a patient refusing such basic care may be particularly unpleasant for the nurses caring for that patient, and for the other patients on the ward. Yet at the same time, a patient who is competent can decide to die slowly by refusing all food. Shouldn't a patient be allowed to make a similar decision through a living will?

A further difficulty with the living will is that a person's view may change over time – what may seem a totally intolerable state of health at 20 years of age may not be regarded as intolerable at all at 75. The lapse of time between the will being initially drawn up and then later interpreted needs to be taken into consideration when applying the will.

Another issue is the applicability of a living will to a woman who later, when the issue of treatment and the validity of the living will arises, is pregnant. It has been suggested that before a living will is made, women of childbearing age should be asked to consider the possibility of becoming pregnant (Law Commission, 1995iii).

Drafting living wills – the role of the nurse

If living wills become commonly used, the nurse may be involved in advising the patient as to how such a will should be drawn up and the implications of it. The BMA (1995ii) has stated that:

Hospital managers and GP practice managers need to consider how to respond to the increasing desire of patients to plan ahead on the basis of accurate health information and advice.

The BMA notes that some hospitals have specialist counsellors who provide support and information regarding living wills, and that home visits are provided. It states that 'hospice outreach services and community nurses may also become involved in carrying out such a role' (BMA, 1995iii). This is in contrast with an earlier statement by the RCN to the effect that the nurse should not be involved in drawing up living wills (RCN, 1992). It is submitted that the RCN approach is preferable. If a patient wishes to draw up a living will, he or she should be able to seek advice for that purpose, but it should come from outside the clinical team. It is important to ensure that any decision is perceived to be wholly independent of any considerations of convenience in resource allocation.

It is likely that the uncertain legal position regarding living wills will continue for some time. In their document *Making Decisions*, the government commented that they had no intention of introducing legislation on advance directives (Lord Chancellor's Department, 1999). They were of the view that the validity of advance refusals was sufficiently recognized in English law. However, this may be questioned. It is arguably the very informality and lack of co-ordination and clear guidelines regarding the use of advance directives at present that has the effect that very little use is made of them.

Continuing powers of attorney

In some situations, although a living will may exist, it may not help the health professional. It may be insufficiently specific, or it may have been made a number of years ago and doubts may be raised as to the extent to which this now reflects an individual's interests. One alternative is for a person to be appointed to make treatment decisions on behalf of the mentally incompetent person. Such a person may be known as a 'treatment attorney' or proxy decision maker. At present, while a person may appoint another person to make decisions about his or her financial affairs, if he or she becomes incompetent, this does not apply to treatment (Enduring Powers of Attorney Act 1985). The Law Commission (1995iv) proposed that the law should be extended to recognize far more extensive use of proxy decision makers and to allow patients to nominate a person to act in their best interests when they themselves become incapable of making a decision. They do, however, comment that the power of any such attorney should be limited and, for example, would exclude the power to authorize the removal of basic care (draft Bill clauses 16(3)(c) and 9(8)). The government has accepted the arguments in favour of the extension of powers of attorney in their document *Making Decisions*. The existing powers in relation to financial affairs will be overhauled, and there will be a new power enabling the appointment of an attorney who will be able to exercise powers in relation to health care and welfare matters as well as financial issues, along the lines proposed by the Law Commission in their report (Lord Chancellor's Department, 1999, Chapter 2). While this may enhance decision making by providing some guidance, recognition of proxy decision making in the health care context may bring its own problems. Not least of these is the fact that ascertaining a person's wishes may be difficult if it is a long time since that person exercised the power of appointment of the proxy decision maker, and decision making is very much dependent upon how aware the proxy is of the patient's current views (BMA, 1995). Nevertheless, it may at least assist in providing some guidance regarding difficult treatment decisions.

'Do not resuscitate' orders

Hospital nurses will be familiar with the practice of placing a 'do not resuscitate' (DNR) order in the patient's notes, but on what basis should this decision be made? A joint BMA/RCN report considered the use of DNR orders (BMA/RCN, 1993). They recommended that a DNR order may be considered if it is believed that cardiopulmonary resuscitation is unlikely to succeed or if it is contrary to the patient's express wishes, or if, were the patient resuscitated, he or she would be unlikely to have a quality of life that the individual would find acceptable. In ascertaining quality of life, the guidelines suggest that as far as possible the patient's views should be obtained, but if this is impossible then the patient's close relatives should be consulted. The guidelines leave the ultimate decision as to whether to make a DNR order in the hands of the consultant, although they do state that patient involvement in these decisions is 'valuable' and 'important'. While discussion is not mandatory, they suggest that careful enquiry should be made of those patients who are thought to be at risk, and that the results of these discussions should be included in the hospital notes.

Does this go far enough to safeguard the patient's interests? There is a danger that a patient is only involved in the process to ensure his or her compliance with the decision. While the guidelines recommend that consultations about DNR orders should be made with members of the clinical team, the ultimate responsibility for the decision is placed in the hands of the consultant, who has the task of assessing an individual patient's quality of life. However, as Schutz (1994) commented:

> ... this is a highly subjective process which requires a depth of relationship that consultants are unlikely to achieve. Even though the consultant has legal responsibility for the patient's treatment in relation to resuscitation, there needs to be more emphasis on the team approach.

Once a DNR order has been made, the guidelines suggest that all members of the health care team should be informed and that the order itself should be subject to a regular review.

The use of a DNR order has now been given judicial approval in principle in the case of *Re R* ([1996] 2 FLR 99). In this case, the court upheld a DNR order in relation to a 23-year-old man who had cerebral palsy, brain malformation and learning difficulties and, while not in PVS, was in what was termed a 'low awareness state'. Evidence was given that he was physically and neurologically deteriorating. The consultant treating R was of the view that it was in R's best interests to allow nature to take its course the next time he had a life-threatening incident. The judge made an order stating that it would be lawful to withhold the administration of antibiotics in the event of the patient suffering a life-threatening infection, and to withhold cardiac pulmonary resuscitation. The DNR order here was drawn up in line with the RCN/DOH guidance.

Despite the guidance regarding DNR orders, a recent study suggested that this is not being followed. In an audit of a hospital in north London, it was found that only 9 per cent of consultants were involved in DNR decisions and there were no records in any case of the issue being discussed with the patient (*JRCP*, 1999). In a report by Age Concern (Age Concern, 2000), there was again considerable concern over evidence that decisions were not made with family consultation. Other countries, such as the USA, have legislation governing DNR orders, but until now legislation on this matter has been rejected in this country. It may be time for that position to be reconsidered. Meanwhile, the nurse may play an important role in monitoring the operation of DNR orders in her or his capacity as patient advocate.

Death

When are health care professionals entitled to declare a patient is dead? There is no statutory definition of death in English law. However, for many years clinical practice has recognized brainstem death as the point at which death occurs (Royal College of Physicians, 1996), and the courts have now confirmed this. In *Re A* ([1992] 3 Med LR 303), the court held that a child who was being supported on a ventilator, and who had been declared brainstem dead, was dead for all intents and purposes, and thus a doctor who had disconnected the ventilator was not acting unlawfully. The House of Lords in *Bland* supported this approach. In that case, their lordships confirmed that those patients in a state of 'cognitive death' with irreversible damage to the upper hemispheres of the brain and who were in a persistent vegetative state were not legally dead.

Certification of death must be undertaken by a doctor (Births and Deaths Registration Act 1953 s22). It is not the role of the nurse to undertake this task. Certain deaths must be notified to the coroner by the doctor who is certifying death, and these include deaths related to suspicious circumstances.

Organ transplants

Transplant technology has developed considerably over the past few decades. A wide variety of transplants of organs and tissues is increasingly undertaken, ranging from kidneys and bone marrow to heart and lungs. The nurse frequently plays an important part in the transplant process. The nurse may work as a transplant co-ordinator, or may counsel patients who are considering whether to undergo a transplant. He or she may also have to attend the patient's body after the removal of organs in the intensive therapy unit or the high dependency unit. In this part of the chapter, the regulation of transplantation is considered.

Cadaver transplants

> A patient has been injured in a car crash and dies later in hospital. It is hoped that the patient's organs can be used for transplantation into a patient urgently awaiting a donor, but can they be lawfully used?

The current law regulating cadaver transplants is contained in the Human Tissue Act 1961. Removal of the organs must be authorized by the person who is 'lawfully in possession of the body' (s1(1) Human Tissue Act 1961). If death has taken place in hospital, this is usually the hospital authorities (s1(7)). The organs may be removed if the deceased person had agreed to the use of his or her organs, whether in writing (through, for example, the use of a donor card) or orally in the presence of two witnesses, during his or her last illness. This will lead to transplants being authorized unless there is reason to believe that the deceased subsequently withdrew such consent.

If there is no donor card, the organs may still be used if this is authorized by the person lawfully in possession of the body. This person must show that he or she has no reason to believe, after making such inquiries as are reasonably practical, that the deceased had expressed an objection to the body being used for transplants, and that the surviving spouse/relative of the deceased does not object to transplantation (s1(2)). The Act requires enquiries to be made of spouse/relative only (s1(2)), and does not take into account the fact that a person may be estranged from relatives and may be in a long-term relationship outside marriage. The legislation does not define what amounts to 'reasonable enquiries'. It has been suggested that it would be reasonable simply to enquire of the spouse or close relative as to whether they or another person has expressed an objection (Skegg, 1984). It is an open question whether, if the organs are needed sufficiently urgently, it would be justifiable to remove them without making any enquiries of the relatives. Despite the technical legal uncertainty surrounding this point, in practice it appears that organs will not be removed unless the donor's relatives have been consulted.

The actual transplant must be undertaken by a doctor who is satisfied that two sets of brainstem death tests have been performed and proved negative. Eyes may be removed by a doctor who has ascertained that life is extinct, or by a person acting on the instructions of a doctor (s4(a) Corneal Tissue Act 1986). The doctor must be satisfied that the person in question is sufficiently qualified/trained to perform the removal completely. The qualified person must either be satisfied that life is extinct by examination, or be satisfied on the basis of a statement to that effect by a doctor.

If it appears that an inquest may have to be held on a body, or a *post mortem* will be required, then organs may not be removed without the coroner's consent (s1(5)). The difficulty with this is that the delay caused in referring the matter to the coroner may render the organs useless. The Home Secretary has issued a circular regulating this issue. It is stated that the coroner's consent should be refused only where there may be later criminal proceedings in which the organ might be required as evidence, or if the organ is/might have been the cause/partial cause of death, or if its removal might impede further investigations.

Commercial dealing in organs

In the late 1980s there was a major scandal when it was discovered that individuals were being offered money to come to this country from Turkey and sell their organs for transplantation. This led to disciplinary proceedings being brought against a number of doctors, with one being struck off the General Medical Council's register. One result of the scandal was the passage of the Human Organ Transplants Act 1989, which made it a criminal offence to pay persons to donate organs or to undertake any other commercial dealing in organs from live donors or from cadavers (s2). There has been some debate as to whether this situation should be altered (Radcliffe-Richards *et al.*, 1998). However, in practice this is unlikely. Bodies such as the World Health Organization

(WHO40 13J) and the Council of Europe, in documents such as the Convention on Human Rights and Biomedicine (Article 22), have come down strongly against the commercialization of the body and its parts.

Live organ donations

If it is sought to use living persons as organ donors, then first, the appropriate consent must be given, and second, certain statutory provisions in the form of the Human Organ Transplants Act 1989 must be complied with. It appears generally accepted that organ transplantation from adults is a type of operation that may be lawfully undertaken (Brazier, 1992). Nonetheless, it is doubtful whether a competent adult is capable of lawfully consenting to the removal of a vital organ with death as a consequence, if only because such removal would lead to the surgeon being prosecuted for murder.

Doubts have also been expressed as to the legality of transplantation of animal organs into humans because of the risk to the intended donor (Mason, 1990). At present such transplants are not being undertaken on humans, but this is now the subject of review by a new body, the Xenotransplantation Interim Regulatory Body (see p. 239 and Fox and McHale, 1997).

In some instances, it may be sought to use a child as a donor. Although child patients are frequently bone marrow donors, use of child patients as solid organ donors is infrequent, and it appears that surgeons are unwilling to use child patients as donors. In the Court of Appeal in *Re W* (*a minor*) ([1992] 3 WLR 758), Lord Donaldson said that the statutory right of children over 16 years to consent to treatment contained in the Family Law Reform Act 1969 did not apply to organ donation. Whether a child is able to consent to his or her organs being donated would have to be decided using the common law. Here, the only guidance available is the *Gillick* test – that a child can consent to a procedure if he or she has sufficient maturity to consent to that procedure. In the case of a very young child, parental consent would be required. In practice, if donation is sought from a child patient of any age, parental consent should be obtained. One particular difficulty may be in ensuring that consent is freely given, bearing in mind the very highly charged emotional situation in which such a decision would be made. If a mentally incompetent adult is proposed as a donor, then the matter should be referred to the court, who will consider whether such a procedure could be said to be in the mentally incompetent adult's best interests (*Re Y* [1996] 2 FLR 791).

What if a child refuses a transplant? As noted in Chapter 6, in the case of *Re M*, a teenager refused a transplant. She was unhappy with the procedure and with living with a transplanted organ from another person inside her. The court nonetheless went ahead and approved the conduct of the transplantation operation in this particular case, overriding her refusal. This case can be contrasted with that of Re *T* (1997; see p. 222), where the court upheld the parents' decision to refuse a liver transplant for their child. In this case the prognosis for the success of the procedure was exceedingly good. Nonetheless, as discussed in Chapter 6, this case may perhaps be distinguished not simply on the basis that the parents were health care professionals with long experience of caring for sick children, but also on the fact that the parents had to come to England for the surgery, which was unavailable in the jurisdiction in which they were working, and there were some suggestions that had a different judicial approach been taken the parents would have gone outside the jurisdiction of the English courts.

Certain other jurisdictions actually prohibit organ donation from mentally incapacitated adults. In addition, the Council of Europe Statement No. R (79) stated that organs could be removed for transplant purposes, but that this was only 'from an adult who is capable of giving his/her consent freely'. The Council of Europe Convention on Human Rights and Biomedicine provides in Article 20 (Protection of Persons Not Able to Consent) that:

1. No organ or tissue removal may be carried out on a person who does not have the capacity to consent under Article 5.
2. Exceptionally and under the protective conditions prescribed by law, the removal of regenerative tissue from a person who does not have the capacity to consent may be authorized provided the following conditions are met:
   i) there is no compatible donor available who has the capacity to consent;
   ii) the recipient is a brother or sister of the donor;
   iii) the donation must have the potential to be life-saving for the recipient;
   iv) the authorization provided for under paragraphs 2 and 3 of Article 6 has been given specifically and in writing, in accordance with the law and with the approval of the competent body;
   v) the potential donor concerned does not object.

The Steering Committee on Bioethics has also been entrusted with the task of preparing a protocol on organ transplantation, which will develop those principles stated in the Convention.

In accord with what is generally recognized practice, the Convention states that an incompetent donor should not be used if there is a competent person available who can act as a compatible donor. It should be noted that this is more restrictive than the current UK position in that it applies only to regenerative tissue. Regenerative tissue is defined in this article as 'that capable of reconstituting its tissue mass and function after partial removal'. As the explanatory notes provide, the most common instance of this at present is bone marrow, but the definition is wider than this to take into account developments in medical science. It may also be regarded as more restrictive than existing English law in that it applies only to those donors who are brother or sister to the donor. As the explanatory notes state (para 128):

> This restriction is intended to avoid both family and doctors going to extreme lengths to find a donor at any price, even if the level of kinship is distant and the chances for a successful transplant are not very likely, because of tissue incompatibility.

Presently the UK is not a party to the Convention but it is undoubtedly the case that this will be very influential in determining reform in this area.

Human Organ Transplants Act 1989

Transplants between related donors

A further repercussion of the Turkish organ scandal was that the Human Organ Transplants Act 1989 placed a number of limitations upon the practice of live organ donation. It is now an offence for a person living in the UK to remove an organ intended to be transplanted into another person or to transplant an organ from one living person to another living person unless the criteria set out in the Act are followed. If the donor intends to give an organ to a relative, it must be shown that the person into whom the organ is to be transplanted falls within a prescribed group. This group is drawn very broadly to include not only parents and children but also, for example, uncles and aunts of the half blood (s2(2)).

Transplants between unrelated donors

While the legislation does allow transplants between unrelated donors, various limitations are placed on such donations (s2(6)). These reflect the concern of the legislators to protect potential donors from exploitation. Transplants between unrelated donors are governed by the Unrelated Live Transplant Regulatory Authority (ULTRA) (s2). The Authority must be satisfied that the donor has received no unauthorized payments. The donor must be given and understand an explanation of the medical procedures and the risks involved in the removal of the organ, and consent must be given freely without coercion or the offer of an inducement. The donor must understand that he or she is entitled to withdraw consent. Both donor and recipient must be interviewed by a person who appears to the Authority to be suitably qualified to conduct such interviews, and this person must make a report to the Authority as to whether the criteria for donation have been satisfied. It has been suggested that, while there is a need to protect unrelated donors, the pressure that related donors are under should nonetheless not be underestimated. The BMA, in a recent document (BMA, 2000b), suggested that all live donors should be subject to rigorous assessment to ensure that consent is truly voluntary, whether this is undertaken by ULTRA or by another body. This suggestion should be supported by legislation – it is important that the interests of both related and unrelated donors be safeguarded.

Reforming the system

There is a grave shortage of organs and long transplant waiting lists – at the end of March 2000, some 5354 persons were on the national transplant waiting list. Many proposals have been made for reform of the present system (e.g. New *et al.*, 1994; BMA, 2000b). These extend from clarification of the provisions of the Human Tissue Act 1961 to legislation allowing automatic removal of organs from the deceased except the person had made an indication to the contrary before death. Below are set out some of the main suggestions for reform.

One option is the introduction of 'opting out' legislation (New *et al.*, 1994; BMA, 2000b). This allows organs to be removed without express permission being obtained, unless a deceased person had expressed an objection before his or her death. There is some evidence that the introduction of such a scheme in countries such as Belgium has increased the supply of available organs. Opting out legislation has recently been given support by the BMA (BMA, 2000b). Nevertheless, proposals to introduce opting out legislation into this country have met opposition. There are fears that persons may feel pressurized into not opting out. Opposition to such legislation may also come from certain religious/cultural groups who are unhappy with transplantation or who do not accept brainstem death. Opting out may also lead to relatives' wishes being ignored. In practice, however, in countries where opting out legislation has been introduced, the donor's relatives are still consulted. Indeed the BMA, in their recent document, suggest that in a situation in which a person has not expressed views on donation while they are alive, but it is apparent in this situation that 'to proceed with the donation would cause major distress to a first-degree relative or long-term partner, the donation should not proceed' (BMA, 2000b). While commendable in the sensitivity to feelings of relatives, such an exception leads to the question of whether the introduction of opting out legislation would lead to a radical increase in supply. The BMA do admittedly see opting out as one part of a wider strategy in relation to donation. They also propose that there needs to be a comprehensive piece of legislation that governs all aspects of organ donation, from live to cadaver. In 1999, the UK government (in response to an earlier call by the BMA for opting out) indicated that it was not in favour of a change of the law to support the introduction of opting out at the present time.

Another alternative is that of 'required request', a practice used in the United States. There, hospitals are obliged to set up procedures enabling routine enquiries to be made of patients and their relatives as to whether organs may be used if the patient subsequently dies. Required request does not appear to have led to any dramatic increase in the number of organs available for harvest in the USA. This may be due, at least in part, to the fact that there have been practical problems with the operation of required request, not least in the fact that in many hospitals the procedures have been badly established and operated. It has, however, been argued that required request can impose considerable burdens on hospital staff in having to make time-consuming enquiries of potential donors and relatives.

In the absence of legislative change, there have been attempts to increase the supply of organs by improving the present system. For many years, members of the public have been encouraged to carry donor cards indicating their willingness to donate organs, although there has been some scepticism regarding the effectiveness of such a scheme (New *et al.*, 1994). A computerized organ donor register was introduced in 1994, the NHS Organ Donor Register, which allows individuals to have their wishes regarding organ donation entered on to computer. Transplant co-ordinators can contact the Organ Donor Register as a means of identifying the donor's wishes. Intending donors may tick a box on their driving licence application form expressing their wish to donate organs, and this information will be entered onto the Organ Donor Register.

One method of facilitating the supply of organs for transplantation, which provoked considerable controversy, is a practice known as 'elective ventilation' (McHale, 1995). Patients with an intracranial haemorrhage, in a hopeless condition and who were regarded as suitable donors, were transferred to intensive care units, where they were ventilated to facilitate use of their organs for transplantation. This procedure was controversial in that when the patient is transferred to the intensive care unit, he or she may not have been declared brainstem dead. This practice was halted because it was stated to be illegal. While medical procedures can be performed upon mentally incompetent patients if in their best interests, the extent to which this is applicable in these cases is uncertain. Elective ventilation is not undertaken for the patient's benefit, but rather to benefit others. Indeed, it may be very much against the patient's interests if, as it has been suggested, it inhibits the patient's right to a peaceful and dignified end. The Law Commission left open the possibility that the question could be addressed in legislation (Law Commission, 1995v). Should consensus be reached on this issue, one option is for a person who is willing to have his or her organs used for transplantation and to be electively ventilated to express this through some form of advance declaration. This could take the form of a donor card similar to the existing organ donor card, but perhaps in a different colour or shape to avoid confusion. It remains to be seen whether elective ventilation will receive sufficient public support to lead to legislative reform.

It has also been suggested that there should be the enhanced use of live organ donors regarding kidney transplantation. Living donor transplantation has better success rates. There are the risks of surgery, although some evidence suggest that kidney transplants have a good safety record

(Nicolson and Bradley, 1999). The BMA (BMA, 2000b) has also emphasized the need for good co-ordination of transplantation, and points, as did the earlier King's Fund report (New *et al.*, 1994), to the success of the Spanish system of national transplant co-ordinators. There has been increased growth in the use of transplant co-ordinators, and there have been calls for the establishment of a national body regulating this area by the UK Transplant Co-ordinators Association and the Royal College of Surgeons (BMA, 2000b).

Transplantation technology in the future

New options have been suggested, which may alter transplantation practice out of all recognition. The first is that of xenotransplantation, the second is the use of cloning of tissues and organs.

Xenotransplantation

At present, xenotransplantation is regulated by the Xenotransplantation Interim Regulatory Authority, which was established following the recommendations of the Department of Health Advisory Group chaired by Professor Ian Kennedy (Fox and McHale, 1997, 1998). This Advisory Group reviewed the acceptability of an ethical framework within which xenotransplantation may be undertaken (this followed an earlier report by the Nuffield Council on Bioethics). The Advisory Group approved the practice of xenotransplantation in principle, accepting that it is ethical to use animals as a source of organs, provided certain conditions are satisfied. The group recognized that animals have rights in a minimal sense, namely that their interests in avoiding suffering must be considered in any assessment of the benefits and harms of any proposed course of action (para 4.22). It regarded xenotransplantation as having the potential for an unlimited and immediate supply of usable organs. However, while xenotransplantation was approved in principle, the group was concerned about the prospect for disease transmission that could result from premature authorization of such transplants. Its caution in delaying animal–human transplants is reflective of heightened public concern regarding the safety of certain animal products following the BSE crisis.

While the Advisory Group regards xenotransplantation as ethical, this view does not command universal support. The ethical issues are complex. In using animal organs, does this mean that we are treating animals in a manner in which we would treat human subjects? If so, does that mean it is morally objectionable? In recognition of the fact that this is an ethically emotive area, it has been suggested that health professionals should be given a statutory right of conscientious objection to participation in such procedures, and they would be able to opt out without subsequent prejudice to career or employment (para 7.26). Were such a measure to be enacted, it would join only two other statutory provisions granting a right of conscientious objection to health professionals – s4 of the Abortion Act 1967, and s38 of the Human Fertilization and Embryology Act 1990.

The Advisory Group stated that xenotransplantation should be the subject of statutory regulation and that a National Standing Committee should be established to regulate such procedures. The government accepted the group's recommendations, and a Xenotransplantation Interim Regulatory Authority was established to approve experiments and monitor progress. This is chaired by the former Archbishop of York, Lord Habgood, who has a background in pharmacology, and has declared a moratorium pending further research. If the Authority is prepared in the future to authorize such transplantations, then a number of other issues require resolution. Currently, there is debate as to whether patients can lawfully consent to a procedure that is clinically risky, such as xenotransplantation (Mason, 1990). If the procedure is ultimately recognized as lawful in principle, then a matter that still has to be addressed is whether particular groups of individuals should become recipients. The Advisory Group was of the opinion that, at least in the first instance, the procedure should be confined to competent adults (para 7.7). It recognized that recipients of xenotransplants should be afforded a high degree of information disclosure and counselling facilities as to the implications of the procedure (para 7.11). The sensitivity of the issue has led to the group recommending that the fact that an individual chooses to refuse a xenotransplant should not inhibit their ability subsequently to become the recipient of a human organ (para 7.15).

The present situation represents a somewhat uneasy compromise. It remains to be seen as to whether such technology will be further developed for clinical applications.

Therapeutic cloning

As discussed in Chapter 9, therapeutic cloning may provide a solution, enabling organs and tissues to be 'grown to order' as replacements. In July 1999 the UK government confirmed that in its view human reproductive cloning is ethically unacceptable, and it has placed a ban on such procedures. A new expert advisory group has been established with the task of assessing the potential benefits of cloning for therapeutic purposes. Tessa Jowell, Minister for Public Health, stated that:

> The government reaffirms its policy that human reproductive cloning is ethically unacceptable and cannot take place in this country. However, we recognize that regulations to allow therapeutic research should be very carefully considered.

The government also said that a 6-month study would be undertaken on the therapeutic applications of cloning, and that cloning would not go ahead straightaway. However, press reports in the summer of 2000 indicated that the government is likely to sanction such technological developments (*Sunday Times*, 30 June, 2000). The development of therapeutic cloning in relation to solid organs may, however, take some time in the light of the fact that the growth of such organs will require exceedingly complex scientific technology.

References

Age Concern England (2000). *Turning Your Back on Us: Older People and the NHS.* Age Concern.

Andrews, K. *et al.* (1996). Misdiagnosis in a rehabilitative unit. *Br. Med. J.*, **313**, 13.

BMA (1995). *Advance Statements about Medical Treatment.* BMA, (i) para 7.4; (ii) para 6.7; (iii) p. 22.

BMA (1999). *Withholding and Withdrawing Life-Prolonging Treatment.* BMA.

BMA (2000a). Physician-assisted suicide; a conference to promote the development of consensus. BMA online http://web.bma.org.uk.

BMA (2000b). Organ Donation in the 21st Century: Time for a Consolidated Approach. BMA online http://www.bma.org.uk/public/

BMA/RCN (1993). *Statement on Cardiopulmonary Resuscitation.* BMA/RCN.

Brazier, M. (1992). *Medicine, Patients and the Law*, 2nd edn. Penguin, p. 274.

British Medical Journal (1997). News: Australian voluntary euthanasia law overturned. *Br. Med. J.*, **314**, 993.

British Medical Journal (1998). Australian euthanasia law throws up many difficulties. *Br. Med. J.*, **317**, 969.

British Medical Journal (1999a). News: GP on trial for murder. *Br. Med. J.*, **318**, 1095.

British Medical Journal (1999b). News: British GP cleared of murder charge. *Br. Med. J.*, **318**, 1306.

British Medical Journal News extra (1999c). New US Act overturns the legality of doctor assisted suicide in Oregon. *Br. Med. J.*, **319**, 1312.

Brody, H. (1999). Kevorkian and assisted death in the United States. *Br. Med. J.*, **318**, 953.

Dworkin, R. (1993). *Life's Dominion: An Argument About Euthanasia and Abortion.* Harper Collins.

Fletcher, N., Holt, J., Brazier, M. and Harris, J. (1995). *Nursing Law and Ethics.* Manchester University Press, p. 210.

Fox, M. and McHale, J. (1997). Regulating xenotransplantation. *NLJ*, **147**, 115.

Fox, M and McHale, J. (1998) Xenotransplantation: the ethical and legal ramifications. *Med. Law Rev.*, **6(1)**, 42–61.

House of Lords Select Committee on Medical Ethics (1994a). HMSO, HL Paper 21-1.

House of Lords Select Committee on Medical Ethics (1994b). HMSO, HL Paper 21-4.

JRCP (1999). *Journal of The Royal College of Physicians*, **33**, 348–50.

Kennedy, I. (1997). Commentary. *Medical Law Review*, **5**, 102.

Kennedy, I. and Grubb, A. (1994). Evidence to the House of Lords Select Committee on Euthanasia, Report 31.

Keown, J. (1991). Euthanasia in the Netherlands. *LQR*, **108**, 51.

Law Commission (1995). *Mental Incapacity.* Law Commission No. 231, (i) para 5.30; (ii) para 5.34; (iii) 5.24; (iv) para 7.1; (v) 6.23–6.26.

Lord Chancellor's Department (1999). *Making Decisions.* LCD.

Mason, J. K. (1990). Organ transplantation. In: *Doctors, Patients and the Law* (C. Dyer, ed.). Blackwell Scientific.

McHale, J. V. (1995). Elective ventilation – some ethical and legal problems. *Professional Negligence*, **11**, 23.

New, B., Solomon, R., Dingwall, M. and McHale, J. V. (1994). *A Question of Give and Take, Research Report No. 18.* King's Fund Institute.

Nicolson, M. and Bradley, A. J. (1999). Renal transplantation from living donors. *Br. Med. J.*, **318**, 409–10.

Nys, H. (1999). Physician involvement in a patient's death: a continental European perspective. *Med. Law Rev.*, **7(2)**, 208–46.

Radcliffe-Richards, J. *et al.* (1998). The case for allowing kidney sales. *The Lancet*, **1950**, 351.

RCN (1992). Living wills: guidance for nurses. *Issues in Nursing and Health*, Ord. No. 00102.

RCP (1996). *Criteria for the Diagnosis of Brain Stem Death*. Review by a Working Group Convened by the Royal College of Physicians. Endorsed by the Conference of Medical Royal Colleges and their Faculties. RCP.

Schutz, S. E. (1994). Patient involvement in resuscitation decisions. *Br. J. Nursing*, **3(20)**, 1075.

Skegg, P. D. K. (1984). *Law, Ethics and Medicine*, Oxford University Press.

UKCC (1996). *Guidelines for Professional Practice*. UKCC, para 32.

Wells, C. *et al.* (1990). An unsuitable case for treatment. *NLJ*, **1544**.

Appendix 1

Guidelines for professional practice

United Kingdom Central Council for Nursing, Midwifery and Health Visiting

The following appendix is reproduced with permission of the UKCC.

Contents

Preamble

The UKCC has produced this booklet to provide a guide for reflection on the statements within the Code of Professional Conduct. For students and those of you who are new to the professions, we hope that you find it useful; others of you may be very familiar with the guidance provided. This booklet has been produced to help reflect on the many challenges that face us in day-to-day practice. This booklet should read as a whole and care should be taken to use each section in the context of all the guidance provided. It is important that time is taken to read and consider the whole document. You may find yourself in a crisis when there is no opportunity to reach for a book. At these times, you may need the guidance offered to make the professional judgment needed for that specific situation.

Once you have read the booklet, you will be able to dip into the relevant sections and we hope that you will use it regularly and reflect on the many subjects covered. Throughout this booklet, many general ethical and legal issues have been covered. However, it is important that you get to know the specific circumstances, safeguards, policies and procedures needed to provide treatment or care relevant to your area of practice.

The development of these guidelines has been a consultative process with input from individuals with different employment, education, consumer and practice backgrounds. It has been produced in order to replace and update the information provided in the following three documents: Exercising Accountability (March 1989, Confidentiality (April 1987 and Advertising by Registered Nurses, Midwives and Health Visitors (March 1985)

With the many challenges facing nurses, midwives and health visitors and the speed in which practice changes, we acknowledge that these guidelines for professional practice will require regular review. We will formally review the contents by June 1998 and, in the meantime, would welcome any comments you have. These should be sent to the Professional Officer, Ethics, at the UKCC's address.

Introduction

1   The UKCC's responsibilities are set out in the Nurses, Midwives and Health Visitors Acts for 1979 and 1992 and our main responsibility is to protect the interests of the public. To do this, we set standards for education, training and professional conduct for registered nurses, midwives and health visitors (registered practitioners). The motto on our coat of arms – care, protect, honour' – reflects these responsibilities. We hope that this booklet will help you to:

- 'care' in a way that reflects your code of professional conduct (the UKCC Code of Professional Conduct, 1992);
- 'protect' patients and clients and
- 'honour' your responsibilities as a registered practitioner.

2   With so many codes and charters about, it is easy to be confused about how they relate to your professional and personal life. The Code of Professional Conduct was drawn up by the UKCC under the powers of the Nurses, Midwives and Health Visitors Act 1979 to give advice to registered practitioners. This code sets out:

- the value of registered practitioners;
- your responsibilities to represent and protect the interests of patients and clients and

- what is expected of you.

3   The role of the UKCC in protecting the public is firstly to maintain a register of people who are recommended to be suitable practitioners and who have demonstrated knowledge and skill through a qualification registered with the UKCC. Secondly, we can remove people from that register either because they are seriously ill or because a charge of misconduct has been proven against them. The code is used as the standard against which complaints are considered.

4   This booklet gives guidance on all sixteen clauses of the code. It deals with areas such as consent, truthfulness, advocacy and autonomy. It cannot deal with every conflict which a registered practitioner may face. We recognise that professional practice and decision-making are not straightforward. The circumstances we work under are always changing. The way we work must be sensitive and relevant and must meet the needs of patients and clients. We must be able to adjust our practice to changing circumstances, taking into consideration local procedures, policies and cultural differences.

Accountability – answering for your actions

5   As a registered practitioner, you hold a position of responsibility and other people rely on you. You are professionally accountable to the UKCC, as well as having a contractual accountability to your employer and accountability to the law for your actions. The Code of Professional Conduct sets out your professional accountability – to whom you must answer and how. The code begins with the statement that:

> 'Each registered nurse, midwife and health visitor shall act, at all times, in such a manner as to: safeguard and promote the interests of individual patients and clients; serve the interests of society; justify public trust and confidence and uphold and enhance the good standing and reputation of the professionals.'

Each clause of the code begins with the statement that:

> 'As a registered nurse, midwife or health visitor, you are personally accountable for your practice and, in the exercise of your professional accountability, must ...'

No one else can answer for you and it is no defence to say that you were acting on someone else's orders.

6   In exercising your professional accountability, there may be conflict between the interests of a patient or client, the health or social care team and society. This is especially so if health care resources are limited. Whatever decisions you take and judgments you make, you must be able to justify your actions.

7   Accountability is an integral part of professional practice, as in the course of practice you have to make judgments in a wide variety of circumstances. Professional accountability is fundamentally concerned with weighing up the interests of patients and clients in complex situations, using professional knowledge, judgment and skills to make a decision and enabling you to account for the decision made. Neither the Code of Professional Conduct nor this booklet seeks to state the circumstances in which accountability has to be exercised, but instead they provide principles to aid your decision-making.

8   If you delegate work to someone who is not registered with the UKCC, your accountability is to make sure that the person who does the work is able to do it and that appropriate levels of supervision or support are in place.

9   The first four clauses of the code make sure that you put the interests of patients, clients and the public before your own interests and those of your professional colleagues. They are as follows:

> 'As a registered nurse, midwife or health visitor, you are personally accountable for your practice and, in the exercise of your professional accountability, must ...
>
> 1   act always in such a manner as to promote and safeguard the interests and well-being of patients and clients;
> 2   ensure that no action or omission on your part, or within your sphere of responsibility, is detrimental to the interests, condition or safety of patients and clients;
> 3   maintain and improve your professional knowledge and competence;
> 4   acknowledge any limitations in your knowledge and competence and decline any duties or responsibilities unless able to perform them in a safe and skilled manner;'

10   The code does not cover the specific circumstances in which you make decisions and judgments. It presents important themes and principles which you must apply to all areas of your work.

Duty of care

11   You have both a legal and a professional duty to care for patients and clients. In law, the courts could find a registered practitioner negligent if a person suffers harm because he or she failed to care for them properly. Professionally, the UKCC's Professional Conduct Committee could find a registered practitioner guilty of misconduct and remove them from the register if he or she failed to care properly for a patient or client, even though they suffered no harm.

12   Lord Atkin defined the duty of care when he gave judgment in the

case of *Donoghue* v. *Stephenson* (House of Lords) (1932). He said that:

> 'You must take reasonable care to avoid acts or omission which you can reasonably foresee would be likely to injure your neighbour. Who, then, in the law is my neighbour? The answer seems to be persons who are so closely and directly affected by my act that I ought to have them in contemplation as being so affected when I am directing my mind to the acts or omissions which are called in question.'

How circumstances can affect your duty of care

13   If there is a complaint against you, the UKCC's Professional Conduct Committee and possibly the courts would decide whether you took proper care. When they do this, they must consider whether what you did was reasonable in all the circumstances.

14   The following examples show how the duty of care changes according to the circumstances. Each example shows a skilled adult intensive care nurse in a different situation.

Example 1
The nurse is on duty in the intensive care unit when a patient suffers a cardiac arrest.
Here, it is reasonable to expect the nurse to care for the patient as competently as any experienced intensive care unit nurse.

Example 2
The nurse is walking along a hospital corridor and finds a woman completely alone giving birth.
In this situation, it is not reasonable to expect the nurse to care for the women as a midwife would. But it is reasonable to expect the nurse to call a midwife or obstetrician and to stay with the woman until appropriate help arrives.

Example 3
The nurse is walking along a street and comes across a person injured in a road traffic accident. In this situation, the nurse does not have a legal duty to stop and care for the injured person. But if she does, she then takes on a legal duty to care for the person properly. In these circumstances, it is reasonable to expect her to care for the person to the best of her skill and knowledge. Although the nurse has no legal duty to stop and give care in this example, she does have a professional duty. The Code of Professional Conduct places a professional duty upon her at all times. However, in this situation it could be reasonable to expect the nurse to do no more than comfort and support the injured person.

What is reasonable?

15 The courts and the Professional Conduct Committee must decide whether your actions were reasonable. The case of *Bolam* v. *Friern Hospital Management Committee* (1957) produced this test of what is reasonable:

> 'The test is the standard of the ordinary skilled man exercising and professing to have that special skill. A man need not possess the highest expert skill at the risk of being found negligent ... it is sufficient if he exercises the skill of an ordinary competent man exercising that particular art.'

16 This test is usually called the *Bolam* test. Although the case concerned a doctor, the *Bolam* test can be used to examine the actions of any professional person. The case of *Wilsher* v. *Essex AHA* (1988) set the standard of reasonable care to be expected of students and junior staff. The standard is that of a reasonably competent practitioner and not that of a student or junior. You have a duty to ensure that the care which you delegate is carried out at a reasonably competent standard. This means that you remain accountable for the delegation of the work and for ensuring that the person who does the work is able to do it. The Code of Professional Conduct provides principles which you can apply to any situation. If you use these principles, you will be able to carry out your legal and professional duty of care.

Withdrawing care to protect the public and yourself

17 There may be circumstances of conflict where the registered practitioner may consider withdrawing his or her care. A situation like this might occur if the registered practitioner fears physical violence or if there are health and safety hazards involved in providing care. There may be other situations where the registered practitioner may seek support or consider withdrawing care, for example due to sexual or racial harassment. Any decision to withdraw care has to be taken very carefully and you should first discuss, if possible, the matter with managers, the patient's or client's family and, if appropriate and wherever possible, the patient or client themselves. In certain circumstances, you may need help to make sure that the public are safe. If possible, you should discuss this with other members of the health care team. However, in areas of practice where violence may occur more frequently, such as in some areas of mental health care and in accident and emergency departments, there must be protocols to deal with these situations. Appropriate training and on-call support arrangements should also be available. In all cases, you should make a record of the fact that you withdrew care so that if your actions or decisions are questioned, you can justify them.

Patient and client advocacy and autonomy

18   Recognising a patient's or client's right to choose is clearly outlined in clauses 1 and 5 of the code. Although the words advocacy and autonomy are not specifically used, it is this section which states the registered practitioner's role in these respects. The code states that:

> 'As a registered nurse, midwife or health visitor, you are personally accountable for your practice and, in the exercise of your professional accountability, must ...
>
> 1   ... act always in such a manner as to promote and safeguard the interests and well-being of patients and clients; (advocacy) ...
>
> 5   ... work in an open and co-operative manner with patients, clients and their families, foster their independence and recognise and respect their involvement in the planning and delivery of care;' (autonomy)

19   The registered practitioner must not practise in a way which assumes that only they know what is best for the patient or client, as this can only create a dependence and interfere with the patient's or client's right to choose. Advocacy is concerned with promoting and protecting the interests of patients or clients, many of whom may be vulnerable and incapable of protecting their own interests and who may be without the support of family or friends. You can do this by providing information and making the patient or client feel confident that he or she can make their own decisions. Advocacy also involves providing support if the patient refuses treatment/care or withdraws their consent. Other health care professionals, families, legal advisors, voluntary agencies and advocates appointed by the courts may also be involved in safeguarding the interests of patients and clients.

20   Respect for patients' and clients' autonomy means that you should respect the choices they make concerning their own lives. Clause 5 of the code outlines your professional role in promoting patient/client independence. This means discussing with them any proposed treatment or care so that they can decide whether to refuse or accept that treatment or care. This information should enable the patient or client to decide what is in their own best interests.

21   Registered practitioners must respect patients' and clients' rights to take part in decisions about their care. You must use your professional judgment, often in conjunction with colleagues, to decide when a patient or client is capable of making an informed decision about his or her treatment and care. If possible, the patient or client should be able to make a choice about his or her care, even if this means that they may refuse care. You must make sure that all decisions are based on relevant knowledge. The patient's or client's right to agree to or refuse treatment and care may change in law depend-

ing on their age and health. Particular attention to the legal position of children must be given, as their right to give consent or refuse treatment or care varies in different parts of the United Kingdom and depending on their age.

Communicating

22   Communication is an essential part of good practice. The patient or client can only make an informed choice if he or she is given clear information at every stage of care. You also need to listen to the patient or client. Listening is a vital part of communication. Effective communication relies on all our skills. Building a trusting relationship will greatly improve care and help to reduce anxiety and stress for patients and clients, their families and their carers. For effective communication, you may need to consult other colleagues with specialist knowledge, or you may need the services of inter-preters to make sure that information is understood. It is important to create an environment for good communication so that you can build a relationship of trust with the patient or client. Employers should recognise the importance of communication when they plan staffing structures and levels.

23   To ensure that you gain the trust of your patients and clients, you should recognise them as equal partners, use language that is famil-iar to them and make sure that they understand the information you are giving. Your records must also be clear, legible and accessible to the patient or client, as outlined in the UKCC's document *Standards for Records and Record Keeping* and under the terms of the Data Protection Act 1984 and the Access to Health Records Act 1990 (*see also Data Protection Act 1998*). Written communication is as impor-tant as verbal communication.

Truthfulness

24   Patients and clients have a legal right to information about their con-dition; registered practitioners providing care have a professional duty to provide such information. A patient or client who wants information is entitled to an honest answer. There may be rare occa-sions when a person's condition and the likely effect of information given at a specific time might lead you to be selective (although never untruthful) about the information you give. Any decision you make about what information to give must be in the best interests of the patient or client.

25   There is potential for disagreement or even conflict between different professionals and relatives over giving information to a patient or

client. When discussing these matters with colleagues or relatives, you must stress that your personal accountability is firstly to the patient and client. Any patient or client can feel relatively powerless when they do not have full knowledge about their care or treatment. Giving patients and clients information helps to empower them. For this reason, the importance of telling the truth cannot be over-estimated. If patients or clients do not want to know the truth, it should not be forced upon them. You must be sensitive to their needs and must make sure that your communication is effective. The patient or client must be given a choice in the matter. To deny them that choice is to deny their rights and so diminish their dignity and independence.

Consent

26   You must obtain consent before you can give any treatment or care. The patient's or client's decision whether or not to agree to treatment must be based on adequate information so that they can make up their mind. It is important that this information is shared freely with the patient or client, in an accessible way and in appropriate circumstances. In emergency situations, where treatment is necessary to preserve life and the patient or client cannot make a decision (for example because they are unconscious), the law allows you to provide treatment without the patient's or client's consent, always acting in the best interests of the patient or client. You should also know that if the patient or client is an adult, consent from relatives is not sufficient on its own to protect you in the event of challenge, as nobody has the right to give consent on behalf of another adult.

27   When the patient or client is told about proposed treatment and care, it is important that you give the information in a sensitive and under-standable way and that you give the patient or client enough time to consider it and ask questions if they wish. It is not safe to assume that the patient or client has enough knowledge, even about basic treatment, for them to make an informed choice without an expla-nation. You must respect the patient's or client's decision, regardless of whether he or she agrees to or refuses treatment.

28   It is essential that you give the patient or client adequate information so that he or she can make a meaningful decision. If a patient or client feels that the information they received was insufficient, they could make a complaint to the UKCC or take legal action. Most legal action is in the form of an allegation of negligence. In excep-tional cases, for example where a patient's or client's consent was obtained by deception or where not enough information was given, this could result in an allegation of battery (or civil assault in Scotland). However, only in the most extreme cases is criminal law likely to be involved.

Who should obtain consent?

29   It is important that the person proposing to perform a procedure should obtain consent, although there may be some urgent situations where another practitioner can do so. Sometimes you may not be responsible for obtaining a patient's or client's consent as, although you are caring for the patient or client, you would not actually be carrying out the procedure. However, you are often best placed to know about the emotions, concerns and views of the patient or client and may be best able to judge what information is needed so that it is understood. With this in mind, you should tell other members of the health care team if you are concerned about the patient's or client's understanding of the procedure or treatment, for example, due to language difficulties.

Types of consent

30   Although the most important aspect of obtaining consent is providing and sharing information, the patient or client may demonstrate their decision in a number of ways. If they agree to treatment and care, they may do so verbally, in writing or by implying (by co-operating) that they agree. Equally a patient or client may withdraw or refuse consent in the same way. Verbal consent, or consent by implication, will be enough evidence in most cases. You should obtain written consent if the treatment or care is risky, lengthy or complex. This written consent stands as a record that discussions have taken place and of the patient's or client's choice. If a patient or client refuses treatment, making a written record of this is just as important. You should make sure that a summary of the discussions and decisions is placed in the patient's or client's records.

When consent is refused

31   Legally, a competent adult patient can either give or refuse consent to treatment, even if that refusal will shorten their life. Therefore you must respect the patient's refusal just as much as you would their consent. You must make sure that the patient is fully informed and, when necessary, involve other members of the health care team. As before, you should make sure that a summary of the discussions is placed in the patient's or client's records.

32   Increasingly, the law and professional bodies are also recognising the power of advanced directives or living wills. These are documents made in advance of a particular condition arising and they show the patient's or client's treatment choices, including the decision not to accept further treatment in certain circumstances. Although not necessarily legally binding, they can provide very

useful information about the wishes of a patient or client who is now unable to make a decision and therefore should be respected.

Consent of people under 16

33 If the patient or client is under the age of 16 (a minor), you must be aware of local protocols and legislation that affect their care or treatment. Consent of patients or clients under 16 is very complex, so you may need to seek local, legal or membership organisation advice. Some of the laws relating to a minor's consent have been referenced at the back of this booklet.

Consent of people who are mentally incapacitated

34 It is important that the principles governing consent are applied just as vigorously to all forms of care with people who are mentally incapacitated as with a competent adult. A patient or client may be described as mentally incapacitated for a number of reasons. There may be temporary reasons such as sedatory medicines or longer term reasons such as mental illness, coma or unconsciousness.

35 When a patient or client is considered incapable of providing consent, or where the wishes of a mentally incapacitated patient or client appear to be contrary to the interests of that person, you should be involved in assessing their care or treatment. You should consult relevant people close to the patient or client, but respect any previous instructions the patient or client gave.

36 In some cases of legal incapacity, such as when a patient is in a persistent vegetative state, certain decisions will need court authority. Court authority may also be necessary or desirable in decisions concerning selective non-treatment of handicapped infants, dealing with certain circumstances of neonate care or sterilisation of a mentally handicapped individual.

Mental Health Acts

37 If you are involved in the care or treatment of patients or clients detained under statutory powers in the Mental Health Acts, you must get to know the circumstances and safeguards needed for providing treatment and care without consent.

Making concerns known

38 Employers have a duty to provide the resources needed for patient and client care, but the numerous requests to the UKCC for advice on this subject indicate that the environment in which care is pro-

vided is not always adequate. You may find yourself unable to provide good care because of a lack of adequate resources. Also, you may be afraid to speak out for fear of losing your job. However, if you do not report your concerns, you may be in breach of the Code of Professional Conduct. You may also have concerns over inappropriate behaviour by a colleague and feel it necessary to make your concerns known. You will need to report your concerns to the appropriate person or authority, depending on the type of concerns. You may feel it necessary to discuss these decisions with other colleagues or a membership organisation.

39   The clauses of the code which relate specifically to these issues are numbers 11, 12 and 13:

> 'As a registered nurse, midwife or health visitor, you are personally accountable for your practice and, in the exercise of your professional accountability, must ...
>
> 11   report to an appropriate person or authority, having regard to the physical, psychological and social effects on patients and clients, any circumstances in the environment of care which could jeopardise standards of practice;
>
> 12   report to an appropriate person or authority any circumstances in which safe and appropriate care for patients and clients cannot be provided;
>
> 13   report to an appropriate person or authority where it appears that the health and safety of colleagues is at risk, as such circumstances may compromise standards of practice and care;'

40   These clauses give advice on the minimum action to be taken. This will help to make sure that those who manage resources and staff have all the information they need to provide an adequate and appropriate standard of care. You must not be deterred from reporting your concerns, even if you believe that resources are not available or that no action will be taken. You should make your report verbally and/or in writing and, where available, follow local procedures. The manager (who may also be registered with us) should assess the report and communicate it to senior managers where appropriate. This is important because if, subsequently, any complaint is made about the registered practitioners involved in providing care, this may require senior managers to justify their actions if inadequate resources are seen to affect the situation.

41   As outlined in clauses 11, 12 and 13 of the code, the registered practitioner's role is to make sure that safe and appropriate care is provided. This means:

- promoting staff support throughout care settings;
- telling senior colleagues about unacceptable standards;
- supporting and advising colleagues at risk;

- reporting circumstances in the environment which could jeopardise standards of practice;
- making sure that local procedures are in place, challenged and/or changed;
- being aware of new codes, charters and registration body guidelines;
- keeping accurate records and
- when necessary, obtaining guidance on how to present information to management.

Working together

42   The UKCC recognises the complexity of health care and stresses the need to appreciate the contribution of professional health care staff, students, supporting staff and also voluntary and independent agencies. Providing care is a multi-professional, multi-agency activity which, in order to be effective, must be based on mutual understanding, trust, respect and co-operation. Patients and clients are equal partners in their care and therefore have the right to be involved in the health care team's decisions.

43   Under clause 6 and clause 14 of the Code of Professional Conduct:

'As a registered nurse, midwife or health visitor, you are personally accountable for your practice and, in the exercise of your professional accountability, must ...

6   work in a collaborative and co-operative manner with health care professionals and others involved in providing care, and recognise and respect their particular contributions within the care team; ...

14   assist professional colleagues, in the context of your own knowledge, experience and sphere of responsibility, to develop their professional competence and assist others in the care team, including informal carers, to contribute safely to a degree appropriate to their roles;'

These clauses emphasise the importance of support and co-operation and also the importance of avoiding disputes and promoting good relationships and a spirit of co-operation and mutual respect within the health and social care team. It is clearly impossible for any one profession to possess all the knowledge, skills and resources needed to meet the total health care needs of society. Good care should be the product of a good team.

44   Good team work is important but co-operation and collaboration are not always easily achieved, for example, if:

- individual members of the team have their own specific and separate objectives or

- one member of the team tries to adopt a dominant role without considering the opinions, knowledge and skills of its other members.

In such circumstances, achieving good team work needs hard work and negotiation between all the health care professionals involved. In all the discussions, it is important to stress that the interests of the patient or client must come first.

45   Discrimination has no place in health care. This means making sure that equal opportunities policies are in place, challenged and/or changed and ensuring that no one has to endure racial or sexual harassment. Each member of a team is entitled to equality and must not be discriminated against because of gender, age, race, disability, sexuality, culture or religious beliefs. There needs to be effective communication and team work to make sure these principles are not neglected.

Conscientious objection

46   In today's developing health service, you may find yourself in situations which you find very uncomfortable. There may be many circumstances in which a practitioner, due to personal morality or religious beliefs, will not wish to be involved in a certain type of treatment or care. Clause 8 of the Code of Professional Conduct states that:

> 'As a registered nurse, midwife or health visitor, you are personally accountable for your practice and, in the exercise of your professional accountability, must ...
> 8   report to an appropriate person or authority, at the earliest possible time, any conscientious objection which may be relevant to your professional practice;'

47   In law, you have the right conscientiously to object to taking part in care in only two areas. These are the Abortion Act 1967 (Scotland, England and Wales), which gives you the right to refuse to take part in an abortion, and the Human Fertilisation and Embryology Act 1990, which gives you the right to refuse to participate in technological procedures to achieve conception and pregnancy.

48   However, in an emergency, you would be expected to provide care. You should carefully consider whether or not to accept employment in an area which carries out treatment or procedures to which you object. If, however, a situation arises in which you do not want to take part in a form of treatment or care, then it is important that you declare your objection in time for managers to make alternative arrangements. In certain circumstances, this may mean providing counselling for the staff involved in these

decisions. You do not have the right to refuse to take part in emergency treatment.

49 Refusing to be involved in the care of patients because of their condition or behaviour is unacceptable. The UKCC expects all registered practitioners to be non-judgmental when providing care. This is one of the issues addressed by clause 7 of the code, which states that:

> 'As a registered nurse, midwife or health visitor, you are personally accountable for your practice and, in the exercise of your professional accountability, must ...
>
> 7   recognise and respect the uniqueness and dignity of each patient and client, and respect their need for care, irrespective of their ethnic origin, religious beliefs, personal attributes, the nature of their health problems or any other factor;'

Confidentiality

50 To trust another person with private and personal information about yourself is a significant matter. If the person to whom that information is given is a nurse, midwife or health visitor, the patient or client has a right to believe that this information, given in confidence, will only be used for the purposes for which it was given and will not be released to others without their permission. The death of a patient or client does not give you the right to break confidentiality.

51 Clause 10 of the Code of Professional Conduct addresses this subject directly. It states that:

> 'As a registered nurse, midwife or health visitor, you are personally accountable for your practice and, in the exercise of your professional accountability, must ...
>
> 10   protect all confidential information concerning patients and clients obtained in the course of professional practice and make disclosures only with consent, where required by the order of a court or where you can justify disclosure in the wider public interest;'

Confidentiality should only be broken in exceptional circumstances and should only occur after careful consideration that you can justify your action.

52 It is impractical to obtain the consent of the patient or client every time you need to share information with other health professionals or other staff involved in the health care of that patient or client. What is important is that the patient or client understands that some information may be made available to others involved in the delivery of their care. However, the patient or client must know who the information will be shared with.

53   Patients and clients have a right to know the standards of confidentiality maintained by those providing their care and these standards should be made known by the health professional at the first point of contact. These standards of confidentiality can be reinforced by leaflets and posters where the health care is being delivered.

Providing information

54   You always need to obtain the explicit consent of a patient or client before you disclose specific information and you must make sure that the patient or client can make an informed response as to whether that information can be disclosed.

55   Disclosure of information occurs: with the consent of the patient or client; without the consent of the patient or client when the disclosure is required by law or by order of a court and without the consent of the patient or client when the disclosure is considered to be necessary in the public interest.

56   The public interest means the interests of an individual, or groups of individuals or of society as a whole, and would, for example, cover matters such as serious crime, child abuse, drug trafficking or other activities which place others at serious risk.

57   There is no statutory right to confidentiality but an aggrieved individual can sue through a civil court alleging that confidentiality was broken.

58   The situation that causes most problems is when your decision to withhold confidential information or give it to a third party has serious consequences. The information may have been given to you in the strictest confidence by a patient or client or by a colleague. You could also discover the information in the course of your work.

59   You may sometimes be under pressure to release information but you must realise that you will be held accountable for this. In all cases where you deliberately release information in what you believe to be the best interests of the public, your decision must be justified. In some circumstances, such as accident and emergency admissions where the police are involved, it may be appropriate to involve senior staff if you do not feel that you are able to deal with the situation alone.

60   The above circumstances can be particularly stressful, especially if vulnerable groups are concerned, as releasing information may mean that a third party becomes involved, as in the case of children or those with learning difficulties.

61   You should always discuss the matter fully with other professional colleagues and, if appropriate, consult the UKCC or a membership organisation before making a decision to release information without a patient's permission. There will often be significant consequences which you must consider carefully before you make a

decision; you should write down the reasons either in the appropriate record or in a special note that can be kept in a separate file (outlined in the UKCC's booklet *Standards for Records and Record Keeping*). You then have written justification for the action which you took if this becomes necessary and you can also review the decision later in the light of future developments.

Ownership of and access to records

62   Organisations which employ professional staff who make records are the legal owners of these records, but that does not give anyone in that organisation the legal right of access to the information in those records. However, the patient or client can ask to see their records, whether they are written down or on computer *(see now the Data Protection Act 1998 and Access to Health Records Act 1990)*.

63   The contracts of employment of all employees not directly involved with patients but who have access to or handle confidential records should contain clauses which emphasise the principles of confidentiality and state the disciplinary action which could result if these principles are not met.

64   As far as computer-held records are concerned, you must be satisfied that as far as possible, the methods you use for recording information are secure. You must also find out which categories of staff have access to records to which they are expected to contribute important personal and confidential information. Local procedures must include ways of checking whether a record is authentic when there is no written signature. All records must clearly indicate the identity of the person who made that record. As more patient and client records are moved and linked between health care settings by computer, you will have to be vigilant in order to make sure that patient or client confidentiality is not broken. This means trying to ensure that the systems used are protected from inappropriate access within your direct area of practice, for example by ensuring that personal access codes are kept secure.

65   The Computer Misuse Act 1990 came into force to secure computer programs and data against unauthorised access or alteration. Authorised users have permission to use certain programs and data. If those users go beyond what is permitted, this is a criminal offence. The Act makes provision for accidentally exceeding your permission and covers fraud, extortion and blackmail.

66   Where access to information contained on a computer filing system is available to members of staff who are not registered practitioners, or health professionals governed by similar ethical principles, an important clause concerning confidentiality should appear within their contracts of employment (outlined in the UKCC's position statement Confidentiality: Use of Computers, 1994).

67   Those who receive confidential information from a patient or client should advise them that the information will be given to the registered practitioner involved in their care. If necessary, this may also include other professionals in the health and social work fields. Registered practitioners must make sure that, where possible, the storage and movement of records within the health care setting does not put the confidentiality of patient information at risk.

Access to records for teaching, research and audit

68   If patients' or clients' records need to be used to help students gain the knowledge and skills which they require, the same principles of confidentiality apply to the information. This also applies to those engaged in research and audit. The manager of the health care setting is responsible for the security of the information contained in these records and for making sure that access to the information is closely supervised. The person providing the training will be responsible for making sure that students understand the need for confidentiality and the need to follow local procedures for handling and storing records. The patient or client should know about the individual having access to their records and should be able to refuse that access if they wish.

69   In summary, the following principles concerning confidentiality apply:

- a patient or client has the right to expect that information given in confidence will be used only for the purpose for which it was given and will not be released without their permission;
- you should recognise each patient's or client's right to have information about themselves kept secure and private;
- if it is appropriate to share information gained in the course of your work with other health or social work practitioners, you must make sure that as far as is reasonable, the information will be kept in strict professional confidence and be used only for the purpose for which the information was given;
- you are responsible for any decision which you make to release confidential information because you think that this is in the public's best interest;
- if you choose to break confidentiality because you believe that this is in the public's best interest, you must have considered the situation carefully enough to justify that decision and
- you should not deliberately break confidentiality other than in exceptional circumstances.

Advertising and sponsorship

70   Clause 16 of the UKCC's Code of Professional Conduct addresses
      the subject of the promotion of commercial goods or services. It
      states that:

      'As a registered nurse, midwife or health visitor, you are person-
      ally accountable for your practice and, in the exercise of your pro-
      fessional accountability, must...
      16   ensure that your registration status is not used in the promo-
            tion of commercial products or services, declare any finan-
            cial or other interests in relevant organisations providing
            such goods or services and ensure that your professional
            judgment is not influenced by any commercial considera-
            tions.'

71   Patients or clients and their relatives or friends are often anxious
      when attending hospitals and other health care facilities. The envi-
      ronment of care should help to promote good health, healing and
      recovery and not be one of commercial advertising.

72   Clause 16 does not intend to prevent registered practitioners
      employed in positions such as the matron of a private nursing home
      or as a representative of a pharmaceutical company, or who are
      offering their professional services privately, from using their regis-
      tration status on items such as business cards and headed note paper.

73   However, if a practitioner has a direct financial or other direct inter-
      est in an organisation providing commercial goods or services, for
      example, a ward sister who is discharging a patient to a nursing
      home owned and run by herself or one of her relatives, then that
      practitioner must make her interests known.

74   It is also unacceptable for registered practitioners to carry comme-
      cial advertising or promotional material on their uniforms.

75   Under the Code of Professional Conduct, registered practitioners
      must protect the interests of patients and clients, be worthy of public
      trust and confidence and avoid using professional qualifications in
      ways which might compromise the independence of professional
      judgments upon which patients and clients rely. The vulnerability of
      patients and clients is reflected by these elements of the code, which
      also indicate the importance of trust between a registered practi-
      tioner and a patient as well as the expectation that the registered
      practitioner will respond to the patient's need unconditionally.

Sponsorship

76   Funding for some posts, projects or services is sometimes offered by
      companies, some of which have a commercial interest in matters
      associated with health care. Sponsorship arrangements which affect

the professional judgment of registered practitioners and patient or client choice should be brought to the attention of those who provide health care services.

77 Students on pre-registration and post-registration courses often need sponsorship to carry out their study, especially for overseas study visits. The decision to accept sponsorship must be made by the individual, taking account of the appropriateness of the support offered.

Receiving gifts

78 You may be offered gifts, favours or hospitality from patients or clients during the course of or after a period of care or treatment. The Code of Professional Conduct states that:

> 'As a registered nurse, midwife or health visitor, you are personally accountable for your practice and, in the exercise of your professional accountability, must ...
> 15 refuse any gift, favour or hospitality from patients or clients currently in your care which might be interpreted as seeking to exert influence to obtain preferential consideration;'

The important principle is not that the registered practitioner never receives gifts or favours but that they could never be interpreted as being given by the patient or client in return for preferential treatment.

Complementary and alternative therapies

79 Complementary therapies are gaining popularity and finding a more substantial place in health care. It is vitally important that you ensure that the introduction of any of these therapies to your practice is always in the best interests and safety of the patients and clients. Clause 9 of the code outlines your privileged relationship with patients and clients:

> 'As a registered nurse, midwife or health visitor, you are personally accountable for your practice and, in the exercise of your professional accountability, must ...
> 9 avoid any abuse of your privileged relationship with patients and clients and of the privileged access allowed to their person, property, residence or workplace;'

The registered practitioner therefore must be convinced of the relevance and accountability of the therapy being used and must be able to justify using it in a particular circumstance, especially when using the therapy as part of professional practice. It should also be part of professional team work to discuss the use of complementary therapies with medical and other members of the health care team caring for the particular patient or client.

80   Some registered practitioners, who successfully complete courses in complementary or alternative therapies not usually associated with their professional practice, quote their registration status when advertising their services. The UKCC believes that a person's registration status should not be needed to support a complementary or alternative therapy course or qualification if the course is valid and credible. However, if it is a registered practitioner's registered status that gives credibility to the qualification, then the registered practitioner must use their own judgment and discretion to make sure that they are not misleading the public.

81   If a complaint is made against you, we can call you to account for any activities carried out outside conventional practice. You should carefully consider the content and status of any courses which you undertake and how you promote yourself.

Research and audit

82   Increasing numbers of registered practitioners are carrying out, or are involved in, research or audit. The results might improve practice, help to audit an aspect of clinical services, inform policy or be part of a graduate or postgraduate qualification. Other practitioners are employed or involved with clinical trials which force on new treatments, new technology or improvements to patient care.

83   If you are involved in these activities, issues often arise which you need to consider. Is the research ethical? Is your role appropriate? Has the Local Research Ethics Committee (LREC) given its approval? Has local management given their approval? What is the make-up of the LREC? Are there registered practitioners on the LREC?

Types of research

84   The range of research carried out varies greatly. Outlined below are some of the types of research that are used in the health care setting.

Projects

85   An increasing number of students are being asked to do project work for diplomas or undergraduate degrees. Many educational institutions recommend that their diploma or undergraduate students do not become involved in clinically-based research.

86   As the number of these projects increases, contact with patients or clients might be refused. This is quite reasonable, as the care and

comfort of patients or clients must always be considered. Projects by registered practitioners may be promoted by developments at clinical level, by involvement in practice units or as a result of participating in clinical supervision.

Higher degrees

87   Research for postgraduate degrees is supervised and guided throughout. It is important to gain approval for research in clinical areas from management in addition to consulting the local LREC before starting the work.

Other research work and clinical research trials

88   Research activities intended to benefit patient care or investigate practice are carried out by a wide range of clinicians, academics and others. Registered practitioners may be involved in this work as part of their job, because of academic interest or in response to a perceived or expressed need.

89   Contracts of employment specify how practitioners must work. They do not always cover concerns about the ethics of research, confidentiality, consent or other issues. Under European Community Directive 91/507/EEC, all elements of clinical trials carried out within the European Union must adhere to the guidelines on good clinical practice for trials on medical protocols in the EU. These guidelines provide a useful framework for nurses, midwives and health visitors to use when they are involved in research work.

90   If there is contact with patients or clients, it is important for you to discuss the benefits of the work with the appropriate manager. You must be certain that approval from the LREC is obtained. Repeated requests for patients and clients to fill in questionnaires or to be interviewed can be intrusive and potentially disruptive to care. For this reason, the views of patients, clients, and their associates will assist in determining prospective compliance.

Criteria for safe and ethical conduct of research

91   You must always refer to the UKCC's Code of Professional Conduct and The Scope of Professional Practice. These documents provide the framework for all actions of registered nurses, midwives and health visitors.

92   As well as using these documents, you need to be sure that the research or clinical trial you are carrying out meets specific criteria. These are that:

  • the project must be approved by the LREC;

- management approval must be gained where necessary;
- arrangements for obtaining consent must be clearly understood by all those involved;
- confidentiality must be maintained;
- patients must not be exposed to unacceptable risks;
- patients should be included in the development of proposed projects where appropriate;
- accurate records must be kept and
- research questions need to be well structured and aimed at producing clearly anticipated care or service outcomes and benefits.

93   You need to consider these criteria before submitting a research proposal to a LREC. You are expected to participate fully in the design process and this includes raising legitimate concerns when they arise. If no LREC exists in your area, it is important to refer to local policy for research.

Audit

94   Audit seeks to improve practice and treatment and to reduce risk by the systematic review of the process and outcome of care and treatment and by the evaluation of records and other data. There are occasions when contact with patients and clients, carers or relatives is necessary and therefore LREC clearance may be required. Consideration of the other points highlighted above is recommended.

Conclusion

95   We have produced this booklet to help you in your professional practice. It would be impossible to discuss all the issues faced by registered practitioners. Answers are not always straightforward. The Code of Professional Conduct and The Scope of Professional Practice apply to all registered practitioners and the interests of the public, patients and clients are of the greatest importance. You should also remember that being accountable and working with those who provide care is the foundation upon which the best standards are achieved. With the many challenges facing nurses, midwives and health visitors and the speed with which practice changes, it is acknowledged that these guidelines for professional practice will require irregular review. We will formally review these guidelines by June 1998 and, in the meantime, would welcome any comments which you may have. Comments on this booklet should be sent to the Professional Officer, Ethics, at the UKCC's address.

96 In producing this booklet, we have been greatly helped by comments from representatives of practice, education, medical, professional, membership and consumer organisations. We have tried to produce the booklet in a form that is easily accessible in order to aid professional judgment and to outline basic principles.

97 If you need further information or advice, please contact our team of professional officers at the:

Standards Promotion Directorate
United Kingdom Central Council
for Nursing, Midwifery and Health Visiting
23 Portland Place London W1N 4JT
Telephone: 0207 637 7181
Fax: 0207 436 2924

Documents relevant to these guidelines

1 *Code of Professional Conduct*, UKCC, 1992
2 *The Scope of Professional Practice*, UKCC, 1992
3 *Midwives Rules and Code of Practice*, 1998
4 *Guidelines for Record Keeping*, 1998
5 *Guidelines for the Administration of Medicines*, 2000
6 *Confidentiality: Use of Computers, Position Statement*, UKCC, 1992
7 *Complementary Therapies, Position Statement*, UKCC, 1995
8 *Acquired Immune Deficiency Syndrome and Human Immune Deficiency Virus Infection (AIDS and HIV Infection)*, UKCC, 1994
9 *Anonymous Testing for the Prevalence of the Human Immune Deficiency Virus (HIV)*, UKCC, 1994

These documents are available on written request from the Distribution Department at the UKCC.

Laws relevant to these guidelines

1 Nurses, Midwives and Health Visitors Acts 1997
2 Access to Health Records Act 1990
3 Family Law Reform Act 1969
4 Age of Legal Capacity (Scotland) Act 1991
5 Children's Act 1989
6 Mental Health (Northern Ireland) Order 1986
7 Mental Health (England and Wales) Act 1983
8 Mental Health (Scotland) Act 1984
9 Abortion Act 1967
10 Human Fertilisation and Embryology Act 1990
11 Data Protection Act 1998

12 Computer Misuse Act 1990
13 European Community Directive 91/507/EEC

These are available from your local branch of Her Majesty's Stationery Office (HMSO).

Appendix 2

The Health Service Ombudsman

England

The following appendix is reproduced with permission of the Health Service Ombudsman.

Section 1 – General guidance

The Health Service Ombudsman investigates complaints about the National Health Service (NHS). Before asking the Ombudsman to look into your complaint, you must first take it up locally with the body you are complaining against. Section 2 tells you how to do that.

If you are not happy with the way your complaint has been dealt with locally, write to the Ombudsman giving all the details. You do not need to employ a lawyer to put your complaint to the Ombudsman. There is a form which you can print and use if you wish.

Section 5 tells you what kinds of complaints the Ombudsman can investigate. There are some complaints which the Ombudsman cannot take up, and Section 6 tells you what they are. It is not possible here to deal with every possibility. If you are not sure whether the Ombudsman can help, you can write or telephone for advice. Section 8 gives the address and telephone number of the Ombudsman's office. There is a printed leaflet which outlines the role of the Ombudsman.

Printed leaflets are also available in large print, tape, symbol summary, and in the following languages: Arabic, Bengali, Chinese, English, Gujerati, Hindi, Punjabi, Urdu, Somali, Sinhalese, Turkish, Vietnamese, and Welsh.

Section 7 explains what happens when the Ombudsman receives your complaint.

The Ombudsman is completely independent of the NHS and the government. There is no charge for the Ombudsman's service. The Ombudsman does not have to investigate your complaint. It is up to the Ombudsman (or staff on his behalf) to decide whether to take up any particular complaint. If your complaint is not to be investigated, you will be told why.

Section 2 – How to make your complaint

The first steps – local investigation

You first need to take up your complaint locally. Your hospital, clinic or surgery can tell you how to do that. You can ask them for a leaflet which will have the details. Most complaints can be settled quickly in this way – by letter or by discussion with you.

If you are not satisfied after that, you can ask for a review of your complaint by an independent panel. If your request is granted, the review will be carried out by a panel, usually of three members. The panel will be chaired by an independent person.

Involving the Ombudsman

The Ombudsman will not normally become involved unless you have taken up your complaint officially and are still unhappy, for example, because:

- it took too long to deal with your complaint locally;
- you were unreasonably refused a panel review;
- you did not get a satisfactory answer to your complaint.

Who can complain to the Ombudsman?

The person complaining can be:
- the patient;
- a relative (normally the closest member of the family);
- someone else, for example someone who works for the NHS or a Community Health Council;
- if the patient is dead, their personal representative (usually their next of kin).

If you complain on behalf of a patient, you must explain why the patient is not doing so. You must also say whether the patient agrees that you may complain on their behalf.

Time limits

You have to send your complaint to the Ombudsman no later than a year from the date when you became aware of the events which are the subject of complaint. The Ombudsman can sometimes extend the time limit, but only if there are special reasons. One reason might be that the local investigation of your complaint took much longer than it should have done.

Section 3 – Putting your complaint to the Ombudsman

You should write and:

- describe what happened, when, where and (if you can) who was involved;
- say why you are complaining. You need to show that there has already been hardship or injustice. The Ombudsman will not investigate something that might cause problems in the future;
- provide all the evidence you can. Send all your letters and any background papers. If you send originals, photocopies will be taken (at no cost to you) and the originals will be returned to you promptly;
- if you can, please include a telephone number where you can be contacted during the day.

You can use the form or just write a letter. The form tells you what information the Ombudsman will need to know.

Before you write, please look at:

- Section 5 – which tells you what the Ombudsman can investigate.
- Section 6 – which tells you what the Ombudsman cannot investigate.

Section 4 – Getting help

Your local Community Health Council will be able to help you. Otherwise you can ask for help from a Citizens' Advice Bureau or from your Member of Parliament.

Telephone numbers and addresses for your local Community Health Council, Citizens' Advice Bureau and Member of Parliament are in the phone book, available in your local library.

Section 5 – What can the Ombudsman investigate?

The Ombudsman can investigate complaints against hospitals or community health services which are about:

a. a poor service;
b. failure to purchase or provide a service you are entitled to receive;
c. maladministration – that is, administrative failure such as:
- avoidable delay

- not following proper procedures
- rudeness or discourtesy
- not explaining decisions
- not answering your complaint fully or promptly.

Where the matters you are complaining about happened after 31 March 1996, the Ombudsman may also investigate:

d. complaints about the care and treatment provided by a doctor, nurse or other trained professional;
e. other complaints about family doctors (GPs), or about dentists, pharmacists or opticians providing a NHS service locally.

Complaints about access to information

You have rights to information about how the NHS operates locally. These are set out in the Government's Code of Practice on Openness in the NHS. Copies of the Code should be available in your local library or from your local hospital. If you ask your Health Authority (Health Board in Scotland) or Trust for information and are not content with the response you first receive, you should write to the chief executive of the Health Authority/Health Board or NHS Trust concerned. If you remain dissatisfied you can complain to the Ombudsman about such things as:

- refusal to provide the information – unless it something you do not have a right to see;
- a delay of over four weeks in getting the information requested;
- the level of any charge you are asked to pay for it.

Such information may be about services available locally, the standards set or achieved, or the details of important decisions or proposals.

Under the Code you can ask for information about the NHS services provided by your local general practitioner, dentist, pharmacist or optician. If you are not satisfied with the reply you receive you may complain to the Ombudsman.

Please note

The Ombudsman does not have to investigate your complaint. It is up to the Ombudsman to decide whether to take up any particular complaint. If your complaint is not to be investigated, you will be told why.

Section 6 – Matters that the Ombudsman cannot investigate

The Ombudsman cannot look into:

a. complaints which you could take to court or an independent tribunal – unless the Ombudsman does not think it would be reasonable for you to do so. If you are seeking damages for what happened, only the courts can decide that. The Ombudsman cannot take up your complaint at all if you have already started legal action;

b. personnel issues such as appointments of staff, pay or discipline. The Ombudsman cannot investigate complaints from NHS staff about their employment. The Ombudsman can look into complaints from staff about the way in which a complaint about them by or on behalf of a patient has been handled by a NHS or Trust or other body;

c. commercial or contractual matters, unless they relate to services for patients provided under a NHS contract;

d. properly made decisions which NHS authority or other body or individual providing NHS services has a right to make even if you do not agree with the decision;

e. services in a non-NHS hospital or nursing home, unless they are paid for by the NHS;

f. complaints about government departments, such as the Department of Health, NHS Executive or the Department of Social Security. Those complaints are for the Parliamentary Ombudsman to consider.

g. complaints about local authority departments, such as social services. Those complaints are for the Local Government Ombudsman to consider.

Section 7 – How will the Ombudsman deal with your complaint?

First stage

When your complaint is received by the Ombudsman, a decision will be made on whether or not an investigation will be carried out. If the Ombudsman cannot look into your complaint or decides not to, you will be told why.

Investigation

If the Ombudsman decides to investigate, you will be sent a statement of complaint. It will set out for you and for the body to be investigated which matters the Ombudsman will look into. The body that is responsible for the matters to be investigated will be asked to send to the Ombudsman their comments and all relevant papers – which might include your medical records (these will be kept confidential).

After those papers have been received and studied a member of the Ombudsman's staff may ask to interview you at a convenient time and place. You can have a friend of your choice with you. The Ombudsman's investigator may then interview others concerned. If your complaint is about treatment provided by doctors, nurses or other professionals, independent professional advisers will be available to help the Ombudsman with the investigation.

Interviews are carried out in private. They are usually informal, although the Ombudsman has the same power as the civil courts to obtain evidence. Because the Ombudsman's investigations are thorough, they can take several months.

The report

At the end of the investigation you will be sent the Ombudsman's report. A copy is also sent to the NHS or other body responsible for the matters you complained about. If your complaint is found to be justified, the Ombudsman will seek an apology for you or another remedy. Sometimes that may include getting a decision changed, or repayment of unnecessary costs to patients or their families. The Ombudsman does not recommend damages. The Ombudsman may also call for changes to be made so that what has gone wrong does not happen again. Where the body you complained about tells the Ombudsman that it will make such changes, the Ombudsman checks that they have done so.

Is there any appeal against the Ombudsman's decisions?

No. A complaint to the Ombudsman is the final stage in the procedure for pursuing a complaint. The Ombudsman's decision on a complaint is final. If completely new information comes to light which could not reasonably have been known about before, the Ombudsman may start a new investigation. That is extremely rare.

Section 8 – Contacts and checklist

The Health Service Ombudsman for England
13th Floor
Millbank Tower
Millbank
London SW1P 4QP

Telephone: 0845 015 4033
Minicom: 0207 217 4066

Before you post your letter, or the completed complaints form, have you:

- said what your complaint is?
- said who is involved?
- said when, and where, what you are complaining about happened?

- enclosed all the correspondence with the NHS or other body locally to whom you have complained, including other papers about your complaint?
- given your address, and if possible, a daytime telephone number?

Index